Hans J. Markowitsch

Intellectual Functions and the Brain

An Historical Perspective

Hogrefe & Huber Publishers
Seattle Toronto Bern Göttingen

I would like to extend my special thanks to Hoechst-Roussel Pharmaceuticals Inc., Somerville, N.J., USA, for their financial support.

Library of Congress Cataloging-in-Publication Data

Markowitsch, Hans J., 1949-
Intellectual functions and the brain : an historical perspective / by Hans Markowitsch.
p. cm.
Includes bibliographical references and indexes.
ISBN 0-88937-081-8 : $78.00. — ISBN 3-456-82157-3
1. Neuropsychology–History. 2. Neuropsychiatry–History.
3. Brain–Research–History. 4. Intellect–Research–History.
I. Title.
(DNLM: 1. Brain–physiology. 2. Memory Disorders–history.
3. Organic Mental Disorders–history. WM 11.1 M3461)
QP360.M348 1992 616.8—dc20 DNLM/DLC
for Library of Congress 92-1482 CIP

Canadian Cataloguing in Publication Data

Markowitsch, Hans, 1949-
Intellectual functions and the brain
Includes bibliographical references and index.
ISBN 0-88937-081-8
1. Brain–Research–History–Sources.
2. Brain–Localization of functions–Research–
Sources. 3. Intellect–Research–History–
Sources. 4. Brain–Disease–Research–Sources.
I. Title.
QP376.M37 1992 612.8'2 C92-093859-0

P.O. Box 2487
Kirkland, WA
98083-2487

Printed in Germany by Hubert & Co., Göttingen

ISBN 0-88937-081-8
Hogrefe & Huber Publishers · Seattle Toronto Bern Göttingen

ISBN 3-456-82157-3
Hogrefe & Huber Publishers · Bern Göttingen Seattle Toronto

Preface

The roots of our present-day knowledge in the field of the neurosciences were laid at the turn of the century; more exactly, an explosion in knowledge of brain-behavior relations occurred in the time period between 1870 and the Second World War. The present book covers relevant research results from this area, as far the subjects have specific relation to the interdependencies between the brain and intellectual functioning.

The book is subdivided into chapters which, on the one hand follow historical dates, and, on the other hand reflect the importance given to the respective subjects. It starts with early attempts from the post-Gall period to specify special features of the brain and cranium which might reflect outstanding intellectual performance. Then frontal lobe-related research is treated, as this part of the brain was regarded to be the intellectual portion par excellence. This chapter is complemented by a further one on the prefrontal cortex, which deals with the topic of psychosurgery which was predominantly done on the frontal lobes. Then I give more general, and more psychology-related approaches for studying memory and amnesia technically, to localize them, and to differentiate them from psychogenic forms of amnesia. Aside from intellectual deterioration related to frontal lobe damage, this was most easily demonstrated in Korsakoff's amnesics. Therefore, a large chapter is devoted to research results on Korsakoff's syndrome. This chapter is supplemented by a further one on non-Korsakoff based diencephalic amnesia. A chapter follows in which the consequences assumed for callosal damage are treated, as the corpus callosum was given a special role by many of the old neurologists. Lastly, before the final remarks, medial temporal lobe amnesia is discussed, though here much less was available at the turn of the century than would be expected on the basis of our present knowledge on the functions of this region.

It is my hope that this small volume will document the most promising results and interpretations in the field of cognitive behavior and the nervous system from the turn of the century. It furthermore aims at providing accurate and detailed information on the respective sources. To accomplish this, all foreign language literature citations have been translated so that the reader can easily evaluate whether the title of a book or article is of interest and worth further looking into. (Furthermore, all references are in agreement with the standards of the American Psychological Association.)

Writing the book was stimulated by meeting Stanley Finger in Berne and later in Bochum. I thank him for fruitful discussions; Dr. C.-J. Hogrefe and J. Flury from Hogrefe and Huber Publishers for always being helpful and interested in the progress of the book; D. Hagenkötter for much secretarial help; P. Calabrese for helpful comments and translations of French and Italian articles; P. Calabrese, C. Lillpopp, and A. Lohmann for assistance with compiling the indexes; and G. Keim and R. Phildius for photographical work. Furthermore, I thank Dr. Louise Dye and especially David Emmans for their help with solving English language problems.

Table of Contents

Preface v

Chapter 1:
Introduction 1

Chapter 2:
Relations Between Brain Morphology and Intellectual Capacity . . 5

Philosophical roots 5
Skull, brain, sex, and character 6
Deviations and exceptional features . . . 6
Holländer 7
Resignation 9
Outlook 11

Chapter 3:
The Frontal Lobes: The Most Recent Attributes of the Brain 13

The Myths of the Frontal Cortex 13

Welt's Cases 14

The Term „Prefrontal Cortex“ 14

Methodological Controversies 16

Intellectual Functions 17

Phineas P. Gage 18

The Turn of the Century 22

Tumors 24
Pfeifer 24
The contributions of H. Smith and of Donath 25
Outlook 25

The Diverse Functions Attributed to the Stirnhirn 26
P. Schuster 26
Forster and others 26
E. Müller 28
Trauma-based cases 28

Animal Studies 30
Comparative work supporting the search for intelligent acts in animals 30
Goltz, Munk and others on the mammalian prefrontal cortex 31
Franz, Bianchi, and Ferrier 33

Final Remarks 34

Chapter 4:
Frontal Lobe Psychosurgery 37

Gottlieb Burckhardt – The First Psychosurgeon 38

The Founders 41

Outcome and Evaluation of Psychosurgery 43

Prospect 45

Implications for Anatomical Knowledge 48

Conclusions 48

Chapter 5:
Memory and Memory Disorders . 51

Early Methods for Memory Assessment . 53
Intelligence and association-psychology . 54
Remembrance and forgetting 56
Albert Gregor's contribution 58
Attempts at quantification 58

Psychogenic Amnesia 61
The Ganser syndrome 62
Fugues 63
Multiple Personalities 63
Dana's case 64
Stevens' case 64

Localization of Mnemonic Abilities . . . 65
Emphasizing the cerebral cortex 65
Amnesia 66
Retrograde amnesia 66
Hanging 68

Retrograde amnesia after cerebral concussion and after shot wounds 70
The case of Grünthal and Störring . . . 70

Chapter 6: Korsakoff's Syndrome 73

Alcohol-related Brain Damage 73

Korsakoff's Descriptions 74

Bonhoeffer's (1901) Book on Alcoholics 76

Korsakoff's Psychosis at the Time of Queen Victoria and King Edward VII . 78
Serbsky, a pupil of Korsakoff 78
Other early authors and single case descriptions 78
Wehrung's survey 79
Boedeker's cases 80
Mathematical abilities versus episodic memory 80
Wizel's case 81
Other cases with unusual mathematical abilities 82

The Search for the Anatomical Bases of Chronic Alcoholism and Korsakoff's Syndrome 83
Gamper's findings 83
Tsiminakis' neuropathological study . . 84
Carmichael and Stern on the neuropathological changes in Korsakoff's patients . 86
Kant's review of the state of the art in 1932 86
Korsakoff's Syndrome in the time before the Second World War 87
Chronognosia 89

Chapter 7: Diencephalic Amnesia 93

Tumors and degenerations 93
Da Fano's analysis of neuronal changes in paralytic and senile dementia and three related reports 95
P. Schuster's contributions to the pathology of the optical thalamus 96
A cyst, tumors, infarcts, and the degeneration of the thalamus: contributions in the fourth decade of this century 97

Chapter 8: The Corpus Callosum 101

Chapter 9: Medial Temporal Lobe Amnesia . . 105

Examples of early studies on the temporal lobe 105
Albert Knapp's contributions 106
Bechterew's case 107

The temporal lobes and memory 108
Artom's documentation 110
The hippocampal formation 111
The discovery of medial temporal lobe amnesia 112

Chapter 10: Final Remarks 113

References 115

Chapter 1: Introduction

Scientific progress leaves much of the work from just one decade ago already appearing outdated, in part even antique. Nevertheless, the time period from after the Second World War is still represented by a few scientists who are active up to the present in their labs and clinics. Furthermore, libraries are usually well equipped with books and journals from the time after the Second World War. I therefore decided to use this epoch in general as a cut-off for the present book (except for the part on psychosurgery, a method of treatment which had its classical period in the 1940ies). For the older literature, and for a quite plastic description of the science of the brain, I would recommend reading E. Clarke and Dewhurst (1972) (see also Patten, 1990, and Yates, 1966). Other sources include Ackerknecht (1985), Brazier (1984), Brooks and Cranefield (1959), E. Clarke and Jacyna (1987), Fulton (1966), Diepgen (1965), Gibson (1969), Kraepelin (1918), H. S. Levin (1991), Lichtenthaeler (1974), McHenry (1969), Morgagni (1761/1967), Pichot (1981), Scholz (1961), Sheer (1966), and Soury (1899). Thompson and Berry (1988) wrote a special chapter on old research in learning and motivation, and in Kolle's (1970) three volume work on great neurologists, portraits of 67 famous scientists are given.

This book is selective – with respect to the languages represented (English and German dominate), with respect to the time epoch covered (mainly the turn of the last century plus/minus 40 years), with respect to the approach which is that of an active neuroscientist, not of an historian, with respect to the contents selected – intellectual functions, and with respect to the species included – principally only mammals with a strong preponderance on humans. Still, in approaching this task, I found that the literature accumulated by the turn of the century is already overwhelming – some of the old monographs contain hundreds or even thousands of citations (e.g., Exner, 1881; Monakow, 1904 [898 references]; Monakow, 1914 [3,174 references]; Nothnagel, 1879; P. Schuster, 1902; A. Stern, 1914). As an example: a phenomenon as exotic as colored hearing ("auditio colorata"), resulted in the appearance of 140 publications by 1896 (Lomer, 1905). Even in much earlier times there had been voluminous books on the brain. A good source for such books and also for references to reviews of previous literature can be found in Pestronk (1989) who lists several text books on the brain from the 16th century and bibliographies from, for example, the time between 1459 and 1799. Also, the field of psychology was covered by a number of substantial text books at the turn of the century (Ebbinghaus, 1902; Jaspers, 1910; Jodl, 1903; Losskij, 1904; Münsterberg, 1900; Pfänder, 1904, Wundt, 1901).

The present book contains a preponderance of German-language articles. Although this could appear to be due to a biased literature search, I find it justifiable when I consider how much of the older literature was written in German (or translated into this language), even when the authors came from the French-speaking part of Switzerland (e.g., Burckhardt, 1891), from Russia (e.g., Korsakow, 1890; Moranska-Oscherovitsch, 1910; Rabinowitsch, 1925), Japan (e.g., Hirosawa & Kato, 1935; Namba, 1958; Watanabe, 1923), Sweden (e.g., Ekehorn, 1901; Retzius, 1902; Henschen, 1923), Denmark (Wimmer, 1926), Italy (Artom, 1923; Mingazzini, 1922), the Netherlands (e.g., Brouwer, 1912), Great Britain (e.g., Holländer, 1900), or the United States (Freeman, 1950; Starr, 1894). (Of course, German-language speaking authors also wrote in English already in the last century: e.g., Hitzig, 1900a; Obersteiner, 1879).

In discussing links between clinical and experimental neuropsychology, Oscar-Berman (1988) recently made an anecdotal note on the preponderance of German language literature in the field of neuropsychology. She remarked, for instance, that Edith Kaplan, while preparing for her language examination in German, found that "apparently the only literature on pure motor agraphia was in German" (p. 574). As many other earlier contributions to the field of the neurosciences were published in German and as this language is no longer so well known in scientific circles as in earlier times, a review of the old literature, with a specific and detailed view on the German language-based contributions, is certainly worthwhile from an historical perspective. (At this point I wish to remark that I have translated all citations from German sources into English in order to provide a more direct flavor of the style and arguments of the respective authors without interrupting the fluency of reading by citing in the original language.)

The principal aim of this book is to provide an accurate review of the sources for the older scientific literature; and for this reason a number of sources are mentioned only cursorily, but may be of value for a scientist interested in the particular topic. The inclusion of relevant work which is not reviewed in detail may sometimes disturb fluent reading; I nevertheless hope my readers will understand that completeness and variety were given priority over elegance in style.

The book is not designed as light reading which accumulates curiosities and integrates them into epic reports, but as a reliable reference book which necessarily emphasizes personal preferences, both with respect to topics and persons. The book was not just planned as a list of mere facts; instead its contents should reveal what technical possibilities existed, how much knowledge was available at a given time, and more importantly, how scientists thought and engaged in scientific study and discussions during the epoch in which they worked.

The importance of carefully studying primary sources cannot be emphasized enough (e.g., Loftus, 1974). As was quite recently documented by Vicente and de Groot (1990), various errors in citing and interpreting an old study (namely de Groot's, 1946, 1965) can be found in more recent literature, thus reminding one of "the inevitable fallibility of human memory" (p. 287, Vicente & de Groot, 1990).

The book provides insights into the way science progressed, especially with respect to those anatomico-functional relations which are considered to be the most complex and complicated anyway – the intellectual functions. The end of the last century marks an epoch of scientific explosion in the studies of brain functions and is a fascinating area with individual scientists following quite divergent lines: from skull measurements (e.g., Clapham, 1878; van der Kolk & Jansens, 1905) over detailed anatomical analyses of the neuronal network (e.g., Golgi, 1883–1884, 1906/67; Tanzi, 1893) to intimate anatomico-behavioral correlations (e.g., Alzheimer, 1904 b; Gudden, 1896; Nissl, 1904), and to the study of the electrical activity of the nervous system (Caton, 1875; Prawdicz-Neminski, 1925; cf. also Karbowski, 1990).

Since the time of Cuvier (1805; cited after Rylander, 1939) the entire brain was considered to be the seat of the mind, though not all parts were considered equipotential. Burdach (1819), for example, favored the frontal lobes as the special workshop of the thinking processes (cf. also Burdach 1822, 1826 and Bast, 1928). This part of the brain, which then became the subject of considerable controversy, and which received major interest also due to the psychosurgery debate after the 1940's (e.g., Hohne & Walsh, 1970; Valenstein, 1980 c), is still among the least understood areas, especially of the human cortex (Fuster, 1989; Markowitsch, 1988 a; Perecman, 1983; Stuss, 1991 a, 1991 b; Stuss & Benson, 1986; Teuber, 1972). Consequently, and as this region still is considered to regulate or influence at least some of our intellectual capacities, a major part of the book is devoted to it.

On the other hand, some regions such as the corpus callosum were given attention as well, apparently due to their special location or appearance in the brain, while for others, such as the basal forebrain and the temporal lobe, little or much less was known and investigated (at least with respect to memory) than nowadays.

Furthermore, for some illnesses the emphasis lay on regions different from those considered central today. As an example, Kohnstamm (1917) considered Korsakoff's disease as principally due to cortical damage, and Pfeifer (1910, p. 653) wrote: "Whether the thalamus has any psychic functions, we ... do not know".

Memory constitutes the basis of our intellectual life and therefore is covered quite extensively. In the description of attempts to find "memory centers" in the brain, the old discussion of the possible existence of a "Landkartensystem" (geographical map-system) (e. g., Gudden, 1886; Meinecke, 1951) is examined more closely (see, e. g., Donaldson, 1891). This discussion reviewed for instance by Lashley (1929) from the psychological viewpoint, is still a matter of controversy up to the present (e. g., John, 1972) and has been influenced by the degree to which the brain is considered as plastic or modifiable, especially after damage (e. g., Sharpey, 1879). It has also been influenced by concepts of time-related changes in neuronal activity and "rewiring" – such as the early concept of diaschisis (Monakow, 1909, 1910b, 1914) which is still dealt with in neurology (e. g., Feeney & Baron, 1986) and psychology (e. g., Teuber, 1975) (cf. Fig. 1). While I do touch on this problem tangentially, I have largely ignored the still controversial topics of brain-mind relations or consciousness and the brain (cf., e. g., Blakemore & Greenfield, 1987; Brücke, 1913; Churchland, 1986; Eccles & Robinson, 1984; Heveroch, 1914; Külpe, 1893; Maudsley, 1873; Oeser & Seitelberger, 1988; Perry, 1904; Semon, 1920; Sperry, 1988; Stodd-

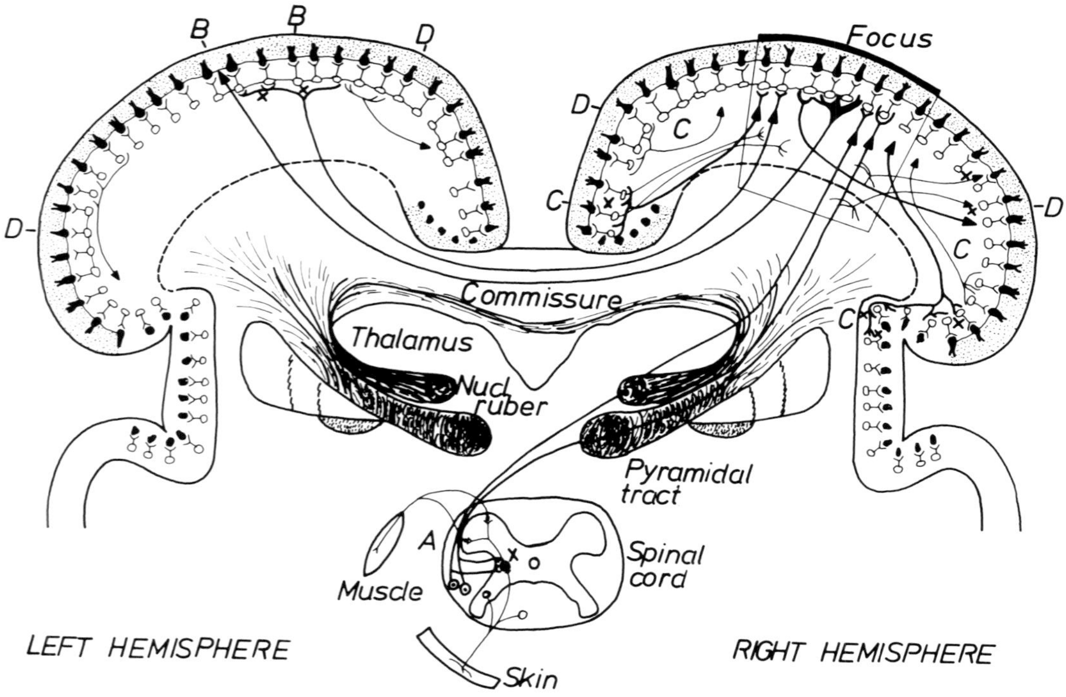

Figure 1. Monakow's (1914) diagrammatic illustration of the effect of diaschisis (translated). After damage to a cerebral cortical area termed "Focus", alterations in the activity of various other brain loci will follow. According to Monakow these can be classified into four groups of pathways: A, diaschisis cortico-spinalis; B, diaschisis commissuralis; C, diaschisis associativa; and D, central pathways of diaschisis (after Figure 1 of Monakow, 1914). 'x'-es denote points of attack for diaschisis.

ard, 1903; Volkmar, 1875, 1876; Wernicke, 1893 a, 1893 b; Ziehen, 1906, 1908 a).

As the book centers on intellectual functions, memory in particular, I have largely omitted research dealing with dementia-like conditions, though, of course, there was ample evidence for this already before the time of Alzheimer (1907). A review, which appeared at the end of the period covered in this book, was written by Grünthal (1930).

I have also not discussed work which has a close relation to the sensory modalities (e.g., Camper & Pringle, 1779), though, of course, the field of language and its disturbances for example has been extensively studied since the first attempts to relate language to the brain appeared (G. Anton, 1898; Berkhan, 1892; Bernhardt, 1885; Bramwell & Edin, 1898; Broca, 1861 a, 1861 b; Dercum, 1907; Gordinier, 1899; Hughlings-Jackson, 1878; J. W. Hunt, 1879; Kussmaul, 1910; Lichtheim, 1885; Liepmann, 1907 a; Liepmann & Quensel, 1909; Mills & Spiller, 1907; Niessl von Mayendorf, 1910; Otuszewski, 1898; Pick, 1903 a, 1905 a; Sachs, 1907; Treitel, 1892; Wernicke, 1874; cf. also the review of Harris, 1991). Some insight into this field is provided by the recent historical review of Sondhaus and Finger (1988), by the somewhat older German-language review of Bay (1961), and by the old monograph of Monakow (1914), who gave more than 1,000 references on aphasic disturbances. "Seelenblindheit" (optic agnosia), the fact that despite the maintained ability to see, the environment cannot be recognized or analyzed by the visual system, is also a topic with a long and interesting background. Milestones were reached in the research on animals (dogs) by Loeb (1884, 1885), in the books of Wilbrand (1881, 1887, 1917) and the articles of Ferrier (1881), Reinhard (1886, 1887 a, 1887 b), G. Anton (1899), Freund (1889 b, 1889 c), Siemerling (1890), Lissauer (1890 a), Moeli (1891 b), Groenouw (1892), F. Müller (1892), Monakow (1892, 1893), Wilbrand (1892, 1907), Hitzig (1900 c), Bechterew (1901), Niessl von Mayendorf (1905), and Bálint (1909).

Within the framework of vision and visual disturbances, Berger's (1900) painstaking cell counts in the occipital lobe of dogs and cats lacking visual stimulation, might be mentioned as well. Berger concluded from his results that the cerebral cortex receiving sensory stimulation-caused engrams, differs significantly from that without such stimulation, and that he considers his results of principal importance, as they show that the stimuli from the environment produce lasting alterations in the cerebral cortex, that is, (as he formulated) in the organ of the psyche (p. 567).

How controversial the discussions on possible anatomico-functional relations were at those times, is exemplified here later. For the visual modality, I refer to the article of Hitzig (1900 b) and especially to Henschen's (1923) article on the "40 years fight on the visual center and its significance for brain research". (It is assumed that Salomon Eberhard Henschen discovered the visual center in the cortex; this scientist wrote a four volume textbook on "The pathology of the brain": Henschen, 1890, 1896, 1903, 1908.)

Altogether, it is hoped that despite the unavoidable selectivity, the condensed form of this volume will still bring out the roots of present-day cognitive neuroscience.

Chapter 2: Relations Between Brain Morphology and Intellectual Capacity

Philosophical Roots

"It is with the brain we feel, and think, and will; but whether there are certain parts of the brain devoted to particular manifestations is a subject on which we have only imperfect speculations or data too insufficient for the formation of a scientific opinion." This was written in the "Quarterly Summary of the Improvements and Discoveries in the Medical Sciences" of the January 1874 number (No. 133) of the journal "Progress of the Medical Sciences" and was based on a paper which David Ferrier gave to the "Medical Times and Gazette" (Sept. 27, 1873).

Calderwood. In his book on "*The Relations of Mind and Brain*" Calderwood (1879), professor of moral philosophy at the University of Edinburgh, defined what in the 19th century was apparently meant by "intellectual functions" (p. 412 f):

We are now, then, to contemplate man as a thinker. In doing so, it becomes needful to distinguish certain departments of thought; the intellectual, or that which is concerned with the understanding of things; the moral, or that which takes cognisance of the regulation of a higher life, in accordance with a higher type of law known to a rational being; and the religious, which has regard to man's relation to an invisible order of things, and to an Absolute Being, as the source and governor of all things finite, equally the visible and the invisible. In all these departments the specific characteristics of human thought are apparent, as they are common to all the three. We find ourselves amongst the generalisations, the conceptions, the inductive and deductive processes, all of which are proved to be familiar to every human mind. The laws which regulate the higher forms of mental activity are the same in all the three departments. There is no distinction to be drawn between them in this respect. Yet are they so different as departments of thought, that some minds concern themselves far more with one of the departments than with the others. Some show an intellectual interest concentrated chiefly on the understanding of things as existing in the material universe, and the most qualified among such thinkers aim at contributing their share to the advance of science. Some who have little familiarity with these regions of research, bestow much thought on the requirements of self-discipline, the management of life as a whole, and the attainment of an excellence towards which approximation may be made, even while bodily strength is failing. Others enlarge this range of thought by considering the relation of practical life to a system of things greater than the visible – seeing the invisible and eternal – and finding a harmony of existence in the absolute excellence of the Deity. In this department also we find a phase of higher mental activity concerned more with the intellectual problems which urge the human mind into fields of speculation, than with the requirements of a moral and religious life.

A similar opinion was held by Ludwig Büchner (1872) in Germany (the brother of the famous poet Georg Büchner) in his book "*Kraft und Stoff*" [Energy and matter] which appeared in at least 12 editions. He furthermore wrote that there was an uninterrupted stepladder from the animal to the highest educated human being, and that in some humans (who might be compared to gods) the intellectual nature predominates, while in others the somatic one does. Even in 1916 an article "Ueber den Seelensitz" [On the seat of the soul] appeared in the *Archiv für Psychiatrie und Nervenkrankheiten* (Kronthal, 1916). The principal conclusion of this article was the following (p. 277): "The soul is a happening [ein Geschehen]; its seat is neither in the brain nor in any other organ. The soul is the sum of reflexes. Therefore, the soul is, where life is." Previously, Arnett (1904), Bain (1881), Flügel (1902), Jaeger (1880), Kern (1907), Lazarus (1876, 1878, 1882), Raue (1850), Rehmke (1891), and R. Sommer (1891) reviewed past and present beliefs on the soul. One of the most recent examples on this matter (at least from a neurological point of view) are the contributions of Bumke (1942) and Laubenthal (1953). Also Forel's book on brain and soul was successful, appearing in 1922 in its 13th edition.

The soul and conscious life of children as well had been intensely studied quite early in neuroscientific research (e.g., Baldwin, 1898; Darwin, 1877/1971; Kussmaul, 1859; Preyer, 1882; Soltmann, 1875).

Skull, Brain, Sex, and Character

Though phrenology had demised in the 19th century (cf. Franz, 1912; Rollett, 1900) there were still numerous attempts to relate skull proportions (e.g., W. Sommer, 1897; Van der Kolk & Jansens, 1905), the brain or portions of it to the subjects' intellectual capacities. This was first done by merely measuring brain weights (cf. e.g. Büchner, 1872; Crichton-Browne, 1879; Dräseke, 1906; Huschke, 1854; Jacobsohn, 1904; Meynert, 1867), sometimes without correcting for body weight or age. W. Sommer (1897), for instance, found a much larger skull volume in "neuropsychopathics" than in normals and reported an asymmetric inner skull for 96% of the "lunatics".

Probably the most extensive work in this field was done by Huschke (1854) (485 cases) and by Matiegka (1902) whose work was summarized by Spitzka in *Science* in 1903. Matiegka, a member of the Bohemian Science Society, was quite careful in his comparisons, listing 15 factors which might influence brain weight. His principal conclusion (summarized in a table in *Science*) was that there is an increase in brain weight from day-laborers over trade-workers and businessmen to scholars, physicians, and other persons of higher mental abilities.

In an extensive study on the brains of criminals (comprised mainly of citizens of the old Austrian-Hungarican-Danube-Monarchy), Benedikt (1879) concluded that "the brains of criminals show deviations from the normal type and that the criminals might be considered as an anthropological variation of its species or at least of the cultured races" (p.110). The view that brain damage such as from prefrontal tumors (Sullivan, 1911) or in specific areas of the brain (frontal lobes, amygdala) might foster a criminal behavior was popularized up to the recent present (Pontius & Ruttiger, 1976; Pontius & Yudowitz, 1980; cf. the chapter on psychosurgery).

A male-female distinction was made by Huschke (1854) who, from his extensive volumetric measurements, concluded that in females the parietal lobe (Scheitelhirn: the brain of the "Gemüth" [feeling or temperament]) and in males the frontal lobe (Stirnhirn: the brain of intelligence) is more voluminous (p.182). A minor development of the female human frontal gyri – which corresponds more closely to the fetal brain prior to its final stage – was also found by R. Wagner (1860, p.89), though he emphasized the existence of a certain variability which allows the appearance of opposite pictures between the sexes (p.90). Sixty years later, Centres (1914) also investigated sex differences. He concluded from his measurements that "with identical body height the cranium volume nearly always is significantly higher in women than in men" (p.1028). He also failed to find any volume differences between healthy and psychiatric cases. Early tracts on the psychology of the female psyche were written by Simmel (1890) and Wendt (1891).

Deviations and Exceptional Features

A number of single case studies were conducted before and at the turn of the century in the search for either deviations from the average or exceptional features (Adler, 1875; Benedikt, 1876, 1880; Bielschowsky, 1915; Binswanger, 1882, 1885; Dwight, 1878; Edinger, 1893;

Elmiger, 1902; Fraenkel, 1886; Giacomini, 1881; Gowers, 1878b; Gudden, 1870a, 1870b; Hermanides & Köppen, 1903; Hoppe, 1908; Jensen, 1875, 1880, 1889; Karplus, 1905; König, 1886; Köppen, 1896; Kotschetkowa, 1901; Leidesdorf, 1865; Matell, 1893; L. Meyer, 1868; Mickle, 1897, 1898; Möbius, 1900; Moeli, 1891a; Näcke, 1893; Probst, 1901a; Rolleston, 1888; Sander, 1868a, 1868b, 1875; Schaffer, 1905; Spitzka, 1901; R. Wagner, 1860, 1862; Waldschmidt, 1887; Weinberg, 1905; Wizel, 1904). J. Marshall (1892/1893), for example, provided comparisons of brain weights for 15 outstanding individuals. Other examples of data on exceptional brains were provided by Bechterew and Weinberg (1909), who studied the brain of a prominent chemist of this period, by Hansemann (1899), who studied the brain of Hermann von Helmholtz, a prominent physiologist, and by Retzius (1898, 1900a, 1900b, 1902, 1904, 1905) who studied a series of exceptional brains (of a prominent astronomer, a female mathematician, a physicist, a statesman, a biologist, and microencephalic brains; cf. also Donaldson, 1890, and Hechst, 1932, for a discussion of microencephalic brains). Muhr (1875), in an extensively detailed case report, presented the brain of a psychotic 47 year old man. He found it to be smaller than average, quite asymmetrical, with a peculiarly deviant cerebellum, and with smaller lobes and asymmetrical telencephalic and diencephalic nuclei and nerves (Figs. 2 and 3). Bechterew and Weinberg (1909) observed a distinct dilation of the left parietal region and furthermore attributed a "luxury outfit" to the prefrontal lobe of their case; similarly, Retzius (1898) and Hansemann (1899) noted some unusual, "secondary" gyri in the prefrontal cortex, and a bilateral dilation in the region of the posterior end of the sylvian fissure (supramarginal and angular gyri), that is, in an area similar to the one which recently was considered to be exceptional microanatomically in Einstein's brain (Diamond, Scheibel, Murphy, & Harvey, 1985).

In a later report, Hansemann (1907) described the brains of T. Mommsen (an historian), R. W. Bunsen (chemist), and A. von Menzel (a picture painter). In parallel to this approach larger and larger series of brains were weighed (Handmann, 1906; Spitzka, 1903; Weigner, 1906). Spitzka (1903, 1907) especially attempted to give a rather complete survey of brains examined from exceptional persons. In his article from 1907 he showed seven brains in particular, but in addition gave short descriptions of more than 130 further ones, studied by various authorities in a number of countries (including brains from 4 women). Several of his illustrations, somewhat exaggerating his interest in constructing definite relations between intelligence and brain morphology, showed brains from an exceptional man, a non-white person (such as a "Bushwoman", "Hottentot Venus", "Papuan from British New Guinea") and an ape (gorilla, orangutan) (Fig. 4). In commenting on these specimens he wrote: "The brain of a first-class genius like Friedrich Gauss is as far removed from that of the savage bushman as that of the latter from the brain of the nearest related ape" (p. 226f).

Similar investigations, though less exaggerated in their interpretation, were given on the brains of an Australian aborigine and Eskimos by Karplus (1902) and Hrdlicka (1903), respectively. A little earlier Marshall (1864) had described the convolutions of a bushwoman's brain and "of the two smallest human idiot brains yet on record, belonging respectively to a microcephalic woman and boy of English parentage" (p. 501). In parallel to these neurological analyses (cf. also Sankey, 1878) other features of the human body such as blood samples (e. g. Bruck, 1867) were studied as well, or exceptional behavioral manifestations (e. g. Christoffel & Grossmann, 1923). (Descriptions of exceptional brains of nonhuman species have also been documented: e.g., Brouwer, 1912; furthermore, weighing brains was also common around the beginning of the 20th century: e.g., Dräseke, 1901; Kohlbrugge, 1901; Ziehen, 1901b).

Holländer

A highly inclusive idea was expressed in the work of Holländer (1900), a "specialist for psychiatry and the nervous diseases", working in London. He reviewed a number of studies on

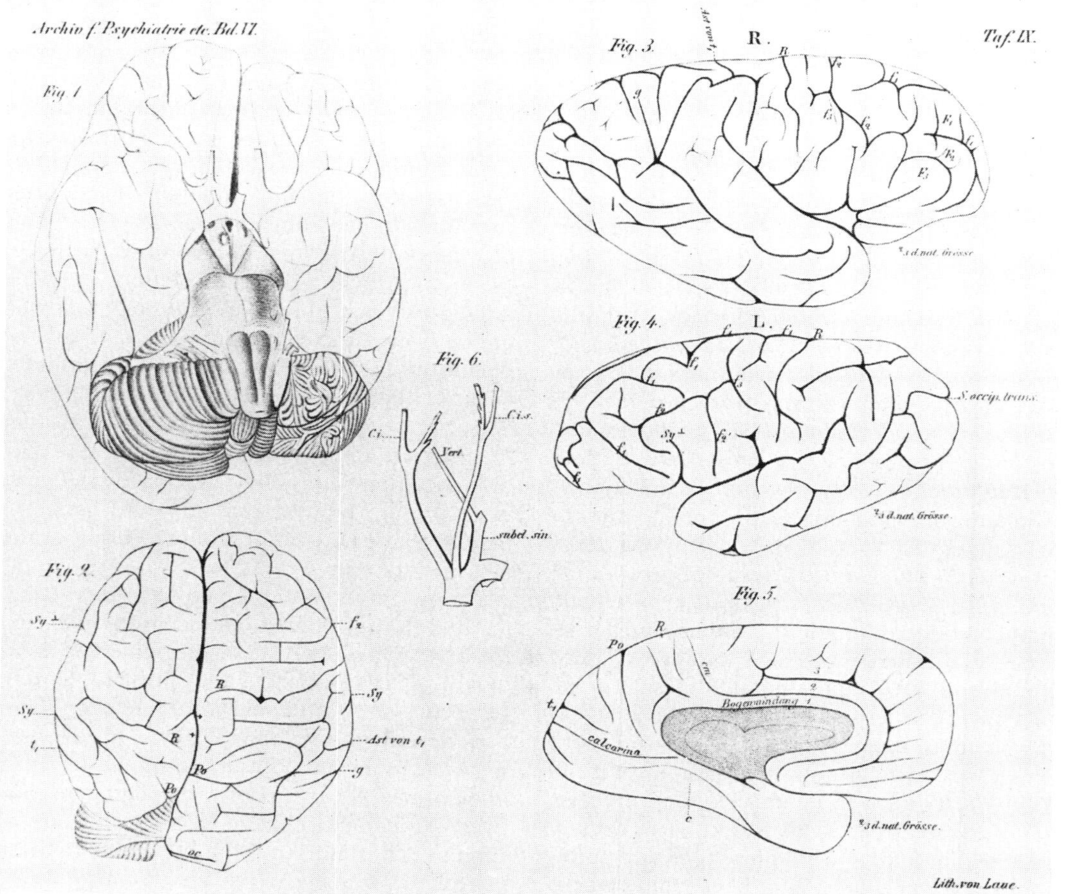

Figure 2. Skull and brain of a person affected by "madness" (from Muhr, 1875). Subfigure 1 shows the inferior surface of the brain. The shortened left hemisphere is visible with the atrophied cerebellum. Subfigure 2 shows a dorsal view of the brain, subfigures 3 and 4 views from the right and left, and subfigure 5 from medial. The arch of the aorta is given in subfigure 6; it shows the ratio of the carotid arteries.

the brain weight of famous persons. While acknowledging the large interindividual variances, he still supposed that a brain which is large in all its parts, indicates not only intelligence, but strong character attributes (of any kind).

It is astonishing how many unique arguments Holländer listed for or against the special role of specific brain areas. On pages 6 and 7, for instance, the controversies about the importance of the occipital lobes for the intellect were listed (cf. in this connection Henschen's, 1923, review on the visual cortex): While Hughlings Jackson, E. A. Schäfer and others stated that the occipital lobes were most important, Holländer argued that (1) in "dementia paralytica" the occipital lobes are spared, that (2) the occipital lobes are better developed in women than in men, and that (3) in criminals the occipital lobes frequently are underdeveloped.

With respect to some other "functions", Holländer gave more accurate (or, for the present, better acceptable) descriptions of possible anatomico-behavioral relationships, for example for aphasic disturbances, acoustic representation, or different representations of numbers and words (Hinshelwood, 1895; Morgan, 1896).

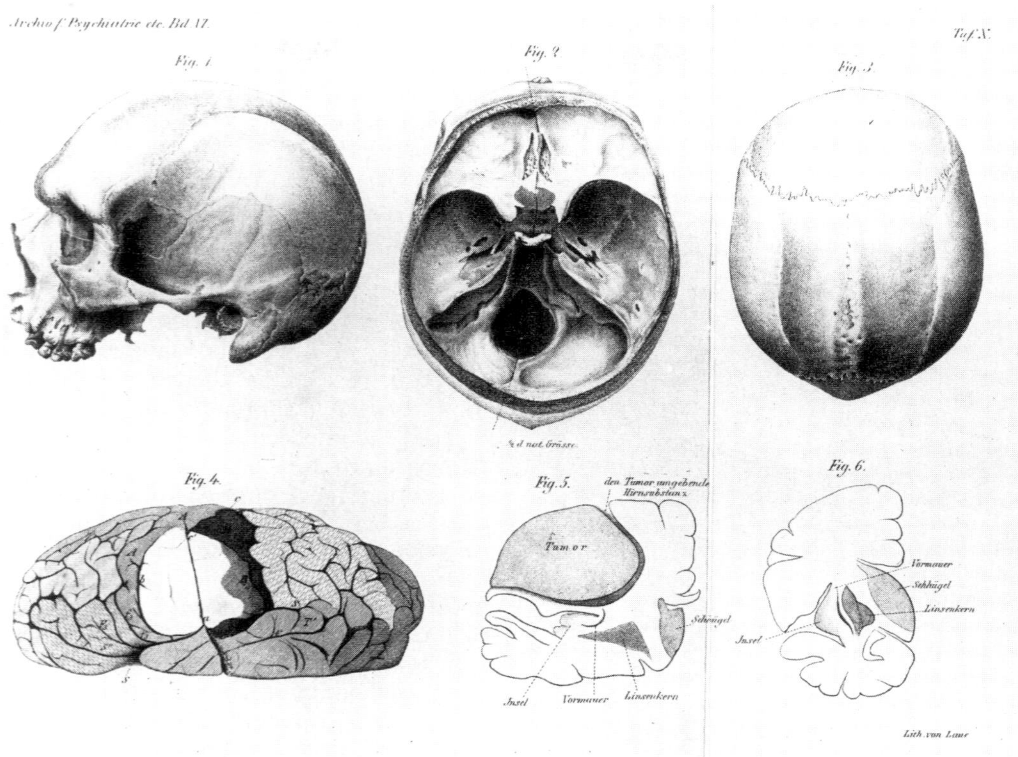

Figure 3. Skull and brain of a person affected by "madness" (from Muhr, 1875). Subfigure 1 gives a lateral view of the skull; subfigure 2 shows the base of the skull with the shortened left brain half. Subfigure 3 is a dorsal view of the skull. Subfigures 4–6 show the area of the tumor from lateral (subfigure 4) and coronal (subfigures 5 and 6) perspectives.

Other relations such as, for instance, a center for "religious hallucinations" in the posterior part of the superior frontal gyrus, or a relationship between the size of the cerebellum and the sexual drive, are no longer seriously considered by present-day neuroscientists.

Holländer concluded that deviations from the normal state can follow if

"(1) a cortical area is normally developed, but highly active, while other regions are poorly developed (and therefore cannot appropriately inhibit the first area);
(2) a cortical area is over-strongly developed in comparison to other, normal, regions; and
(3) a cortical area is pathological so that the fundamental psychic activity localized there shows an exaggerated manifestation." (p. 32).

Resignation

While most studies of brains from "exceptional" persons noted some special features, such as "luxury outfits" of the prefrontal lobe, "secondary gyri", or a "special development of the occipital lobe" (Krücke, 1963, on the brain of the neurologist L. Edinger), the overall outcome of this kind of research remained disappointing. This was also recognized by Retzius in his later investigations in which he appeared less enthusiastic with respect to the possibilities of detailing distinct neuromorphological characteristics of his cases, though he still emphasized some enlargements or a greater richness of convolutions in parietal and prefrontal areas. It is astonishing how frankly authors in-

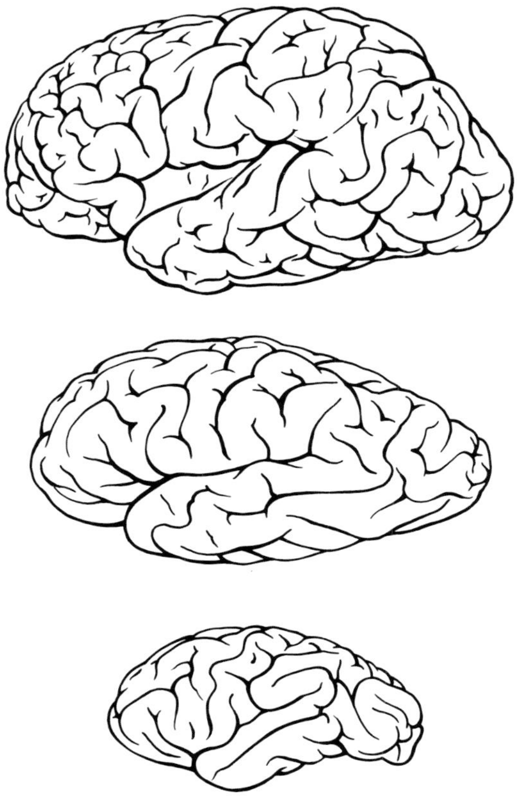

Figure 4. Brains of Helmholtz, a Papuan from New Guinea, and a gorilla. Copy of Figure 11 of Spitzka (1907).

terpreted data when these ran counter to their expectations. Matiegka (1902) described the results of authors who had found the heaviest human brains ever described in "an epileptic idiot" (2850 g) and in a newspaper boy (2400 g) who was considered to have been "more or less an idiot" (p. 30). Matiegka argued that while such relations are perplexing on the first glance, they are not convincing because "who would equalize the functionless brain mass of a lunatic with the active brain mass of mentally distinguished persons" (p. 30).

A few years later, Stieda (1908) described the brain of a scientist who had been able to speak 40 to 50 languages. Though his analysis of the brain was at least as detailed as those of Retzius, his conclusions were rather cautious, or even negative as to the possibilities of relating psychological characteristics and gross neuromorphological features. He emphasized that there is indeed a wide variation in the patterns of sulci and gyri, but denied a functional role for them.

Much earlier, in 1860, R. Wagner had already come to conclusions that were quite advanced for the time he lived in: "The result, though not based on a very large number of weighted brains, shows that the relative weight of the hemispheres compared to the rest of the brain is even larger in women than in men, and this supports the idea that there is no simple relation between hemispheric weight and intelligence and intellectual work" (p. 92). In 1862, R. Wagner confirmed his view stating that within a certain range of brain volume there is no relation between the expression of the psychic functions and the brain's volume.

Hansemann (1907) and Stieda (1908) gave particularly thorough discussions; Hansemann pointed out that it might be more worthwhile and rewarding for future investigations to examine the brains of humans with mediocre intellect, but exceptional abilities in a certain field, and Stieda (1908) considered it probably more fruitful to look at fine neuronal and biochemical variations in the brain and not at gross morphology (cf. also Auerbach, 1906, and Wallace, 1905). This idea was followed by Kaes (1905, 1909 a, 1909 b) and Brodmann (1908 b, 1909 a) and, somewhat later, by O. Vogt (1929) who studied I. Lenin's brain and found it to contain huge pyramidal neurons in the third layer which led him to term Lenin an "Assoziationsathleten" (cf. also the review in Kleist, 1934 b). All in all, this method of investigating relations between brain morphology and the subject's intellectual capacities became less and less attractive.

With increasing medical research and an increasing accumulation of case descriptions, it became more the case that relations between brain pathology and intellectual deficiencies became more and more translucent (but see the cautious notes of Monakow, 1909, 1910, 1914). Aside from the more general affections of the brain such as commotio cerebri (e.g., Bollinger, 1891; Mayer, 1929) and dementia

(Alzheimer, 1907, 1911; Bielschowsky & Brodmann, 1905; Bolton, 1903 a, 1903 b; Ciarla, 1915; Hübner, 1910; Pick, 1892, 1893, 1901, 1906; Probst, 1903; W. Scholz, 1923; Spatz, 1937; Stockert, 1932; Stransky, 1905 a, 1905 b, 1905 c; Yoshikawa, 1905), insights into the machinery of the nervous system in cognitive information processing (see chapter on "Memory and Memory Disturbances") came from work on specific degenerative diseases such as multiple sclerosis, Huntington's chorea, and Parkinson's syndrome (e.g., Adler, 1901; Freund, 1891; Hallervorden & Spatz, 1922; Jolly, 1913; Marburg, 1906; Parkinson, 1817; Raecke, 1906; Redlich, 1898; F.C. Rose, 1989; Seiffer, 1905; Stier, 1903; cf. Tyler & Tyler, 1986, and Yahr, 1978 for a description of Parkinson's life and personality), on genetic-based diseases (Down, 1886, 1887; Fraser & Mitchell, 1876; cf. Wilkins & Brody, 1971), and on the alcoholic Korsakoff syndrome (Boedeker, 1905; Brodmann, 1902, 1904; Gregor, 1902; Kalberlah, 1904; Korsakoff, 1889, 1890; Korsakow, 1890, 1891; Korsakow & Serbski, 1892; Krauss, 1904; Kutner, 1906; E. Meyer & Raecke, 1903; Pick, 1915; Serbsky, 1907; Thomsen, 1890; Wehrung, 1905), and on distinct brain damage, especially of the temporal lobes and of diencephalic structures (e.g., Bechterew, 1900 a; Bonhoeffer, 1901, 1904; Freund, 1889 a; Gianelli, 1897; Gudden, 1896; Holländer, 1900; Kaplan, 1898; A. Knapp, 1905, 1906; Knauer, 1909; Kraepelin, 1886 a, 1887 a, 1887 b, 1900; Liepmann, 1910, 1913; Meynert, 1884; Monakow, 1881; Nothnagel, 1879; Phelps, 1894; Pick, 1886; Rieger, 1889, 1890; Siemerling, 1887; W. Sommer, 1880; Sterz, 1910; Thomsen, 1888; Viedenz, 1903; Wernicke, 1889; Zingerle, 1912 a). A number of old references, especially from English literature, can be found in Macmillan's (1986) "journey through skull and brain" and examples of early books on the possible anatomical loci of complex functions include the contributions of Campbell (1905), Flechsig (1896 a, 1896 b) and Luciani and Seppili (1886) (cf. also F. Walsh, 1964).

With respect to experimental literature, studies on animals with brain damage contributed substantially to an understanding of the brain's management of intellectual processes (e.g. Bianchi, 1894, 1895, 1922; Ferrier, 1874, 1875, 1886; Goltz, 1877, 1881 a, 1881 b, 1884, 1888, 1892, 1899; Goltz & Ewald, 1899; Gudden, 1870 b; Hitzig, 1874 b, 1876, 1900 b, 1901 a, 1903 a, 1903 b; Munk, 1881). More recently they have provided a number of comparative studies on differences and similarities between the human and the nonhuman primate brain of which I will cite only a few examples, namely the earlier works of Grünthal (1936 a) and the more recent ones of Ettlinger (1971), MacPhail (1982), and Passingham (1981, 1982).

Outlook

Today the search for correlations between specific features of brain morphology and psychotic disorders has been revived, especially due to the advent and progress of neuroimaging techniques. Here, morphological changes have been found in uni- and bipolar affective disorders (Dupont et al., 1990; Sackeim et al., 1990), schizophrenia (Altshuler, Casanova, Goldberg, & Kleinman, 1990; Andreasen et al., 1990; Bruton et al., 1990; Buchsbaum et al., 1990; Hawton, Shepstone, Soper, & Reznek, 1990; Lewis, 1990; Minabe, Kadono, & Kurachi, 1990; G. P. Reynolds, Czudek, & Andrews, 1990; Waddington et al., 1990), and even in depression (Zubenko et al., 1990). But improved conventional stereological methods are also in use again (e.g., Pakkenberg, 1990). The opposite case, in which traumatic brain disease may result in mental diseases, was frequently discussed in the old literature; for examples see Browne (1872), Guder (1886), Hay (1875), Herzog (1842), and Souplet (1871). I wish to mention here in particular Guder's (1886) book in which a number of examples of early brain surgery (with frequent recovery) are listed, including sources from English and French literature of the last century.

Chapter 3: The Frontal Lobes: The Most Recent Attributes of the Brain

The Myths of the Frontal Cortex

In 1908 Niessl von Mayendorf already termed the prefrontal cortex the most mythical part of the brain ("der mythenreichste der Gehirnteile"; p. 1175; cf. also Schiller, 1985). Since the beginning of modern brain research in the second half of the 19th century, intellectual functions such as planning, foresight, decision making, and related acts have been attributed especially to this brain region (G. Anton & Zingerle, 1902; Bianchi, 1894, 1895; Biro, 1910; Ferrier, 1874; Ferrier & Yeo, 1884; Fritsch & Hitzig, 1870; McBurney & Starr, 1893; Mingazzini, 1901), or Brodmann's (1909 b, 1912) 'regio frontalis' (cf. also Nissl, 1919). In 1854 Huschke claimed: "The frontal lobe is the brain of intelligence, the parietal lobe that of temperament" (p. 180) and indicated that he had made this same statement as early as in 1821.

The dominant view at the turn of the century is exemplified in the following citation from Mills and Weisenburg (1906, p. 338):

> The evidence afforded by studies in human and comparative morphology and anatomy of the cerebral surface in favor of the view that the prefrontal lobe, and especially the left prefrontal lobe, is the seat of the highest mental faculties, is of much value. Already a considerable number of the brains of notable men presenting special fissural and gyral arrangement and development of the prefrontal region indicative of high or unusual endowment have been put on record. Reference need only be made to the classical cases of Gauss, Helmholtz and Grote and to the more recent studies of E. A. Spitzka on the brains of the two Seguins, Cope, Harrison Allen, Major Powell and others. If the anatomical and morphological characteristics of such brains are placed side by side with those of criminals, paranoics, negroes and other human beings of low individual or racial development (as studied by Dr. Mills and others), the psychophysiologic importance of the prefrontal region becomes apparent. It might be remarked in passing that morphological and anatomic studies do not always seem to give to the left prefrontal lobe the preponderance in higher mentality attributed to it by some. Spitzka, for instance, found in the brain of Major Powell a preponderant development of the mesial surface of the right frontal lobe. In studies of this kind a comparison should always carefully be made between the fissural and gyral characteristics of the prefrontal and parieto-temporo-occipital areas. A superior development of the latter is not always accompanied by an equally superior pattern of the former. In rare cases the former may largely outclass the latter.
>
> Morphological studies of the brains of imbecilles, such as have been made by Willmarth and others, are corrobarative of the view of the higher psychic functions of the prefrontal region. These brains are, as a rule, characterized by unusual simplicity in fissural and gyral arrangement.

In 1922 this view was corroborated on the basis of results from more than 300 cases of veterans from World War I. Pfeifer stated that with respect to intellectual qualities prefrontal damaged patients performed worst. This held for the processes of thinking, logic, discriminating, complicated acts of will and attention, affect, general memory, and the ability to memorize, and was most severe in subjects with left prefrontal damage. (The relation of the "mental faculties" to "exclusively" the left prefrontal lobe was stressed by Phelps, 1902, 1906, who gave detailed accounts on about two dozen patients.)

The link between the prefrontal cortex and the intellectual faculties of the personality was emphasized throughout the last century. A number of neurological and psychiatric diseases received attention at the same time (or even earlier) which have at least some affinity to the frontal lobes. These included Alzheimer's disease (*Alois Alzheimer 1864–1915*; Alzheimer, 1907, 1911; N. Hoff & Hippius, 1989), Parkinson's disease (*James P. Parkinson 1755–1824*; Parkinson, 1817; Schiller, 1986; Yahr, 1978), Pick's disease (*Arnold Pick 1851–1924*; Pick, 1878, 1886, 1892, 1893, 1901, 1906; Braunmühl, 1930; Pötzl, 1942; Spatz, 1937), multiple sclerosis (*Jean-Martin Charcot 1825–1893*; Compston, 1988; Goetz, 1987), Huntington's chorea (*George Sumner Huntington 1851–1916*), schizophrenia (*Eugen G. Bleuler 1857–1939*), and Korsakoff's syndrome (*Sergei S. Korsakoff 1854–1900*; Korsakoff, 1889, 1890; Korsakow, 1890, 1891; Korsakow & Serbski, 1892).

Welt's Cases

Welt (1888) held a view of the prefrontal cortex which differed from the dominant view at the end of the last century. The first case she described was that of a 37-year old Swiss craftsman who fell from the fourth floor of a house and received damage to the left frontal lobe (case I). She gave a very clear, detailed description of changes in the character of this patient. Prior to the trauma he had been a cheerful, relaxed man of good humor, but afterwards he became very critical and annoying to his co-patients. For, when the professor of the clinic urged him to behave himself and told him that he received good meals and the best wine in the hospital, the patient answered that the other patients and the hospital staff were at fault and, concerning the wines, that he was used to drinking Chateau Laffite and other French wines but not the "sour stuff" provided in the clinic. Figure 5 provides a view of the prefrontal damage seen in this patient. (For a critique of Welt's interpretation of this case see E. Müller, 1902 b.)

Welt added further case descriptions, one of which was the "crowbar case" (see below); she noted that character changes in different patients might go from better to worse, or vice versa, someone who was originally taciturn might develop a lively, merry, and alert character. Her report is furthermore of value because of the detailed tables she gave on roughly 50 cases taken from older literature (dating from 1819) in which frontal lobe damage was unaccompanied by character changes. From comparing locations she concluded that changes in character most likely followed damage to the (right) medial orbital surface of the frontal lobes. A detailed behavioral and anatomical analysis of a 39-year-old woman, who developed personality changes (including religious delusions) after massive prefrontal degeneration, can also be found in Voegelin (1897), and the case of a young soldier with basal prefrontal damage and bizarre social behavior was given by Knörlein (1865).

The Term "Prefrontal Cortex"

While 'lobus frontalis' or the German 'Stirnhirn' were coined by Chaussier (1807) and F. Arnold (1838), respectively (cf. Eberstaller, 1890), the term prefrontal cortex was apparently first used in a book by Owen (1868) on the anatomy of mammals (Divac, 1988). Its subsequent use was frequent (e. g., Bianchi, 1895; J. M. Clarke, 1898; Eberstaller, 1890; Ferrier, 1886, 1889; Ferrier & Yeo, 1884; Flechsig, 1896 a, 1896 b; Fritsch & Hitzig, 1870; Hadden, 1888; Hitzig, 1874 a, 1874 b, 1874 c; Horsley & Schäfer, 1888; Luciani & Tamburini, 1878; Soltmann, 1875; Welt, 1888; Williamson, 1896). As late as 1890 Eberstaller criticized the use of the term because he considered that separating a lobus praefrontalis from a lobus postfrontalis involved only an 'arbitrarily drawn dividing line' ("willkürlich gezogene Trennungslinie")

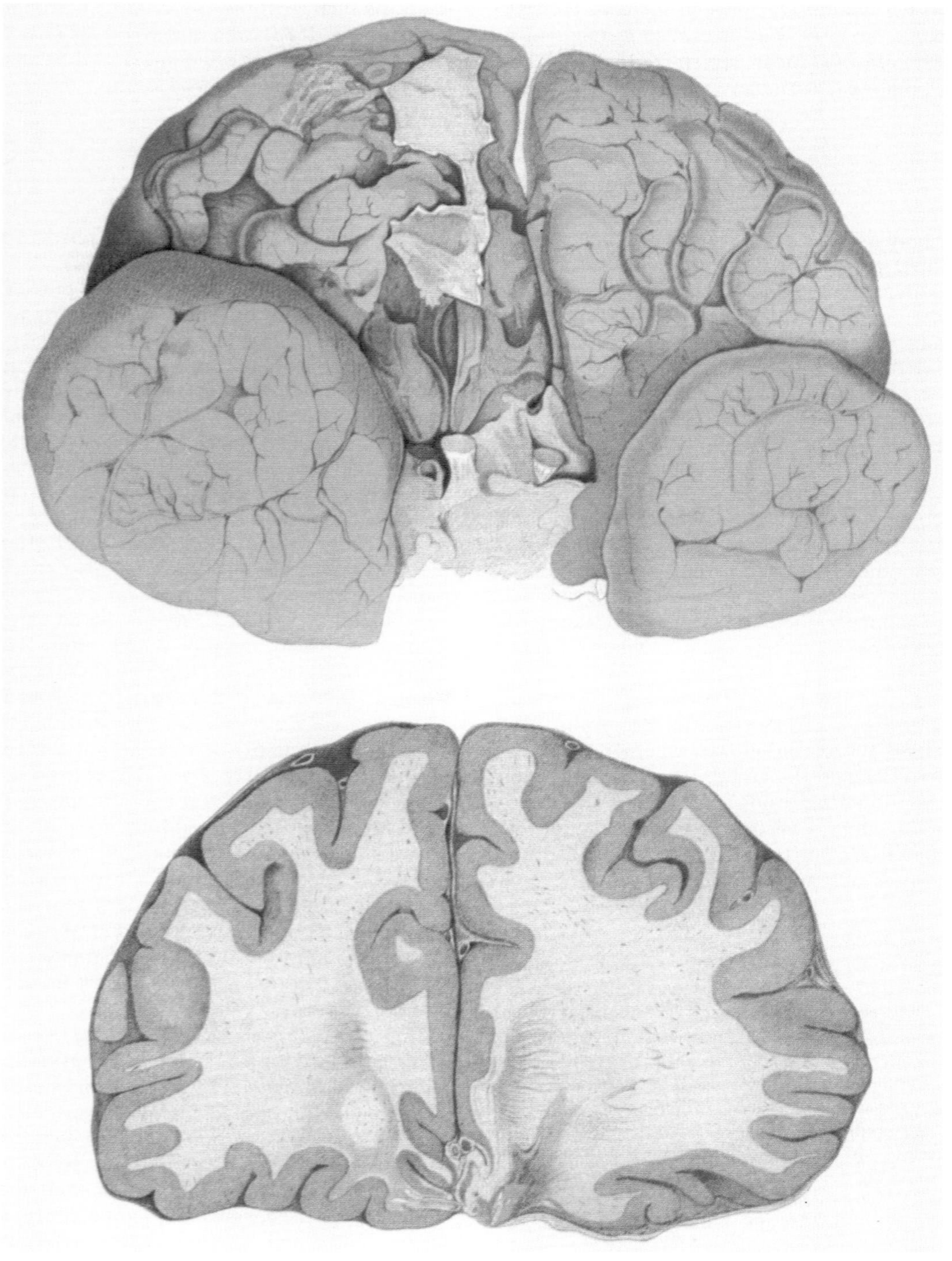

Figure 5. The appearance of the basal prefrontal cortex (top) and of the case from the Zurich-clinic, discussed by Welt; the bottom part of the figure shows a coronal section through the frontal lobe of this case made 3 cm posterior to the tip of the frontal brain (From the Table VII of Welt, 1888.)

which would vary between subjects. However, while the latter view prevailed throughout the 19th century (and in part still does; cf. e. g. Stuss & Benson, 1986), there were some well-known scientists such as Munk (1877, 1881, 1882) and Goltz (1884, 1888) who suggested more profane, motor-related, functions for this most anterior part of the (human) brain.

Methodological Controversies

Many of these controversial opinions were related to the particular methods used by the individual scientists, their dominant views on the action and interaction of nervous tissue, and the animal(s) studied (cf. discussions of this issue by Dodds, 1878; Exner, 1881; Feuchtwanger, 1923, p. 179 f; Goltz, 1877; Hitzig, 1876; Jastrowitz, 1888; Loeb, 1885, 1886; Pfeifer, 1910; Richter, 1918; C. Vogt, 1900; O. Vogt, 1897, 1900 a, 1900 b; and Klebanoff, 1945; S. A. K. Wilson, 1931). Statements of Goltz (1877, 1888) and Munk (1882) illustrate this point: 'Similar to Hitzig, I will also pass over the stimulation experiments of Munk. I share Schiff's [1880] opinion that "it is difficult to suppress laughing at those who want to discover nerve centers using galvanic currents"' (Goltz, 1884, p. 486).

Criticizing Munk's lesion experiments and Wernicke's support of Munk's results, Goltz (1888, p. 452) questioned whether Munk ever had lesioned the gray matter in toto as Munk stated that his lesions had been 3 mm deep at most while – according to Goltz – the gray matter in a dog brain is up to 10 mm deep at the bottom of some deep sulci:

> Nevertheless Munk maintains to have ablated the total of the gray matter of the visual sphere which is indeed 10 mm at several loci, by removing a layer of only 3 mm depth. Wernicke, an admirer of Munk, made no objections to this mysterious performance; for advocates of modern localization hypotheses use a strange double-entry mental bookkeeping. If confronted with observations which do not conform to their opinion, they wear double pairs of spectacles, to find confirmatory evidence, even if this is nonexistent. On the other hand, if they are confronted with work where the authors salute the 'Lokalisationslehre' [theory of localization of brain functions], then the most adventurous things are accepted in blind faith.

The in principal identical argument revelled at Munk was made by Loeb (1886, p. 332).

Munk (1882, p. 773) argued against Ferrier's results thus: "The question of just how Mr. Ferrier was able to ascribe the apathy, sleepiness, nervousness, etc. in the monkeys to the loss of function in the frontal lobe (instead of considering them the obvious results of only the mechanical lesioning and of the encephalomeningitis, commensurate with what occurs after other larger brain injuries in unfortunate experiments) would not be understandable at all except by realizing that Mr. Ferrier interprets whatever he observes after his extirpation experiments without criticism for his own set opinion." (Also, Carville [cited after Bartholow, 1874], Dupuy [cited after Bartholow, 1874], Goltz, 1877, Hitzig, 1874 b, and Bianchi, 1895, stated that Ferrier had made premature conclusions; Bianchi stated that he "was too much impressed by the phenomena observed immediately after the operation"; vice versa, Ferrier, 1878 a, had strongly criticized Munk before: "Herr Munk does not appear to have paid any attention to such precautions, ..." [p. 230].) In another article Munk (1877) had criticized that "modern representatives of the physiology of the central organs leave centers [in the brain] to germinate and increase as generously as funguses in modern pathology" (p. 4).

Gudden (1886) and Monakow (1902), on the other hand, were more careful in considering the value of individual techniques and the results obtained by applying them. Nevertheless, Monakow (1902) also pointed to the fact that some researchers – such as Ferrier – were too quick in drawing conclusions from their first studies, while the conclusions of others, such as Hitzig – based on long experience – were quite reliable (p. 582). (See also Hitzig's, 1887, sharply formulated attack against Loeb which included comments such as 'An apostle of lawlessness arose with Mr. Loeb in the field of brain physiology, ...'.)

An example taken from Monakow (1902, p. 587) can suffice to show how great the difference of opinion was on the action of the brain: 'Consider only the first mutilation experiments (by rinsing out brain substance), undertaken for example by Goltz (about 24 years ago). Such an "operation method" can only be tolerated by someone who takes the brain as a homogenous mass.'

Seen in the light of this Sturm und Drang period when most methods for studying the brain had just been developed and hence were rather crude, it is not surprising that some authors were skeptical of techniques which they did not apply themselves, and this all the more so, because little was as yet known about the anatomy and physiology of the brain and of the consequences of its being damaged (cf. e.g., Forel, 1887; Jacobsohn, 1904). Dodds in 1878 divided the available methods into "the method of electrical stimulation" (p. 343) and "the method of destruction" (p. 358).

Intellectual Functions

Returning to the frontal lobes and the question of their role in guiding intellectual behavior, Goltz (1888), especially, vigorously attacked the views of his colleagues. In order to give an impression of his style, a paragraph is cited here in which he discussed Munk's 'invention of the body sphere ("Rumpfsphäre")':

> One of the most amazing outgrowths of the unlimited drive to localize functions of the brain is Munk's invention of the body sphere. After locating the sensitive areas for the arms and legs and the head within the excitable zone, it was necessary to attribute to a little area, left over in the cortex, responsibility for the (central) body. Munk [1881, p. 61] writes: "For a year and more the frontal lobe was able to withstand every attempt at understanding its function", etc. Now it has finally been stamped as the sensitive area for the body. One might expect therefore that Munk would attempt to substantiate this hypothesis by demonstrating a disturbance in the skin of the body after extirpation of the frontal lobe. The opposite is the case: Munk explicitly states that sensation is never influenced by frontal lobe destruction. Nonetheless he considers it "precisely proven" that the frontal lobe is the sensitive area for the trunk. This means a sensitive area for an area that has nothing to do with feeling. For the humble understanding of a normal person this is only intelligible with difficulty, but when one is fully determined to complete a map of the brain with a new discovery, one can easily get past such small obstacles in logic.

Munk was also the target of a vehement and detailed attack by Hitzig (1903 b): "I would not believe that he [Munk] would defend himself with insults and hateful and malicious suspicions, as well as by making unfounded contentions and accusations, ..., I thought at least he would have been more intelligent" (p. 605f). And: "I will harmonize my tone with his, but otherwise do not care about him, and especially will not put my drawn sword back into its sheath as long as I might need it for defense and am able to use it" (p. 629).

Hitzig (1876) also made a rejoinder to Goltz in which one of his criticisms was that experiments with frogs might not allow a transfer to the situation in hemiplegic humans (cf. also the similar critique of Fritsch, 1884).

Based on Fritsch and Hitzig's (1870) observations that the frontal lobes were electrically non-excitable and that extirpation of them resulted neither in any form of paralysis nor in loss of perceptual abilities, but, rather in defects of intelligence, Fritsch and Hitzig (1870) simply termed the frontal lobes the 'organ for abstract reasoning'. Later, in 1884, Hitzig completed these observations by reporting that frontal lobectomies may – temporarily – lead to visual disturbance in the contralateral eye, indicating a direct connection between the frontal lobe and the visual system. Ferrier (1874) principally agreed with Fritsch and Hitzig's descriptions, though he emphasized attentional deficits in addition to those of intelligence. He considered the frontal lobe to be an inhibitory center with the result that damage there would disinhibit movements which in the intact brain could be merely imagined without having to be executed.

In several publications Bianchi (1894, 1895, 1922) basically confirmed Hitzig's and Ferrier's interpretations that the frontal lobes were electrically non-excitable and were involved in higher mental processes so that their damage led to loss of critique and careful planning, and to apathy, intellectual bluntness, and motoric restlessness. In 1895 he added temporary motor disturbances as a consequence of frontal extirpation to his list of findings. Integrating his results, he concluded that the frontal lobes provide the "*psychical tone*" to the individual by fusing perceptions and emotional states. Removal of the frontal lobes would "disaggregate the personality, and incapacitate it for serialising and synthesizing groups of representations" (p. 522).

The non-excitability of the prefrontal region and its distinction from the motor cortex was also emphasized by Grünbaum and Sherrington (1902, 1903) who furthermore distinguished a 'frontal eye field' from the motor cortex in the chimpanzee (Fig. 6) (see also Ferrier, 1875, 1886; Horsley & Schaefer, 1888; Mott & Schaefer, 1890, for observations on the frontal eye field). Additionally, relations between prefrontal cortical damage and movement disorders, including apraxia, were documented by F. Hartmann (1907).

Grünbaum and Sherrington's map raises the question of the delineation and definition of the prefrontal cortex (cf. Brodmann, 1909 b, 1912; Cole, 1911; Goldman-Rakic, 1987; Markowitsch, 1988 a). It should be noted in this connection that Flechsig (1896 a) introduced three large association centers for the human cerebral cortex, a frontal, a parietal, and an occipito-temporal one (Fig. 7). (Paul Emil Flechsig formulated the theory that the development of function follows the same sequence as myelination and is dependent on it; cf. Barker, 1897; Flechsig, 1894.)

Furthermore, it seems appropriate on this occasion to refer to Hitzig's (1874 a) rather early statement that "there is little missing in the well-developed human brain when we consider our closest cousin, the chimpanzee" (p. 47). Hitzig made this statement especially with reference to the frontal lobe (cf. his Figs. 3 and 4).

Phineas P. Gage

It is astonishing that the literature between 1870 and 1920 frequently omits references to the so-called crowbar case (exceptions: Calderwood, 1879; Ferrier, 1886; Goltz, 1888; Jastrowitz, 1888; Welt, 1888; Wundt, 1908, 1910, 1911 a). Harlow gave two reports on the case (1848, 1869) and Bigelow (1850) a further one, on the man whose maxillary bone was pierced by an iron rod of more than one meter in length and roughly 6 kg in weight, which passed behind the left eye, through the frontal lobe, and exited at the beginning of the right upper cranium. Harlow (1848) described the man as "Phineas P. Gage, a foreman, engaged in building the road, 25 years of age, of middle stature, vigorous physical organization, temperate habits, and ... of considerable energy of character" (p. 20). Harlow (1848, p. 20) gave a particularly graphic and vivid description of the accident and of the movement of the iron rod through the head (Fig. 8):

It appears from his own account, and that of the by-standers, that he was engaged in charging a hole, preparatory to blasting. He had turned in the powder, and was in the act of tamping it slightly before pouring on the sand. He had struck the powder, and while about to strike it again, turned his head to look after his men (who were working within a few feet of him), when the tamping iron came in contact with the rock, and the powder exploded, driving the iron against the left side of the face, immediately anterior to the angle of the inferior maxillary bone. Taking a direction upward and backward toward the median line, it penetrated the integuments, the masseter and temporal muscles, passed under the zygomatic arch, and (probably) fracturing the temporal portion of the sphenoid bone, and the floor of the orbit of the left eye, entered the cranium, passing through the anterior left lobe of the cerebrum, and made its exit in the medial line, at the junction of the coronal and sagittal sutures, lacerating the longitudinal sinus, fracturing the parietal and frontal bones extensively, breaking up considerable portions of the brain, and protruding the globe of the left eye from its socket, by nearly half its diameter.

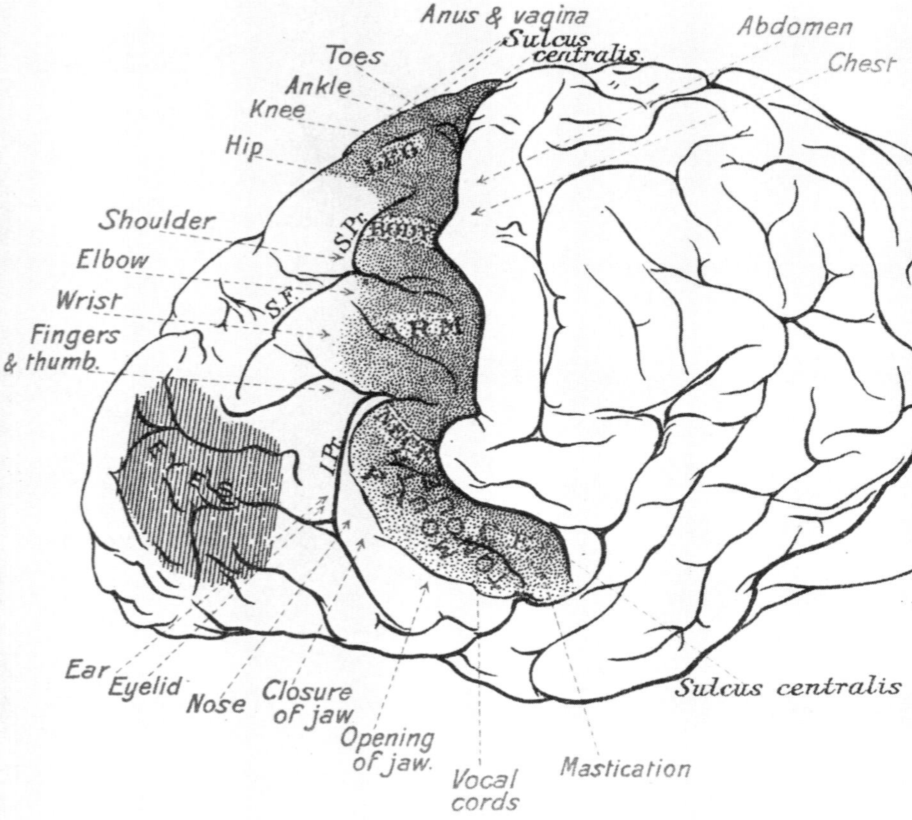

Figure 6. Brain of a chimpanzee. Copy of Plate 4 of Grünbaum and Sherrington (1902). The extent of the "motor" area on the lateral surface of the hemisphere is indicated with the position of the frontal eye field ("eyes" written in the left part of the figure) and the representation of the eyes in the occipital lobe area ("eyes" written in the right part of the figure; primary visual cortex). Grünbaum and Sherrington remarked: "The names printed in large ... on the stippled area indicate the main regions of the 'motor' area; the names printed in small ... outside the brain, indicated broadly by their pointing lines the relative topography of some of the chief sub-divisions of the main regions of the 'motor' cortex. But there exists much overlapping of the areas and of their sub-divisions which the diagram does not attempt to indicate. The shaded regions marked 'Eyes' indicate in the frontal and occipital regions respectively the portions of cortex which, under faradisation, yield conjugate movements of the eyeballs. But it is questionable whether these reactions sufficiently resemble those of the 'motor' area to be included with them. They are therefore marked in vertical shading instead of stippling as in the 'motor' area. S. F. = superior frontal sulcus. S.Pr. = superior precentral suclus. I. Pr. = inferior precentral sulcus." (p.208).

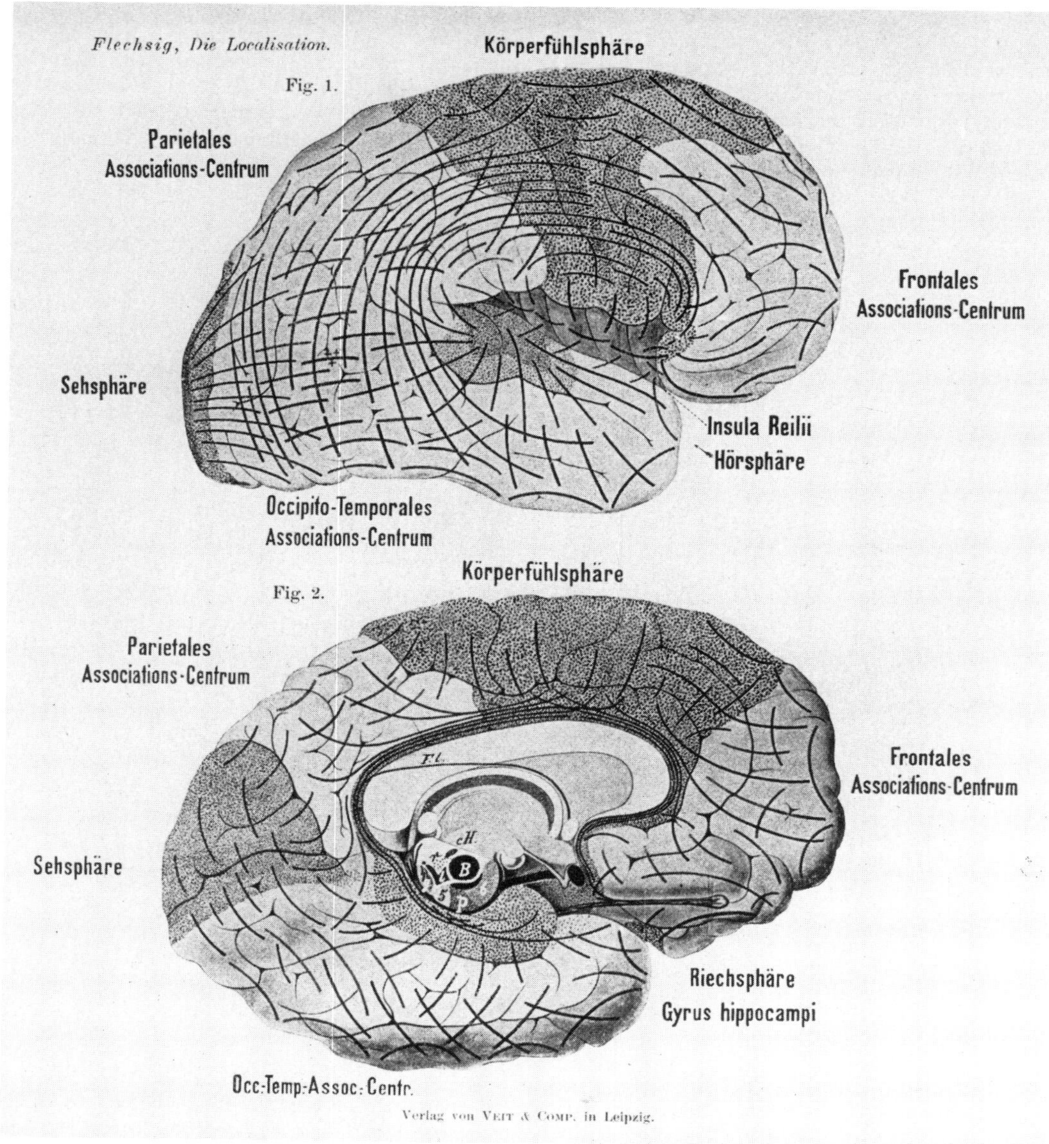

Figure 7. Association areas, course of fibers, and cortical description as given in the Plate of Flechsig (1896a).

An opening of about eight cm in diameter was observed by Harlow. The patient's state worsened at first and he lay in a semi-comatose condition for more than two weeks, but then improved during the next month. The report ended with a remark to the editor of the *Boston Medical and Surgical Journal*: "Should you think these notes of sufficient importance to deserve a place in your Journal, they are at your service."

Twenty-one years later Harlow (1869) published a report on this case which seemed rather unbelievable to his fellow surgeons. He documented the case as having occurred "in an ob-

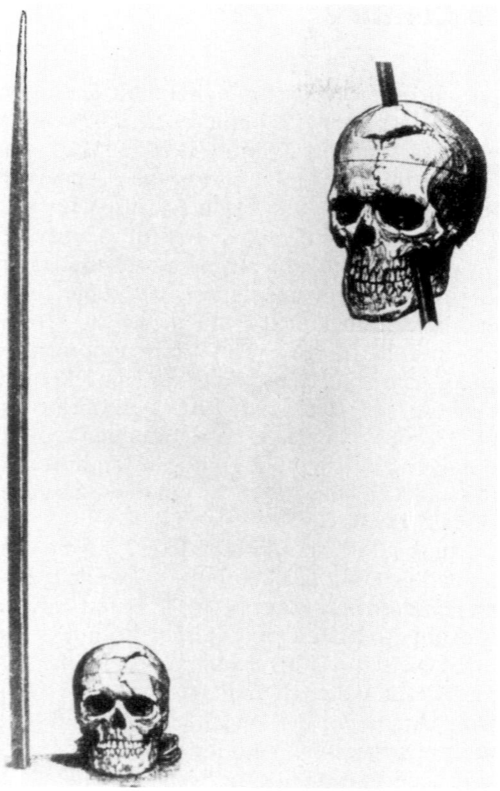

Figure 8. Views of the skull and of the iron bar, traversing the brain of Phineas Gage (after Figs. 1 and 2 of Harlow, 1869).

scure country town (...), ... attended and reported by an obscure country physician, and ... received by the Metropolitan Doctors with several grains of caution, insomuch that many utterly refused to believe that the man had risen, until they had thrust their fingers into the hole of his head, and even then they required of the Country Doctor attested statements, from clergymen and lawyers, before they *could* or *would* believe – many eminent surgeons regarding such an occurrence as physiological impossibility; the appearances presented by the subject being variously explained away." (p. 3).

About three months after the accident the patient had lost his vision in the left eye but was in good physical condition. His personality, however, had changed radically so that his friends said that he was "no longer Gage" (p. 14). In the years following the accident he worked in a livery stable and then in Chile "to establish a line of coaches at Valparaiso" (p. 14), where he remained for nearly eight years, before returning to the United States. He died after several epileptic fits "twelve years, six months and eight days after the date of his injury" (p. 15 f).

This case demonstrated that after substantial damage of the prefrontal cortex a person can still survive for years, engage in responsible work and therefore appear to be functioning on only a slightly subnormal intellectual level; nonetheless it seems that the case description remained largely unknown for a considerable time and/or was regarded as atypical. It did show that the frontal lobes were – in accordance with the observations of many scientists at the turn of the century – not directly involved in sensory or motor acts and could be lost to a substantial degree without being vital for life to the subject (but see the case of G. Berman, described in Kussmaul & Nothnagel, 1873, p. 52). On the other hand, the case of Phineas Gage also revealed that frontal lobe damage may result in personality changes and especially the loss of foresight and persistance in following through ideas or intentions. In Harlow's (1869, p. 13) words: "The equilibrium or balance, so to speak, between his intellectual faculties and animal propensities, seems to have been destroyed. He is fitful, irreverent, indulging at times in the grossest profanity (which was not previously his custom), manifesting but little deference for his fellows, impatient of restraint or advice when it conflicts with his desires, at times pertinaciously obstinate, yet capricious and vacillating, devising many plans of future operation, which are no sooner arranged than they are abandoned in turn for others appearing more feasible. A child in his intellectual capacity and manifestations, he has the animal passions of a strong man". (See also Macmillan, 1986, and Steegmann, 1962).

A similar evaluation of the consequences of frontal lobe damage was given several decades later by Fanny Halpern (1930) who stated that prefrontal damage makes man more similar to animals with respect to attitude and movements.

The Turn of the Century

After the controversial debates of the 1870's and 1880's, more modest tones dominated at the turn of the century (but see, e.g., Flechsig, 1898). Still, emphasis for the functions of the prefrontal cortex was placed more on the intellectual side (e.g., G. Anton & Zingerle, 1902; Bolton, 1903 a, 1903 b; Breukink, 1907; Cramer, 1899; Flechsig, 1896 a, 1896 b; Grosglik, 1895; Phelps, 1902, 1906). From the observations on a large number of cases, Bolton (1903 b) termed the prefrontal cortex "the part of the cerebrum concerned with the highest functions of mind, namely *attention and general orderly coordination of psychic processes*" (p. 560). In his second article (Bolton, 1903 a) he elaborated on this saying "that the anterior centre of association of Flechsig is the region concerned with attention and the general orderly coordination of psychic processes, and that the cellular elements throughout the cortex which are especially concerned in the performance of associational functions are those of the pyramidal layer of nerve-cells" (p. 236 f).

Flechsig (1896 a) also emphasized attentive processes and their consequences for personality ('active attention, contemplation, goal-directed ego'; p. 63); furthermore he (Flechsig, 1896 b) considered the frontal association center (Fig. 9) as responsible for the control of drives, saying that animals and human infants with their still underdeveloped association areas are merely "Affectwesen" [affective creatures] (p. 103) (cf. also Flechsig, 1901).

G. Anton und Zingerle (1902, p. 185) considered 'the voluntary active fixation of attention, the voluntary concentration necessary for thinking' as the central function of the frontal lobes. (While Flechsig argued in favor of the phylogenetic development of the prefrontal cortex, Ziehen (1911) remarked that frequently in microencephalic idiots the 'Stirnhirn' in particular is more markedly developed than the other lobes [p. 465].)

G. Anton, who gave a thorough survey on the state of the art in 1906, reflected Flechsig's opinion on the frontal lobes describing them as the crucial components of the consciousness of a person, as necessary for higher ethic feelings as well as regulators for impulses to act. A similar view was held by Wundt (1908, 1911 b), who termed the prefrontal cortex the "Apperzeptionszentrum" of the brain (cf. also Henning, 1926). For Wundt, "apperception" is a psychological act which, objectively means that a conscious event becomes clearer, and, subjectively, entails certain feelings which may be termed "attention" (p. 381). The term apperception and its explanation by Wundt (cf. his schematic diagram, Fig. 105, and the description on pp. 378–385) are not easily understood, although an entire monograph was dedicated to the subject by the end of the nineteenth century (Kodis, 1893).

Munk (1882, footnote on p. 757 f), who read an earlier edition of Wundt's "*Grundzüge der Physiologischen Psychologie*", stated that he was able to understand neither Wundt's schematic picture nor his explanations; in his opinion Wundt had no clear image of what he meant with 'Apperception' and had combined quite diverse processes. Wundt's original intention had been to simplify the term intelligence so that a relation between intelligent actions or processes and the activity of the frontal lobes could be justified (cf. also Exner, 1894, or Ziehen, 1909, for early discussions of the term intelligence).

Such an intention was also expressed by Monakow (1904) who discussed the contemporary views on the functions of the prefrontal cortex and concluded (p. 106): "Intelligence is a complicated inference of an enormous sum of singular processes which are acquired successively over years by the action of the senses and of the muscular apparatus. But by now the most primary psychic processes which follow the acts of each singular sense are already such complicated things occurring under the collaboration of the total cortex that such processes can only be considered rather reluctantly under the viewpoints of localization with respect to gyri and cortical islands". Monakow (1904) also pointed to the high development of the frontal lobes in ungulates such as horses (amounting

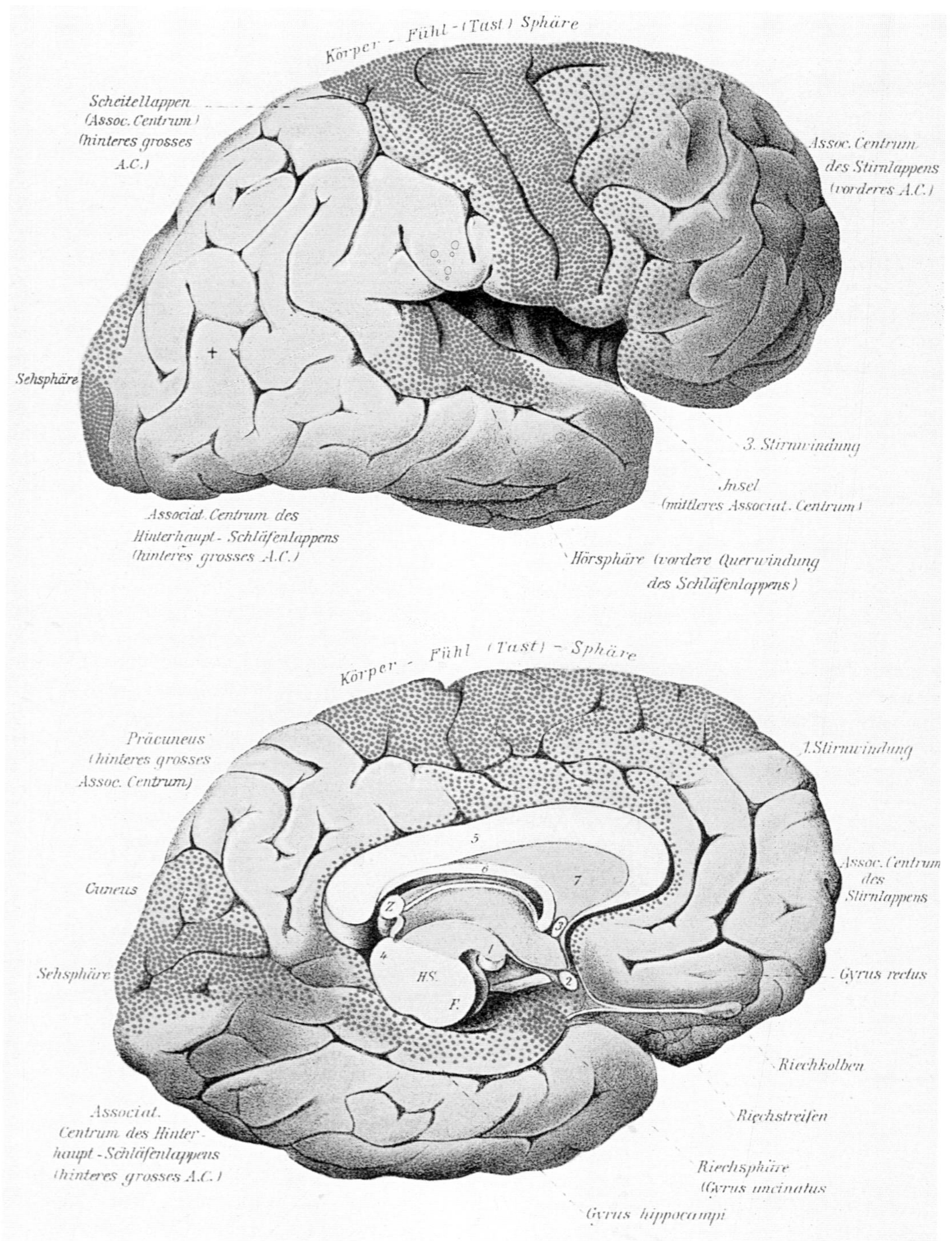

Figure 9. The partition of the lateral (top) and medial (bottom) aspects of the human cerebral cortex after Flechsig (1896b). Note extent and position of the frontal association center.

up to 30% of the cortical volume) such that in his view this fact contradicts the theory that there is a parallel development between the differentiation and improvement of the frontal lobes and intellectual activity. However, it must be acknowledged that Monakow erred more towards the 'anti-localizationists' than to the 'localizationists' (cf. Prince, 1910). In interpreting lesion data he emphasized such methodological problems as the existence of inflammatory processes in the brain, of the lack of aseptic precautions during surgery, and of the action of diaschisis (distant and time-dependent effects of local damage) (Monakow, 1910a, 1910b, 1914; cf. also Hitzig, 1903c).

Tumors

At the turn of the century, interpretations of the functions of the human prefrontal cortex were based largely on single case descriptions of tumor patients, usually by autopsy. In addition, cases with degenerative diseases, such as Pick's disease (Pick, 1901, 1906) or similar forms (e.g., Richter, 1918) also received some attention. Since these patients usually became dementic, this was used to support the involvement of the frontal lobes in the highest of mental functions.

Case descriptions of tumors removed from the frontal lobe region (or detected post mortem), produced contradictory results (Auerbach, 1902; Batten & Collier, 1899; Bayerthal, 1903; Beevor, 1898; Bickel, 1903; Bostroem, 1921; Bramwell, 1899; Bruns, 1892, 1897, 1898; Campbell, 1909; Cortesi, 1908; Cowen, 1902; Dercum, 1910; Donath, 1912, 1923; Elder & Miles, 1902; Frazier, 1936; Freud, 1891; Friedrich, 1902; Grimm, 1868; Gürtler, 1923; Herter, 1916; Höniger, 1901; Jastrowitz, 1885; Jefferson, 1937, 1950; Lannois & Paviout, 1902; Liepmann, 1907a; Mann, 1898; R.M. Marshall, 1909; Oppenheim, 1890a, 1890b, 1891, 1902, 1907; Petrina, 1912; Pfeifer, 1910; Pitt, 1898; Sharkey, 1898; H. Smith, 1906; A. Stern, 1914; Stewart, 1906; Veraguth & Cloetta, 1907; Wernick, 1918; Williamson, 1891, 1896).

For example, Cortesi (1908) gave quite a number of arguments for taking each frontal lobe patient as a completely individualized person who might be quite distinct in symptoms and consequences from other cases with similar brain damage. He argued further that no specific symptom can be seen as characteristic for frontal lobe pathology. Cortesi's argumentation sounds quite similar to that of Symonds (1937), three decades later. (Symonds' most frequently cited sentence may well be: "The symptom picture depends not only upon the kind of injury, but upon the kind of brain"; p. 464.)

As another example, Elder and Miles (1902) removed a tumor from a patient's left dorsal prefrontal lobe and after examining his postoperative behavior they concluded that one should discard the idea that the prefrontal lobes are 'silent regions' as a language deterioration had in fact resulted. They went on to state that it "seems probable that the processes involved in judgement and reason have for their physical basis the frontal lobes. If so, the total destruction of these lobes would reduce man to the state of an idiot, while their partial destruction would be manifested by errors of judgement and reason of a striking character" (p. 366).

A related discussion about characterizing the prefrontal cortex as silent was carried on by Ridewood and Jones (1903) who discussed a case with a cerebral tumor. They wrote "that a special form of 'reasoning insanity' is associated with neoplasms of this region; but others consider the frontal lobes to be 'tolerant and silent' in regard to symptoms".

Pfeifer

A collection of 13 prefrontal cases with considerable data can be found at the beginning of the 180-page long article of Pfeifer (1910). From reading Pfeifer's work one gets the impression that he included cases which document nearly all the attributes given previously and even today to frontal lobe damaged subjects; he concluded, however, that affective disturbances were the main ones, while those of intelligence were rare (and if so mainly with respect to memory; cf. also Morsier, 1929, and Morsier & Rey, 1945). Later, Pfeifer (1922) apparently changed his mind as he noted that prefrontal damaged patients demonstrate by far the most severe deficits of all brain-damaged in the field of intellect, with respect both to their way of thinking and to logical thinking, discriminability, and combinatory judgement.

The Contributions of H. Smith and of Donath

H. Smith (1906) described a woman from whom a tumor situated mainly over the middle frontal convolution was removed and who afterwards improved considerably in various cognitive and sensory functions. Donath (1923) reviewed a number of cases with prefrontal tumors and pointed to the importance of the site and extent of the tumor which apparently determine the effects on behavior to a considerable degree.

A particularly thorough review was made by Donath in 1912; he distinguished between local and distant symptoms of frontal lobe damage and grouped cases with specific symptoms. He was of the opinion that even in cases with no obvious psychic disturbances, some such disturbance could have been found after close examination; and thus, like other authors earlier, he attributed the locus of the highest intellectual functions to the prefrontal cortex.

In his article "On the symptomatology of gross lesions (tumors and abscesses) involving the prae-frontal region of the brain", Williamson (1896) analyzed the symptoms of 50 cases and frequently noted mental symptoms (Table 1).

Outlook

As an outlook, S. I. Schwab emphasized in 1927 the changes in personality after tumor development in the frontal lobes, and some years later Lemke (1937) gave detailed descriptions of four cases with bilateral frontal lobe tumors. In one case, he noted loss of interest and initiative and also a strong disturbance in thinking and reasoning and a loss of memory which he equated with a Korsakoff syndrome. Memory loss was also found in about half of the 314 cases with frontal lobe tumors, examined and compared by Voris, Adson, and Moersch (1934). In 1937 Jefferson came to a conclusion different from Lemke's; he failed to find sufficient changes after unilateral removals of the frontal lobe, and so he interpreted his findings in the following way "Whilst, therefore, a considerable amount of caution must be exercised in drawing conclusions from them which would tend to the formulation of a dogma, they illustrate the more plastic conception of cortical activities current to-day" (p. 206). (Worster-Draught,

Table 1

Mental changes in 50 cases with tumor or abscess of the frontal lobes (from page 361 of Williamson, 1896)

Cases*	
A condition of mental decadence; a dull mental state; loss of power of attention; loss of memory; loss of spontaneity; the patient taking no notice of his surroundings; sleeping during the greater portion of the day, or semi-comatose	32
Loss of memory, mental failure, but patient cheerful	6
Patient suspicious; suffered from delusion, and occassionally violent	1
Patient irritable and violent	1
Patient generally asleep; irritable when awake	2
Patient ambitious, excitable, memory lost	1
Slowness of mental processes; patient simple and childish	1
Mental anxiety; childishness; hallucinations; suicidal tendencies	1
Mental conditions not stated	5
	50

* In two of these it is noted that the patients were in a perplexed mental condition, and constantly appeared to be searching for something.

1931, termed this "the psychological make-up" and Symonds, 1931, in the same symposium, related mental changes to the amount of white matter destruction rather than to its precise localization.) Jefferson's view confirmed that of Serog, who in 1911 had already stated that both "Witzelsucht" and Korsakoff's psychosis are not caused after frontal lobe damage by the lesion locus per se, but by a (nonspecific) increase of intracranial pressure, and thus they were general symptoms. (The role of intracranial pressure increase in frontal lobe tumors had already been emphasized by Ruckert, 1909.) Serog also pointed out that 'intelligence' has no prefrontal locus, but is the product of the total cerebral cortex. (In the United State, Strauss and Keschner, 1935, held this view also at the time when Jefferson published his article, while Halstead, 1947, somewhat later adhered to a different opinion.)

The Diverse Functions Attributed to the Stirnhirn

A reduction or loss of attention and interest and apathetic behavior were most frequently noted as characteristic for frontal lobe damage (e.g., Herzfeld, 1901; Höniger, 1901). P. Schuster (1902), who subdivided the psychic changes in frontal lobe damaged patients in nine groups (p. 75), noted as most frequent symptoms 'simple, general mental paralyzation, irritability, hypomania, and 'Witzelsucht' (This last term, which Blumer & Benson, 1975, translated as 'facetiousness', was coined by Oppenheim in 1891 and not, as Blumer & Benson stated, in 1889; in fact Oppenheim in 1891 only wrote "Sucht zu witzeln" [p. 57]).

P. Schuster

In the first 77 pages of his monograph, P. Schuster (1902) summarized in detail what was known at that time on the 'Stirnhirn'. He gave a well-balanced review of the pros and contras on the involvement of the prefrontal cortex in psychic functions, citing the work of the important neurologists of the time (e.g., Bianchi, Ferrier, Flechsig, Goltz, Hitzig). In the clinical part of this chapter he listed altogether 147 cases of his own and others, 47 of which, he thought, could be classified as having had tumors limited to the region of the prefrontal cortex. In conformity with other authors of that epoch, P. Schuster noted that in comparison to the effects of unilateral lesions in other cortical areas those in the prefrontal region had less marked consequences on behavior, and when behavioral deteriorations were observed after unilateral frontal damage, they most frequently were on the emotional level (hypomania). Psychic disturbances were more closely related to damage in prefrontal gray matter than in white matter. As a final conclusion, P. Schuster was of the opinion that intelligence defects were more closely related to left frontal and affective disturbances to right frontal damage.

In this connection Berger (1920, 1923) made some rather pronounced statements that should be mentioned. He was of the opinion that damage to the medial, inferior and posterior half of the prefrontal regions inevitably resulted in psychic disturbances and that this is also the case after unilateral lesions only (Brodmann's, 1909 b, area 11, or O. Vogt's, 1910, regio unistriata euradiata tenuifibrosa [Fig. 10]; cf. also Spatz, 1937, who generally confirmed Berger's arguments and also followed the nomenclatures of Brodmann and O. Vogt).

Forster and Others

Forster (1919 a) gave a good deal of detail on a case involving a gunshot wound through the dorsal convexity of the left frontal lobe showing lack of drive, but no specific deterioration of intelligence (this case was also included in the review article of Forster, 1919 b). On the other hand, intellectual deterioration may be determined at least to some degree by attention-related loss and apathetic behavior (cf. Schob, 1921). Flechsig (1896 a, p. 63) noted that 'posi-

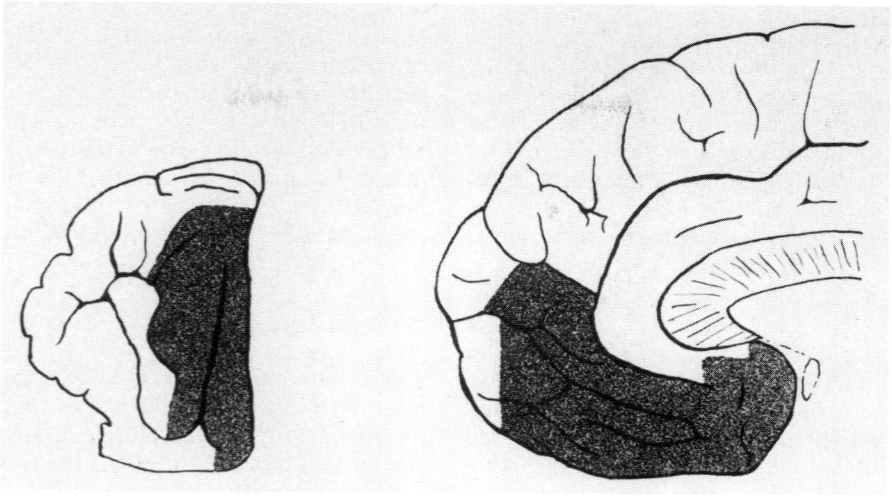

Figure 10. The area of the prefrontal cortex which according to Berger (1923) has "psychic" functions. (After Figures 21 and 22 of Berger, 1923.)

tive knowledge is not affected per se after frontal lobe damage, but its appropriate use or realization'.

Aside from Breukink (1907), Hans Berger (1923) (who became famous for discovering the electroencephalogram; cf. Berger, 1929, 1938; R. Jung, 1963; Karyofilis, 1974) described the perseverative tendency after prefrontal damage (Fig. 11). Related symptoms were frequently attributed to disturbances in motilation or to "psychomotoric" disturbances (Heilbronner, 1905 a, 1905 b, 1905 c; Pick, 1921; Sölder, 1895), or to a delay in shifting ("Verzögerung der Umstimmung"; Stein, 1931, p. 629).

Already at the turn of the century authors such as Bayerthal (1903), Bernhardt and Borchardt (1909), and Monakow (1904) noted that cases with brain tumor are inappropriate for a precise determination of the functions of the frontal lobes.

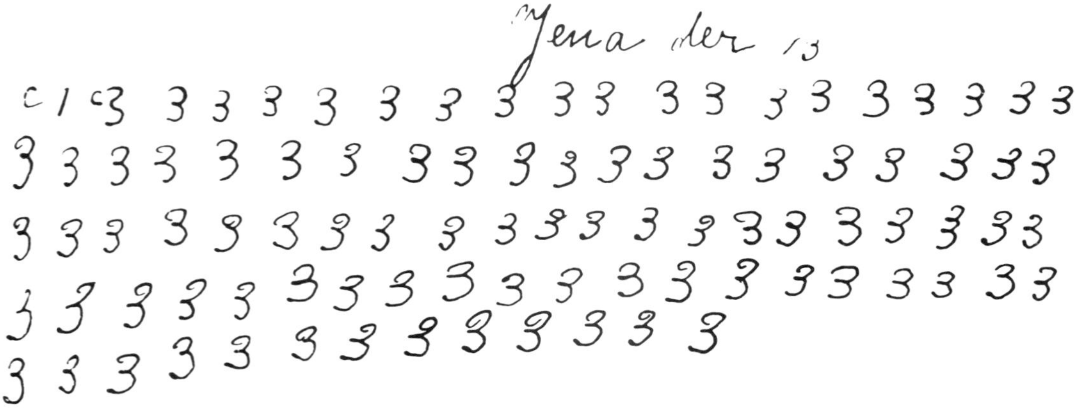

Figure 11. Perseveration in a patient with prefrontal damage (after Figure 20 of Berger, 1923).

E. Müller

E. Müller (1902 a, 1902 b, 1902 c, 1903) was one of the psychiatrists who at this period also rather vividly argued against evidence for higher, psychic functions as being "Herdsymptome" (E. Müller, 1902 a) of the frontal lobe, but he also opposed the validity of other views on prefrontal functions involved with character or Witzelsucht. Because his main interest was in tumors of the frontal lobes, his arguments were in the same direction as those of Monakow (1904) and others: He pointed to possible interactions of a tumor and psychic disturbances, to symptoms usually accompanying the growth of a tumor such as increased brain pressure, disturbed blood circulation, possible metabolic changes, and genetic predispositions (Müller, 1902 b). Based on the evaluation of 164 cases he (1902 a, 1902 c) focused on the frequent behavioral recovery and disappearance of prior symptoms after tumor removal, emphasized how large frontal tumors frequently are, and classified many of the so-called frontal lobe symptoms as generalized symptoms after tumor growth in the cerebrum. In his contribution "Zur Symptomatologie und Diagnostik der Geschwülste des Stirnhirns" Müller (1902 c) provided a list of all the 164 cases he had used in his statistics and made a thorough systematical review on the frequency of particular symptoms or concomitants in cases with frontal lobe tumors (e. g., general structure of the body, nourishment condition, skin temperature, epilepsy, hysteria, ataxia, sensory disturbances, tremor, changes in somatic sensibility, aphasia, agraphia, vomiting, pulse changes, dizziness, visual and visuo-motor changes, brain nerves, urinary changes, sexual behavior, or changes in the functions of bladder and rectum).

In his last article of this series (E. Müller, 1903) he discussed the etiology of frontal tumors and concluded that frontal tumors, in comparison to those in the cerebellum or any other brain regions, have a higher likeliness of occurring later in life with the peak frequency being in the fourth decade of life. (However, this last finding has to be related to the life expectancy in Europe at the end of the last century.) (See also A. Gordon's, 1917, report on functional similiarities between prefrontal and cerebellar lesions and Sarbo's, 1925, relation between frontal and cerebellar neurological signs.) The list of the 164 cases was repeated in Müller's publication from 1903 and six more recent cases were added to that list. A controversial discussion between Auerbach (1904) and E. Müller (1904) followed this last report.

Trauma-based Cases

The results on soldiers wounded during and after the First World War and other gun shot reports (e. g., Allers, 1916; Dziembowski, 1916; Engerth & Hoff, 1930; Gerstmann, 1916; Glass, 1911; Grage, 1930; Kramer, 1915; Leszynsky, 1909; Ratig, 1923; M. Rothmann, 1914; Schob, 1921; A. Stern, 1915; Wyeth, 1904; cf. also Spatz, 1941) then revealed insights into the consequences of acute and sometimes quite circumscribed frontal lobe damage and shifted interest more to attentive and emotional (and sometimes even motoric: Engerth & Hoff, 1930) than to intellectual components of personality change (Allers, 1916; Axhausen & Kramer, 1920; Brodmann, 1915; Choroschko, 1923; Feuchtwanger, 1923; Forster, 1919 a, 1919 b; Goldstein, 1910, 1923, 1927; Goldstein & Reichmann, 1920; Grünthal, 1936 b; Holmes, 1901; Kleist, 1934 a; Poppelreuter, 1915, 1917, 1918; Rosenfeld, 1917; Schultz, 1915, 1917; Sittig, 1916), though Poppelreuter (1918) emphasized intelligence defects as well (p. 177: "dementia or intelligence defects, concerning higher factors of thinking, combining, determining, reasoning, ..."), and Schlesinger (1916) found pronounced retrograde amnesia without any other concomitant changes in one soldier hit in the frontal lobes. Occasionally, short case descriptions can be found of persons who shot themselves in the head (e. g., Lindsay, 1904).

The most extensive work in this period was the monograph of Feuchtwanger (1923) who compared a wealth of data from 200 soldiers with definite frontal lobe damage with those of 200 other brain-damaged soldiers who most likely had no frontal lobe damage. He further subdivided the 200 frontal lobe patients into 153 with pure prefrontal damage and 47 in whom other brain regions (e. g., Broca's area, precentral cortex) were affected in addition. "Moria" (a term coined by Jastrowitz, 1888; also to be found in the chapter written by Jastrowitz in the book of Leyden & Jastrowitz, 1888; cf. Oppenheim, 1891, p. 55), meaning a grossly non-serious ("unernst") behavior with respect to one's own conditions of life, was observed nine times as often in frontal as compared to non-frontal damaged patients and was that symptom which most clearly differentiated between the two groups. According to Oppenheim (1891, p. 55) Jastrowitz formulated: "I have seen a certain form of mental disturbance, namely a dementia with a peculiar cheerful excitement, the so-called moria, purely and simply in cases with tumors of the frontal lobes".

Table 2, which is translated from Feuchtwanger's Tabelle 1, gives a summary of the frequency of occurrence of other symptoms.

Choroschko (1923), in full agreement with Feuchtwanger's analysis, formulated what at that time (and probably even up to today) was considered to be the most reliably extractable attributes from the analysis of prefrontal patients (p. 302): "We consider the relation of the frontal lobes to the psyche as proven. This relation is primarily observed with respect to the function of active attention and the expressions of will per se (drive, initiative, arbitrariness)" (cf. also Klebanoff, 1945).

A really deep and broad analysis of intellectual functions in prefrontal damaged subjects apparently still waits to be performed, though around the turn of the century detailed tests were already described or suggested; however, they were apparently never used for prefrontal patients (Gregor & Hänsel, 1909; Rieger, 1889, 1890; cf. the section on "Early Methods for Memory Assessment" in the chapter 'Memory and Memory Disorders').

Table 2

Overview of the symptoms observed in 200 frontal lobe and 200 non-frontal lobe damaged patients (after Table XX of Feuchtwanger, 1923)

	Frontal lobe cases		Non-frontal cases	
	Abs. no.	%	Abs. no.	%
All cases	200	100	200	100
Cerebral disturbances of movement and sensation	38	19	92	46
Disturbances in balance	88	44	72	36
Cerebral language disturbances	22	11	62	31
Cerebral perceptual disturbances	2	1	45	23
Gnostic disturbances	–	–	27	14
Disturbances in remembering	60	30	71	36
Disturbances in learning	72	36	102	51
Disturbances in thinking	21	11	32	16
Disturbances in attention	117	59	93	47
Excitement and euphoria	119	60	72	36
Hastiness	8	4	3	2
Fatigue	35	18	52	26
Witzeln	9	5	1	1
Depression	54	27	30	15
Slowness and apathy	76	38	30	15
Epileptic attacks	43	22	55	28
Psychogenic disturbances	42	21	56	28

Animal Studies

Though in the humanistic tradition intellectual functions were necessarily related to the human brain, there were nevertheless numerous attempts to use animals for studying at least the more rudimentary or elementary concomitants of intellectual activities. This was all the more the case, as on the one hand the techniques for studying interactions between brain and behavior were limited anyway, and as on the other hand the creative ideas for studying behavior and nervous tissue in animals were fairly well developed.

Comparative Work Supporting the Search for Intelligent Acts in Animals

Attempts to study "intelligence" in animals were frequent but also divergent: Kolbe (1903), who defined intelligence as autonomous acts of the soul, such as thinking and the conscious performance of acts (p. 1), wrote a general article "Ueber die psychischen Funktionen der Tiere" and cited numerous early works on the 'soul' or the 'life of the soul' ["Seelenleben"] in animals (e.g., Lubbock, 1889). While he attributed "Verstand" [intellect] even to ants, he denied the existence of "Vernunft" [reason] ('intelligent insight into the relations between cause and effect') for nonhuman animals. Nevertheless he cited one example which at least showed that ants can perform "zweckdienliche Handlungen" [purposeful acts]: The Swiss neurologist August Forel had brought Algerian ants to his Zürich property and noted that due to the frequent attacks by Swiss ants the Algerian ones changed their nests gradually by narrowing the entrance so that they became much safer against attacks (cf. Forel, 1901, 1903).

Ants (and bees) anyway were quite attractive research subjects at that time as is reflected by titles such as 'The psychic talents of ants' (Wasmann, 1899), 'More on the psychic qualities of ants' (Bethe, 1900), 'May we attribute psychic qualities to ants and bees?' (Bethe, 1898), or 'Comparative studies on the life of the soul of ants and higher animals' (Wasmann, 1909; cf. also Volkelt, 1914, and Ziehen, 1908b). A major report on the behavior, including "the mental powers" of spiders, was given by Porter (1906b). Chicken, sparrows, and other birds, were other animals in which mnestic functions were investigated (Kroh, Götz, Scholl & Ziegler, 1927; Porter, 1904, 1906a; Volkelt, 1914; Ziehen, 1908b, p. 39). In mammals such as cats and dogs "memory types" such as a "visual" or "kinesthetic memory" were inferred from their performance in maze situations (Szymanski, 1913); the behavior of rhesus monkeys in captivity was studied in detail (Kinnaman, 1902a, 1902b). For animals such as hedgehogs and moles, Gudden (1870b) stated that most of their psychic life is limited to smelling (p. 697). A small monograph on comparative psychology was written by Dahl (1922). In this book he acknowledged that even worms may have consciousness, at least during the process of mating (p. 26). Furthermore, he wrote separate chapters on memory and consciousness in animals and included a large amount of literature in his statements.

Comparative studies were performed in order to determine at what level of brain development behavior was principally guided by the cerebral cortex (see Soemmering, 1796, p. 52, for a very early comparative brain analysis; later: Loeb, 1899). In this context, of course, the experiments on mammals without the cerebral cortex or with other significant neural tissue removals were spectacular (Berger, 1900; Dresel, 1924; Edinger & Fischer, 1913; Exner & Paneth, 1888; Goltz, 1888, 1892; Goltz & Ewaldt, 1899; Holmes, 1901; Jakob, 1931; Munk, 1890, 1894; H. Rothmann, 1911, 1923; Karplus & Kreidl, 1912; Rademaker & Winkler, 1928; Poltyrew & Zeliony, 1930; Zeliony, 1929). The relation of sensory functions to the cerebral cortex was also investigated with surprising accuracy by Luciani (1884) (cf. also Rabagliati, 1878, 1879) (Figs. 12, 13, and 14). The prefrontal cortex soon constituted an area of major interest. Though the boundaries for this area – or, for some species, even its location, were

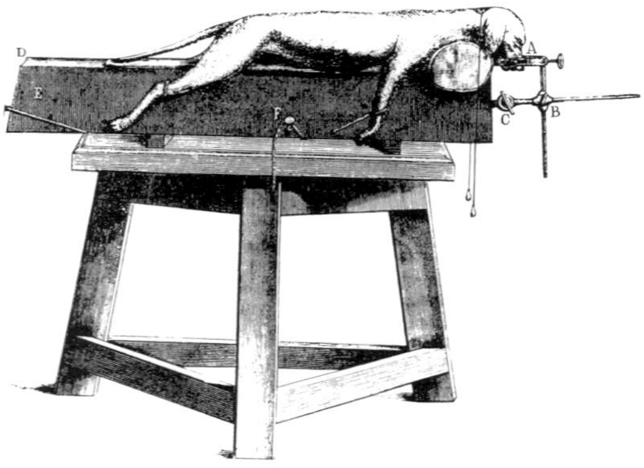

Figure 12. The stereotaxic arrangement for investigating the functions of the dog brain, used by Luciani and Seppilli (1886) (their Fig. 1).

hardly known – experimenters were rather free in relating observed behavioral deficits to prefrontal damage (Bianchi, 1895; Franz, 1906, 1907; Goltz, 1899; Weber, 1907), as well as in transfering results to brain-behavior relationships in humans (cf. e.g., Burckhardt, 1891; Busch, 1957; Chapman, Livingston & Livingston, 1949; Heimann, 1963; Horsley, 1887; Hutton, 1943; A. Meyer & Beck, 1954; Moniz, 1936, 1948, 1956).

In 1899 Goltz already stated that a dog with but one cerebral hemisphere has only slight deficits in intelligence and its "personality" remains principally stable, and this fact should encourage surgeons to risk removing even large tumors, as long as they remain within one hemisphere. He then cited Horsley (1887) as one of the surgeons who had already started such endeavors. (Pearce, 1982, reviewed even earlier attempts of surgical interventions within the cranium.)

Goltz, Munk and Others on the Mammalian Prefrontal Cortex

However, the overly naive topological homologization of 'pre-frontal' areas and the lack of theoretical help from neuroanatomy (at least before the time of Brodmann's 1904/05, 1908 a, 1909 b, 1912, publications; cf. Nissl, 1919) led to quite diverse behavioral out-

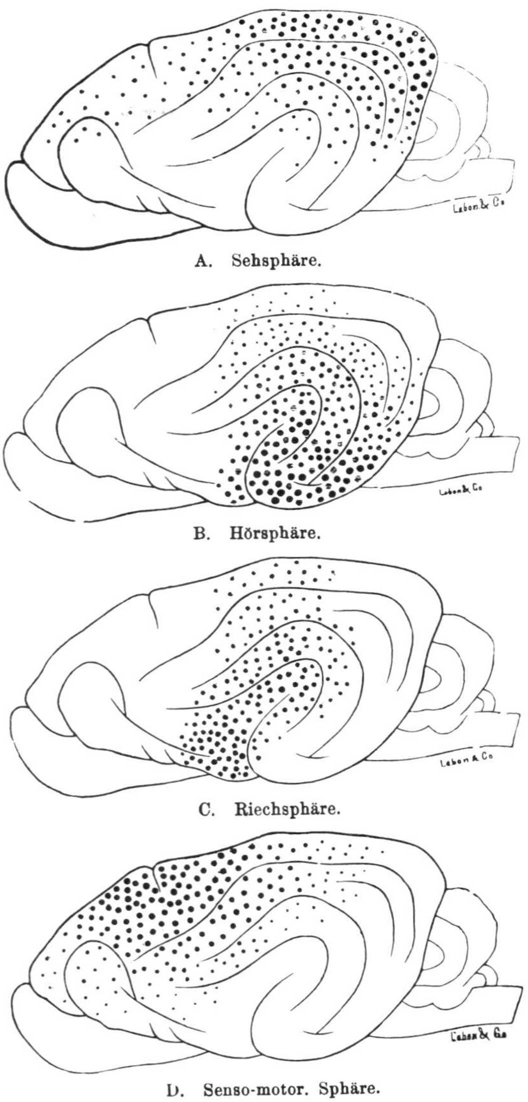

Figure 13. Summary picture from Luciani and Seppilli (1896) showing the areas of the dog's cerebral cortex sensitive to the different modalities. (A. Sehsphäre = visual sphere; B. Hörsphäre = auditory sphere; c. Riechsphäre = olfactory sphere; D. Senso-motor. Sphäre = senso-motor sphere.)

comes. This was noted for instance by Feuchtwanger (1923) who referred to the incomparability of the stimulation-based results of Weber in cats and of Munk and Sherrington in dogs and monkeys (p. 183). In addition, opinions could diverge even within a single given species. While some authors such as Hitzig (1884) adhered to the conception that in dogs the area anterior to the cruciate sulcus (that is, the prefrontal area) is responsible for intellectual behavior, Goltz (1888) and his pupil Kriworotow (1883) pointed to a somatosensory hyperreactivity of prefrontal lesioned dogs.

Early research was, of course, performed to investigate the functions of the cerebrum in general and mentioned the frontal lobes only insofar as animals with frontal as opposed to other cerebral cortical lesions were found to differ (Fritsch & Hitzig, 1870; Goltz, 1877; Gudden, 1870 a, 1870 b; Munk, 1881). Nevertheless, it seems that, especially at the beginning of systematic brain research when necessarily little was known, controversial attacks were again common (see Ferrier, 1878 a, 1888, Schäfer, 1888 a, 1888 b, and the citations of Goltz, Hitzig, Monakow, and Munk at the beginning of this chapter, or the rejoinders of Erb, 1880, Mayser, 1879, Takács, 1880, and Westphal, 1874). Another citation of Goltz (1877, p. 28) being: "The brain map of Ferrier's dog contains as many centers as Thuringia has political entities". Motor symptoms observed following frontal lobe stimulation in dogs were attributed to current spreading too far over the cortex or to having unwanted posterior ablations, and neither of these arguments could be rejected easily.

While Goltz (1877, 1881 a, 1881 b, 1884, 1888, 1892, 1899) clearly was an early "anti-localizationist", he nevertheless made observations in prefrontally lesioned dogs (as well as on rabbits and monkeys; see Goltz, 1899) which interestingly resemble similar behaviors of human sub-

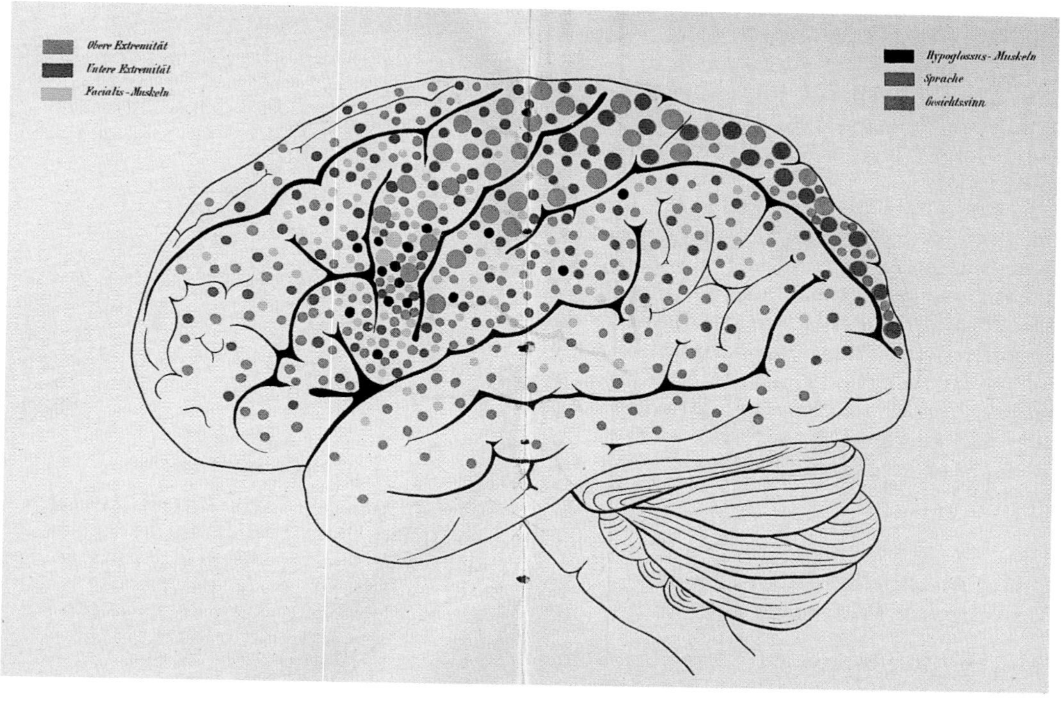

Figure 14. Summary picture from Luciani and Seppilli (1896) showing the areas of the left human cerebral cortex involved in motor, language, and visual functions. "Obere Extremität" = dorsal extremity; "Untere Extremität" = ventral extremity; "Facialis-Muskeln" = facialis muscles; "Hypoglossus-Muskeln" = hypoglossal muscles; "Sprache" = language; "Gesichtssinn" = visual sense.

jects with prefrontal damage, though his results were not taken up by later researchers on the nonhuman prefrontal cortex. In fact, Goltz' (1888) interpretation of the behavioral observations in his prefrontally lesioned dogs very closely resemble the interpretations made much later in human patients with prefrontal damage.

Thus, for example, he found that his prefrontal dogs were unable to perform certain acts appropriately, a behavior which reminded Goltz of some mild forms of aphasia: "There are aphasics who state quite credibly that they have the correct picture of the word(s) in front of their eyes, but are unable to write it down as the executing nerve-tools do not obey their will" (Goltz, 1884, p. 475).

Goltz (1888) furthermore noted a marked irritability and excitedness of prefrontally lesioned dogs. He and Munk held the opinion that "intelligence is situated everywhere in the cerebrum and nowhere specifically; for intelligence is the embodiment and resultant of all images which result from the sensory experiences. Every lesion of the cerebrum damages intelligence, all the more, when the lesion is extensive, and this is always due to the loss of that group of simple and complex images, which the sensory experience of the respective pathway has as basis" (Munk, 1878, p. 547).

Munk (1881) made important statements on possible mechanisms of recovery of function following brain damage. New learning, redundancy, vicariation, and functional restituion were all discussed in his complete edition. With respect to intelligence, he mentioned that magnitude, duration, extent, and kind of damage determine the degree of disturbance.

Grosglik (1895) also used dogs with prefrontal lesions and noted somatosensory, visual, and intellectual disturbances. He pointed to concomitants of frontal lobe damage which might be confounded with intellectual behavior (depression, nonchalance, lack of attention). Electrical brain stimulation in cats was used by Weber (1907) to determine the function of the "Stirnhirn" (cf. also Hitzig, 1874 d).

Franz, Bianchi and Ferrier

Extensive studies on the functions of the frontal lobes in cats and dogs were performed by Franz (1902, 1906, 1907), who cited Gall, Spurzheim, Flourens, Rolando, Fritsch and Hitzig, Ferrier, Goltz, Horsley, Munk, Schäfer and Sherrington, as those of his predecessors who contributed most to the understanding of localization of functions in the brain. Citing studies of Munk and Ferrier, he discussed the frontal lobes as motor centers; referring to Schäfer's (1900) work he discussed "the frontal lobes as centers of inhibition", and finally, based on the views of Broca and Hitzig and "many others" he considered "the frontal lobes as centers for intellectual states" (Franz, 1907, p. 16 ff.). He gave a thorough overview of the English- and German-language literature available with accurately cited references (a rare instance at that time).

Franz then cited Bianchi's and Hitzig's work on animals before introducing his own technique for experimenting with prefrontally lesioned cats and monkeys. His interest in the psychological topic of "habit training" was based on the experiments of prominent learning psychologists of those days such as Thorndike and Lloyd Morgan (cf. Franz, 1902).

In 1912, Franz' speech as president of the Southern Society for Philosophy and Psychology was published in *Science*, entitled "New Phrenology" (a similar term, "modern phrenology" had already been coined earlier by Goltz, 1885). With respect to the "old phrenologists", Gall and Spurzheim, Franz argued that "the conception of one function for one part of the brain was too simple and too alluring to be dispensed with" (p. 322). After reviewing the work of the better researchers of the time he concluded that "although it is apparent that mental states are not to be found spatially associated with definite areas distinguished from one another by histological and macroscopical characteristics, for practical purposes we must admit a close connection between the brain and mental processes" (p. 327), and finally (p. 328):

What memory means physiologically we do not know; where memories are stored we do not know. All that we do know is that certain disturbances of the brain are accompanied by certain mental abnormalities, and that similar mental abnormalities are produced by or accompany diverse lesions. We have no facts which at present will enable us to locate the mental processes in the brain any better than they were located fifty years ago. That the mental processes may be due to cerebral activities we may believe, but with what anatomical elements the individual mental processes may be connected we do not know. ... We should be willing to stand with Brodmann, believing that mind is a function or an attribute of the brain as a whole, or is a concomitant of cerebral operations, but I at least am unwilling to stand with the histological localizationists on the ground of a special mental process for special cerebral areas or for special cerebral cell groups.

Leonardo Bianchi's (1922) 348 paged volume constitutes a detailed, scholarly written review of the state of the art of the frontal lobes at that time, interpreting and commenting on the work of his contemporaries from various countries. It is especially interesting to find a discussion on the possible functions of the frontal lobes, as published by workers especially from Germany, Italy, the United Kingdom, the United States, and France. Bianchi refused to accept the simplification of the frontal lobes being the centers of inhibition, and instead assumed that they determined the "psychical tone" (Bianchi, 1895, p. 521) of the individual. Frontal lobe damage "disaggregate[s] the personality, and incapacitate[s] for serialising and synthetizing groups of representations" (Bianchi, 1895, p. 522).

In the book of Bianchi, the references to different authors and their studies are not very exact. Sheperd Ivory Franz was referred to as "Ivory Sheperd" (p. 88) or "Sheperd" (p. 124). In the third chapter on the "Evolution, Morphology, and Structure of the Frontal Lobe", a picture of the dolphin brain is given (Fig. 31) and the anatomy of the frontal lobes of sheep, horses, and a number of other mammals is discussed.

David Ferrier, "Physician of the National Hospital for the Paralysed and Epileptic" in London, was probably as famous a professor as was Bianchi at the turn of the century, though his results and interpretations were attacked on the other side of the channel (cf. above). He principally worked with monkeys, using the methods of "electrical irritation" and "extirpation" of brain areas (Ferrier, 1875, 1886; Ferrier & Yeo, 1884). Two of his contemporaries were Victor Horsley and Edward Albert Schäfer, who employed "electrical stimulation" and "ablation" as well (Horsley & Schäfer, 1888). These authors were especially interested in the motor functions of the cerebral cortex, situated posterior to the frontal cortex (cf. their Diagrams I and II and pages 6 and 10, resp., which give a topographical map of the cortical representation for the leg, arm, head, trunk, and face). Especially after Pavlov's (Pawlow, 1953) success in training dogs, more psychology-oriented techniques were also established (e. g., Nicolai, 1908).

Final Remarks

Interest in the frontal lobes continued in the 20th century and was revived by the various procedures of surgical intervention. In parallel to these latter descriptions, numerous others were published which confirmed or refined knowledge of the consequences of prefrontal damage or degeneration (e. g., Pick's disease: cf. Braunmühl, 1930; Lüers, 1950; Lüers & Spatz, 1957; Spatz, 1937). Emotional changes (Sachs, 1930), disinhibition (Jarvie, 1954), loss of the feeling for decency (Jefferson, 1937, 1950; Kretschmer, 1949, 1954), sexual disinhibition and exhibitionism (Lauber, 1958), and loss of memory for recent events (Jefferson, 1937; Sachs, 1927), were among the common characterizations. Lidz (1949) summarized findings that "thinking is finished more quickly and with greater satisfaction and assurance than in normal persons" (p. 26). " ... it may be that symbols, although readily available, are deprived of their full associative value, and ... this limitation may affect the liability to utilize other assets" (p. 26). Detailed reviews of psychological changes after frontal lobe damage were also given by Donath in 1923, by Duus and by Ruffin in 1939, by Klebanoff in 1945, and by Leonhard in 1959.

Donath (1923) first commented on the motor areas of the frontal lobe, but then argued on the more complex functions controlled by portions of the frontal lobe. He was of the opinion that engrams are stored in the frontal lobe, which initiate motor acts by interacting with impulses of will, which (according to him) likewise are to be found in the frontal lobes. It was also Donath's opinion that different kinds of engrams are compared in the frontal lobe (that is, apperception would take place here), judgements are made and compared, and conclusions are drawn in this part of the anterior cerebrum. Donath concluded that while other centers, particularly parietal, temporal, and insular regions, participate in the control of higher intellectual functions, the major burden would be lying in the prefrontal areas, which consequently were "the seat of the highest mental activity" (p. 301).

Duus (1939) gave a short survey of research on the frontal lobes, especially their orbitofrontal section. He collected 25 cases with tumors from the literature to which he added five of his own. Welt (1888) and P. Schuster (1902) were among the authors from whom he borrowed case descriptions. While Müller (1902 a, 1902 b, 1902 c) had criticized Welt's (1888) proposed link between orbitofrontal brain damage and character changes, Duus re-emphasized the existence of character changes which, in accordance with Kleist's (1934 a, 1934 b) nomenclature, manifest themselves as deteriorations in the "self-" and the "community-ego", as changes in arousal and as an expanding dominance of the lower stages of the ego involved in body, drives, and emotions (cf. also the similar view on character and temperament changes in frontal lobe patients held by Wimmer, 1926).

Duus (1939) stated:

> The initially inconspicuous patients become childish, superficial, foolish, show a tendency for mocking others and "witzeln", are restless and unsteady, frequently egotistic, malicious, tactless and shameless, do not take moral matters sincerely, are explosive and sometimes even criminal. These character weaknesses are frequently coupled with a heightened mood, self-confidence and somatic condition, especially at the onset of the illness when no serious complaints exist. At other times when complaints are more obvious, the cheerful mood turns into a dissatisfied, dysphoric, and nervous one. The patients become ill-humored, suspicious and bagatelles can bring them into rage. A tendency for masturbating, drinking, and excessive eating can be observed as further indices of a heightened condition of drive. These factors at this stage are frequently coupled already with a deteriorating memory.

Duus summarized that changes in character dominated at the beginning of the illness, but with time they were more and more covered by dorsolateral and diencephalic symptoms so that they would not be easily diagnosed at a later stage (cf. also Duus, 1980).

Klebanoff (1945) listed a number of old sources starting with Fritsch and Hitzig (1870) and Ferrier (1886) and ending with Ruffin (1939) and Duus (1939) (erroneously spelled Duss in Klebanoff's article). He discussed traumatic lesions, frontal lobe tumors, and ablations, and compared such findings with those after damage to the temporal, parietal, or occipital cortex. On the question of whether there is an "organic psychological syndrome" he gave the following answer: "Intellectual deterioration, memory defects, impaired abstract-thinking ability, loss of initiative, difficulties in sustaining attention, alterations in the general personality structure, and changes in psychomotor tempo and mood tone are particularly characteristic of tumors and other lesions of the frontal region of the cortex." (p. 615).

Sperling in 1957 commented on changes in character as a consequence of prefrontal damage and also discussed the two divergent possibilities, views that either different prefrontal subregions are of differential value (cf. e.g., Hassler, 1948, 1950; Kleist, 1934 a, 1934 b), or there is only a "difference according to quantity" (cf. e.g., Kalinowski, 1952).

The present state of frontal lobe research is reflected in three recent books (Stuss & Benson, 1986; Fuster, 1989; Levin, Eisenberg, & Benton, 1991; Perecman, 1987). Bowen (1989) gave a review of two of these books (Stuss & Benson, 1986; Perecman, 1987). He pointed out that the question on the role or roles of the prefrontal cortex is still open for debate and quoted Mesulam (1985) as saying: "The identification of the behavioral specializations of the human prefrontal cortex remains one of the most enigmatic areas in behavioral neurology".

Stuss and Benson discouraged the use of animals for unravelling prefrontal functions; they only considered human case descriptions as valid, as in their eyes the human prefrontal cortex differs in anatomy and functions considerably from that of nonhuman species (but see the remarks on the ape's prefrontal cortex given in Markowitsch, 1988 a). All this work, however, demonstrates the need for ongoing investigations of the contributions of the frontal lobes to the processing of intellectual functions.

In my view, Feuchtwanger's (1923) monograph still represents the modern state of the art. His summary of the psychological sector, given on pages 174 and 175, reads in translation:

"The various forms of damage in frontal lobe patients have in common the fact that their psychic disturbances are within the fields of emotion and performance, and not in the field of concrete actions, as with damage in more posteriorly situated parts of the cerebral cortex. Disturbances of concrete functions (perception, memory, thinking, movement, etc.), which can be found in pure prefrontal damage, are in the cases investigated not primarily, but secondarily caused by the emotional or topical deficits."

Feuchtwanger listed such emotional disturbances as those in the areas of basic mood, affect, the value system, and disinhibitions; as topical disturbances he gave those of attention, concentration, will, and motivation. Characteristic, he found, is furthermore the blending of the main defects with minor defects, especially as they are related to emotions, attentiveness, and will.

Chapter 4: Frontal Lobe Psychosurgery

According to Lüers (1950) T. Meynert had written already 100 years previously that psychiatry would more and more result in a study of effects of the frontal lobe and its connections (cf. also Rosenfeld, 1928). And just this was the case during the epoch of psychosurgery. With the rise of psychosurgery – an operative intervention performed in order to influence experience and behavior, at a time when there was not yet much evidence for the reliability of functional improvement (Adler & Saupe, 1979) – the historical limit set for this monograph – World War II – has been reached.

For clarity I wish to point out that this chapter is limited to psychosurgical approaches to the frontal lobes and to the time period from the late 19th century. For reviews of the precursors in psychosurgery I refer the readers to the chapters in Lisowski (1967) and Valenstein (1980a). Common expressions from this period are "leucotomy" (originating from "leucotome", the instrument used for fiber cutting), and "lobotomy" ("cutting a lobe") for the technique of separating the frontal cortex from the rest of the brain by cuts, and "lobectomy" for those instances when a lobe actually is removed.

There are a few examples of isolated work on psychosurgery from early times: Burckhardt (1891) and Ludwig Puusepp* (who according to Valenstein [188a, p. 20] "made knife cuts between the frontal and parietal brain lobes in three manic-depressive patients" (cf. Puusepp, 1914). Donath's (1899) osteoplastic trepanation is another case in point (an operation which apparently resulted in an end to his patient's fugue states, and there is also the work of H. Hoff and Pötzl (1932) who tried to change the psychic conditions of three schizophrenics by directly damaging basal ganglia or thalamic regions. They gave up, however, as none of the cases improved (cf. also Stengel, 1949, p. 446f). But mainstream frontal lobe psychosurgery for therapeutic purposes did not start until the first operation done by Egaz Moniz in 1935 together with Lima (Moniz & Lima, 1936).

Moniz based his decision to introduce psychosurgery on results which Fulton and Jacobsen (1935) had obtained in apes and presented during a congress he attended (their congress report from 1935 is cited in Fulton, 1951), and on the results of a patient on whom a bilateral frontal lobectomy had been performed in 1930 and whose behavior had been documented on the same congress (cf. Brickner, 1939, 1952). Fulton (1947) gave a vivid description of Moniz' reactions during the International Neurological Congress in London in 1935 on hearing about the findings on "Becky" and "Lucy", two chimpanzees with frontal lobe removal tested by Jacobsen (1935) (cf. also Crawford, Fulton, Jacobsen, & Wolfe, 1948; Jacobsen, 1936; Jacobsen & Nissen, 1937; Jacobsen, Wolfe, & Jackson, 1935). Subsequently, in his first operation Moniz injected alcohol into the human subcortical white matter, but thereafter used a leucotome (Moniz & Lima, 1936; see also: Moniz, 1937, 1948, 1956).

In the United States Freeman and Watts (1939, 1942b) popularized this technique which soon resulted in the treatment of large numbers of patients (world-wide up to 20,000 such operations by the beginning of the 1950's ac-

---

* The name of Ludwig Puusepp is written differently in different publications. In the year 1900, the medical student L.M. Pussep as guest of a scientific session gave a talk "On the influence of ligating or compressing of the abdominal aorta on the spinal cord"; and Artom (1923) cited a French-language publication which gives Puusepp's name as 'Poussep', and an Italian-language one in which he is written as 'Pouseppe'.

cording to Flor-Henry, 1975, and more than 1,000 alone in British hospitals by 1945: Frankl & Mayer-Gross, 1947; later 15,000 operations were estimated for Great Britain by 1962 and 50,000 for the "first wave" of lobotomy in the United States: Valenstein, 1980a). This period has been documented in a number of reports from Freeman and Watts (Freeman, 1941; Freeman & Watts, 1939, 1941, 1942a, 1943, 1944, 1945, 1946b, 1946c, 1947a, 1947b; Freeman et al., 1941; Watts & Freeman, 1938, 1945, 1948a, 1948b) and in monographs and edited books (e.g., Freeman & Watts, 1942b; Fulton, 1951; Fulton, Aring & Wortis, 1948; Greenblatt, Arnot, & Solomon, 1952; Mettler, 1949; A. Meyer & Beck, 1954; Partridge, 1949; Tow, 1955). The diversity of the techniques used can be seen in Figures 15-19. (See also the discussions on the surgical methods given by Beck, McLardy, & Meyer, 1950; Dal Bianco, 1950; Dax & Ridley-Smith, 1943; Freeman & Watts, 1942b; Heimann, 1963; Hofstatter, Smolik, & Busch, 1945; Liberson, Scoville, & Dunsmore, 1951; Reitman, 1946, 1948; Riechert, 1950; and Worchel & Lyerly, 1941.)

Psychosurgery (Adler & Saupe, 1979; Hohne & Walsh, 1970; Valenstein, 1980c) was applied as a cure for anxiety (Babcock, 1947), tics, drug addictions, alcoholism, "sex perverts" (Scoville, 1971), schizophrenia (A.E. Bennett, Keegan, & Wilbur, 1943; Jenkins, Holsopple, & Lorr, 1954; Robin, 1958; Rothschild & Kaye, 1949; Watts & Freeman, 1948b), manic-obsessive (Bridges & Goktepe, 1973; Cohen, Novick, & Ettleson, 1942; Ederle, 1951; G.N. Jones & McCowan, 1949) or obsessive-compulsive disorders (Sargant, 1951; Tan, Marks, & Marset, 1971), criminal behavior, pain (Bartsch, 1953; Bonner, Cobb, Sweet, & White, 1952; Freeman & Watts, 1946a, 1948; Grantham, 1951; King, Clausen, & Scarff, 1950; Kolb, 1953; Koskoff, Dennis, Lazovik, & Wheeler, 1948; Krüger, 1953; Le Beau, 1951; Le Beau & Petrie, 1953; Rowe & Moyar, 1950; Scarff, 1950), neurotic behavior (Le Beau & Choppy, 1956; Sargant, 1951; Sargant & Stewart, 1947) and the like, but has created an ongoing debate up to the present, as in (at least the majority of) these cases apparently non-pathological tissue was removed or damaged in order to alter the personality and as changes in other personality dimensions were not uncommon (e.g., Allison & Allison, 1954; Crown, 1951, 1952).

Though psychosurgery was reduced drastically from the 1960's onwards (concomitant with the rise in use of drug treatment), the long term consequences of these surgical interventions were evaluated even in the 1970's and 1980's (e.g., Freeman, 1971; Hussaein, Freeman, & Jones, 1988; Hohne & Walsh, 1970; Miller, 1985; Miller & Milner, 1985; Robin & Macdonald, 1975; Pakkenberg, 1989; Stuss et al., 1982, 1983, 1986; Stuss & Benson, 1983; Stuss, Benson, Kaplan, Weir, & Della Malva, 1981) and in refined forms psychosurgery is performed up to the present (e.g., Bridges, 1972; Kiloh, Smith, & Johnson, 1988; Mitchell-Heggs, Kelly, & Richardson, 1976; Sachdev, Smith, & Matheson, 1990; J.S. Smith & Kiloh, 1980; E. Turner, 1973).

Gottlieb Burckhardt – The First Psychosurgeon

Gottlieb Burckhardt, director of the Insane Asylum in Prefargier (Neuchâtel) in Switzerland, was born in 1816 as a son of a medical doctor and was described by Bach (1907) as both scientifically engaged and as a highly capable practitioner. His book from 1875 on the physiological diagnosis of nervous diseases (Burckhardt, 1875) became rather well-known at the time. In 1888 he was the first who performed psychosurgery (in six cases with schizophrenic and further symptoms). But while Adler and Saupe (1979) stated that Burckhardt's work was practically never cited, I found that his early contribution was acknowledged by a number of workers, including Ederle (1948), Freeman (1942, 1971), Freeman and Watts (1942b), Fulton (1949), Haddenbrock (1949), Partridge (1949), Pool (1951), Scoville (1972), Stengel (1949), and E. Turner (1973) (cf. also C. Müller, 1960).

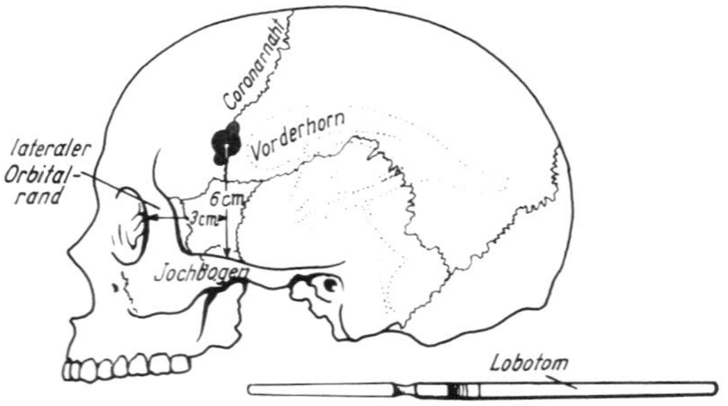

Figure 15. Lateral view of the skull with the ventricular system projected onto it and the topography of the bore-hole for standard leucotomy. (Reproduced from Fig. 6 of Heimann, 1963; with permission from the author and Springer Press.)

Burckhardt (1891) wrote only one – though a comparatively large – article on his results with psychosurgery (cf. Bach's, 1907, necrologue on Burckhardt). His aim had been to find new aids for curing otherwise untreatable psychoses. He explicitly pointed out that the indications for his surgery were purely psychiatric in all cases and that the rationale for performing the operations rested in part on acknowledged experimental and clinical results and in part on his own conclusions, which might not be obvious from the beginning. For this reason he gave a thorough review of the literature and then inferred that "affects are cortical in nature" and are "transposed into movements by the motoric cortical areas" (p. 475). Consequently he assumed that "agitation and impulsiveness are evoked because stimuli of an enormous number, quality, and intensity impinge on the motoric areas so that an improvement can only be reached by introducing resistance between the two" (p. 478). As the only and less fortunate alternative, Burckhardt mentioned the removal of either the sensory or the motor cortical areas with all consequences. Thus, the goal he decided on was to remove bilaterally a cortical strip of 2 cm width posterior to the motor cortex, possibly entering the temporal lobes as well (p. 478).

Burckhardt's first patient was a female farmer of about 51 years with "agitated dementia ... of considerable danger". Four operations in succession were done by Burckhardt, the first

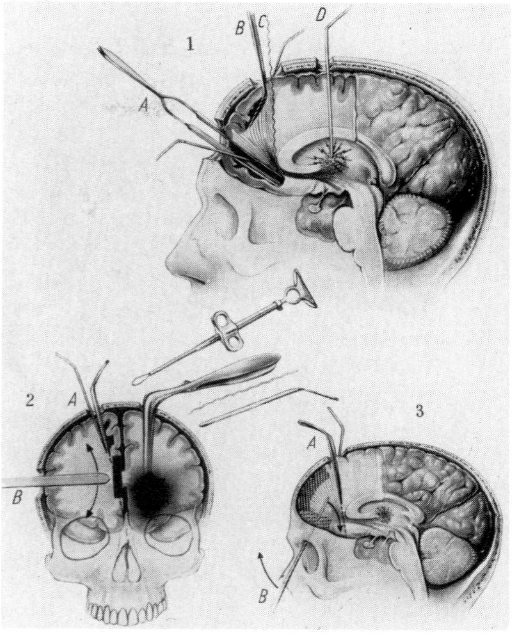

Figure 16. Various selective techniques of leucotomy. 1: A. orbital undercutting; B. undercutting of the dorsal convexity; C. electrocoagulation of the lower medial quadrant; D. stereotaxic electrocoagulation of the thalamic mediodorsal nucleus. 2: A. undercutting of the cingulate gyrus; B. standard lobotomy; C. lobotomy of the lower medial quadrant, diverse techniques. 3: A. overt standard lobotomy; B. transorbital lobotomy; punctuated and striped area: topectomy inferior and superior, resp. (Reproduced from Fig. 9 of Heimann, 1963; with permission from the author and Springer Press.)

on December 29, 1888, which lasted four hours and resulted in the removal of 5 g cortex. As the patient's behavior improved only partly (she was still somewhat agitated and aggressive), Burckhardt performed a second operation about two months later with the intention of elongatating the cortical ditch laterally. Another 2.5 g brain tissue were removed, after which the patient appeared more cheerful than before. As her condition had not changed otherwise since the operation, Burckhardt did a third one at the end of May (i.e., exactly 5 months after the first), now intending to remove a strip from the left parietal cortex. After this operation the patient had apparently lost

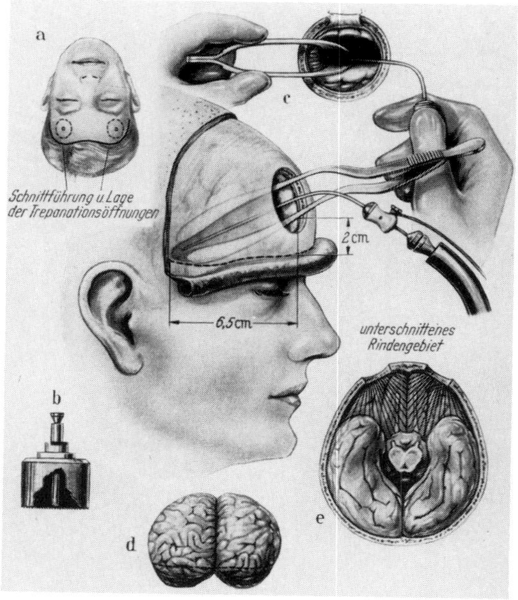

Figure 17. Orbital undercutting after W. B. Scoville. a: position of the trepanation holes; b: middle figure: topography of the operation with position of the instruments; c: view through the trepanation hole into the undercut area; d: position of the sectional plane in the brain; e: undercut cortical area.
(Reproduced from Fig. 10 of Heimann, 1963; with permission from the author and Springer Press.)

some of her visual and auditory hallucinations and also some of her agitatedness.

To fulfill his original plan, Burckhardt stated that the motoric language area should be his "next object of attack" ("Ich schloss weiter, dass, in Verfolgung meines anfänglich aufgestellten Planes, die Gegend der motorischen Sprachcentren das nächste Angriffsobject bilden müsse."; p. 490). Though he acknowledged the risk of making the patient aphasic, he considered the operation worth the attempt and performed it about 13 months after the first now removing 1.5 g cortex. After the operation Burckhardt concluded that "Frau Borel has changed from a dangerous and agitated dementic into a calm dementic" (p. 493). She did not improve in intelligence, but in Burckhardt's eyes, she did show some progress in other areas in comparison to the preoperative condition. From the descriptions given, the patient still had insight into her environment and sometimes might make appropriate and logical comments so that in my eyes she was not clearly severely dementic.

Considering the intention for his brain surgery, Burckhardt felt that this was supported by the outcome. Nevertheless, he acknowledged that "the ways of cerebral events are manifold and intermingled. Things need not necessarily be as we imagine them. This, however, cannot hinder us to at least imagine them" (p. 494).

Burckhardt's second case was considered to be dementic as well and to suffer from megalomania. He was placed in the psychiatric clinic at an age of $31^1/_2$ years. He had been a talented pupil, but "he started with masturbation at an early age and had overindulged quite early in Venere et Baccho" (p. 494).

Burckhardt removed the first and second prefrontal gyrus, but while the patient improved somewhat, the operation resulted in the occurrence of epileptic attacks which led Burckhardt to refrain from a second operation. He stated that while others considered the area of cortex removed as the "center for agraphia", the patient on the contrary was able postoperatively to write a postcard to his mother (dictated by a nurse).

The third, fourth, and fifth cases had auditory hallucinations; the auditory cortex was then removed with "considerable impairment" in cases III and IV and "considerable appeasement and reduction of the hallucinations" in case V (case V was operated on twice). The last of Burckhardt's reported cases had a number of complex psychiatric deviations. After removal of the "acoustic word area" (p. 533) he had convulsions four days thereafter and died on the sixth postoperative day.

Burckhardt concluded from his results that "every new surgical intervention had to find its indications and methods and every path, which led to new achievements is paved with crosses of death" (p. 547). Although the results were not very encouraging he considered psychosurgery as a worthwhile method. Of the two categories of medical doctors, those adhering to the motto "primum non nocere" and those favoring "melius anceps remedium quam nullum", he stated that he followed the second.

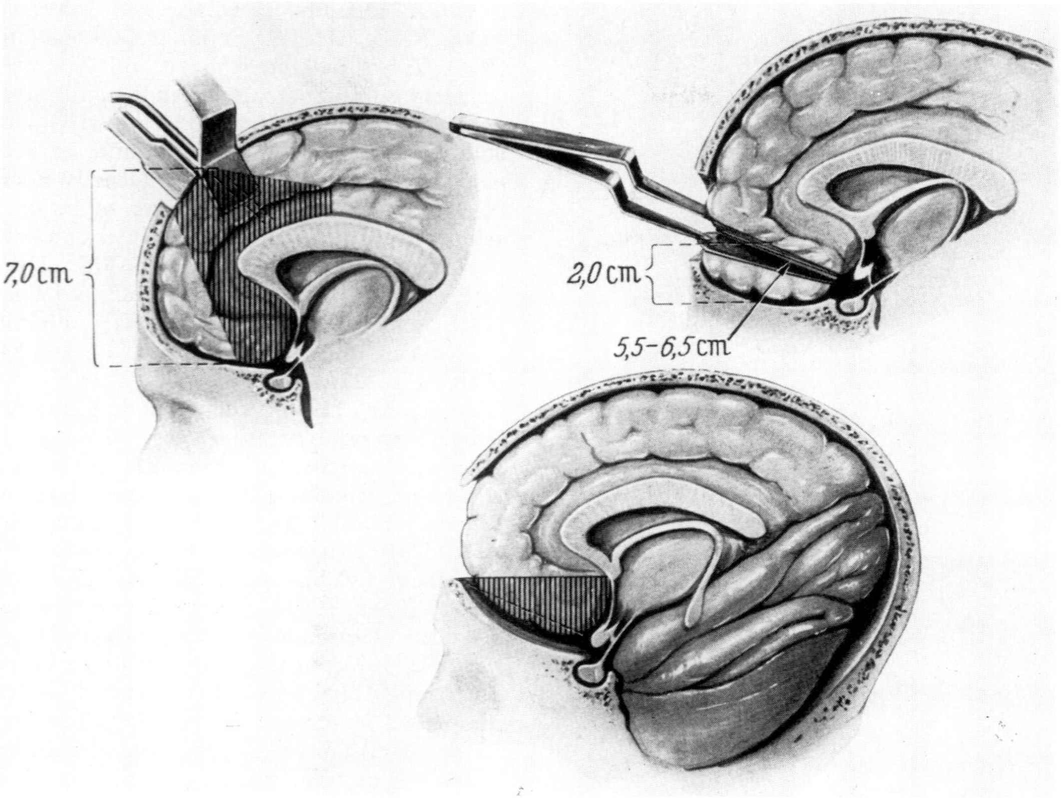

Figure 18. Top left: the striped area shows the cortical areas which (with W. B. Scoville's surgical technique) are separated from the gray matter; top right: topography of orbital undercutting in a medial view; bottom: an overly deep cut, ending in the septal areas and leading to loss of consciousness, convulsions, and finally to a state of confusion. (Reproduced from Fig. 11 of Heimann, 1963; with permission from the author and Springer Press.)

The Founders

While surgical removal of parts of the frontal lobe had been done several times before the 1930's (e. g., Ackerly, 1935; Bailey, 1933; Brickner, 1936, 1939, 1952; Dandy, 1925; Penfield and Evans, 1935; H. Smith, 1906; Starr, 1894), Moniz really gave the firing signal for psychosurgery. American surgeons such as Freeman and Watts (1942 b) soon popularized the technique which spread all over the world (e. g., Govindaswamy & Balakrishna, 1944). Its popularity was reinforced by the lack of alternatives at that time and probably also by the relative simplicity of the method. (Freeman in fact was dissatisfied with Moniz's technique and adopted the one described by Fiamberti in 1937; cf. Freeman, 1971).

Gardner (1957) stated for example "...that the psychiatrist who makes an adequate study of the surgical anatomy and technique of this operation can readily qualify for its use. This is because of its comparative safety and the inherent simplicity of the technique. In our series the operative mortality rate to date is 1.2%." (p. 140). Barahona-Fernandes (1953) gave a

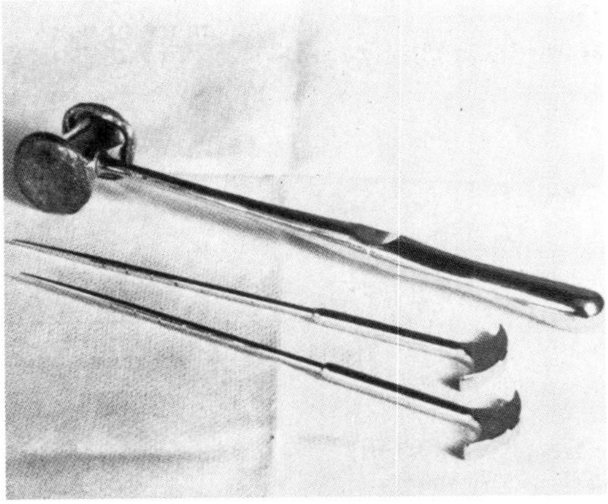

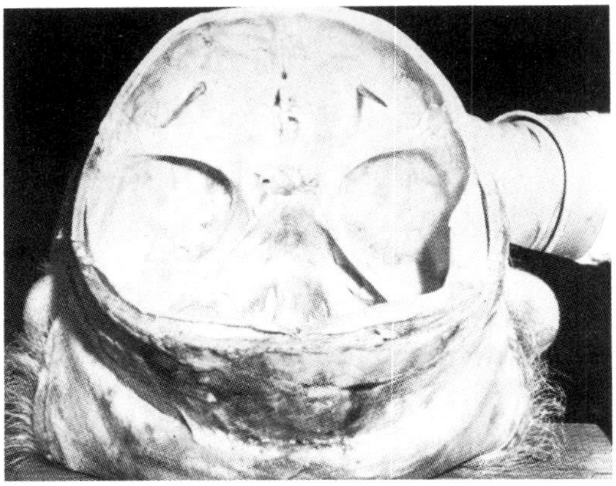

Figure 19. The transorbital leucotomes and mallet used for Freeman's transorbital approach (top). The "geometrical precision with which the instruments can be placed" is given in the bottom part of the figure. (Reproduced from Figs. 1 and 2 of the article of Jones & Shanklin, 1950).

quite positive view of the consequences of prefrontal leucotomy. He stated that there are good chances for being cured, and that the patients gain a life in peace and calm at home, instead of in a hospital.

Nevertheless, at least a certain possibility for surgery-evoked convulsions does exist (S. Levin, Greenblatt, Healey, & Solomon, 1950; N. L. Paul, Fitzgerald, & Greenblatt, 1956). Even without convulsions or other sequelae substantial anterograde and retrograde degeneration has to be reckoned with, in addition to the disruption of frontal cortical neuronal activity. Le Beau (1951) listed a number of other factors which have to be considered when performing leucotomies or topectomies (cf. also Beck, McLardy, & Meyer, 1950; McKissock, 1943, 1951) and Heath and Pool (1948) referred to the possibility of death due to severing an artery, edemas, or trophic changes (p. 427).

Freeman's (1948) transorbital lobotomy (sometimes referred to as "ice pick surgery") especially was quite easy, done in a few minutes, and was consequently adopted quickly. Freeman himself had performed (or supervised) 3,000 transorbital lobotomies before his retirement (Valenstein, 1980 a; cf. Freeman, 1953 a, 1953 b, 1957). Other methods, such as Scoville's "selective cortical undercutting" (Scoville, 1973; Scoville, Wilk, & Pepe, 1951), posterior cuts (A. Meyer & McLardy, 1948), or the orbital leucotomy described by Tow and Lewin (1953) gained less popularity or were not developed until later, such as the stereotactic approach for the orbital cortex (Herner, 1961; Knight, 1964) (cf. also Freeman, 1949 a, and the methodological descriptions on topectomy given in Pool, 1949, 1951 and the reports of Boehlke, 1952, Corsellis & Jack, 1973, and Newcombe, 1973).

As psychosurgery is intended to serve as a method for improving behavior, and as the method by definition interferes with preoperative personality features, its outcome has been given particular attention. Especially the earlier reports tended to emphasize positive results (e. g., Anderson, 1949; Banay & Davidoff, 1942; Egan, 1949; Fleming, 1944; Grassi, 1950; Halstead, 1947; Halstead, Carmichael, & Bucy, 1946; T. Hunt, 1942; R. E. Jones, 1949; Köbcke, 1947; Mixter, Tillotson, & Wies, 1941; Puusepp, 1937; Schrader & Robinson, 1945; Strecker, Palmer, & Grant, 1942; Ström-Olsen, Last, Brody & Knight, 1943), though in some instances intellectual deterioration (Babcock, 1947; Heilbrunn & Hletko, 1943; Malmo, 1948;

Porteus, 1952; Porteus & Kepner, 1942, 1944; Porteus & Peters, 1947; M.F. Robinson, 1946; J.S. Smith & Kinder, 1959; Stämpfli, 1952; Wittenborn & Mettler, 1951) or impairments in the ability for abstracting were remarked (Goldstein, 1944, 1949; Yacorzynski, Boshes, & Davis, 1948); Elithorn, Piercy and Crosskey (1954) mentioned autonomic changes (cf. also Chapman, Livingston, & Livingston, 1949; Delgado & Livingston, 1948; Livingston, Chapman, Livingston, & Kraintz, 1948; Livingston et al., 1948). Even with the Porteus maze, leucotomized subjects behaved worse than controls (M.F. Robinson, 1946). Postsurgical behavioral impairments were usually attributed to methodological inadequacies, in particular when so-called "blind approaches" (cf. Figs. 16–19) had been used (cf. the discussion in Heath & Pool, 1948, p.427f). In such instances, even suicide apparently may follow as a long term consequence of the intervention, as Evans exemplified with two cases as late as 1971. (Nonetheless, for a recent report of a patient who after psychosurgery held a very high and responsible position in the Japanese government see Hirose, 1979, and for an older one see Rylander, 1950, who reported that a student with a postoperative IQ of 146 started university studies eight months after leucotomy in "mathematics and the difficult Finnish language", p.304.)

Outcome and Evaluation of Psychosurgery

In 1938 Johannes Lange stated that after Brickner's (1936) case no surgeon would dare to eliminate bilaterally "the huge apparatus of inhibition" nature had given to man with the frontal lobes. But then this hope was totally discouraged by the psychosurgeons who became active immediately after J. Lange's last publication (cf. Spatz, 1950).

Finesinger (1949) and Frankl and Mayer-Gross (1947) suggested that more long term follow-ups should be made which should include an assessment of the patient's prepsychotic personality, changes due to the illness up to the operation, and a comparison of these changes with postoperative performance (up to two years after surgery). The authors gave some examples of the changes found in patients after psychosurgery. Rothschild and Kaye (1949) evaluated 100 lobotomized cases who had had schizophrenia, partly since periods beyond 20 years. They found a postoperative improvement in most of them, but suggested to preferably perform surgery in cases who had been ill for 4 or 5 years or longer. A similar view was held by Constantinides and Stroussopoulos (1954) who had evaluated 103 cases with leucotomy, and by Strecker, Palmer, and Grant (1942) who had results on 22 cases of frontal lobotomy.

Frequently, it was found that patients treated by psychosurgery were more 'easy going' postoperatively, with "sports and light entertainment" (p.821) dominating, whereas prior to surgery "serious interests in arts, literature, religion, or politics" (p.821) had been noted (Frankl & Mayer-Gross, 1947). Changes in biological rhythms and other vegetative changes were reported Bochnik (1952) and by Rinkel, Greenblatt, Coon, and Solomon (1947).

With respect to family life, 48 patient records were collected, showing a considerable number of difficulties, mainly due to "(1) shallowness of feeling and lack of affection and of consideration for others, even for children; (2) domineering manner, self-willed stubbornness, and inaccessibility to reason; and (3) outbursts of temper and irritability" (Frankl & Mayer-Gross, 1947, p.822).

But in 1947 and one year later in 1948, Paul Glees (1947, 1948a) still encouraged the application of prefrontal leucotomy as a therapeutic action (cf. also Glees, 1948b). He emphasized the successive behavioral changes during surgery: As the operation was usually done under local anesthesia, it was possible to talk with the patient and the discussion with him or her did not change as long as only two of the four prefrontal quadrants have been sectioned. Following transection of the third quadrant, answers became shorter and emotionally flatter, but only after complete transection of all four quadrants did the patient become silent, with his or her face expressionless; he or she could lose orientation, even denying that surgery was being done. Nervousness was lost, blood pressure and pulse rate reduced. But recovery usually followed soon and rehabilitation of the personality was frequent. Glees seems to have adhered to the view that disinhibition and "Witzelsucht" (euphoria) were the dominant consequences of orbitofrontal removals or transections, while intellectual changes could be neglected. (Similar opinions were held by many earlier authors [e. g., Feuchtwanger, 1923; J. Lange, 1938; Rylander, 1939, 1943], while Hebb and Penfield, 1940, and Hebb, 1939, 1941, 1942, 1945, found no significant effects on personality or intellect.)

In a 500 paged volume, Partridge (1949) gave "a survey of 300 cases [with pre-frontal leucotomy] personally followed over $1^1/_2$–3 years". His interpretations seem more balanced which is reflected in a sentence like this: "... pre-frontal leucotomy, like most other surgical operations, is capable both of conferring benefit and of doing harm" (p. 467). For Partridge, prefrontal leucotomy should remain the treatment of last choice, provided that such choice is not delayed beyond the limits after which recovery became impossible.

The bibliography included in Partridge's book is rather exhaustive for that time and subdivided in the following manner: (a) reviews of the literature, (b) references in the text, (c) clinical observations, (d) operative techniques, and (e) anatomical, physiological, and pathological observations. Shortly after the Second World War, in 1947, the Association for Research in Nervous and Mental Disease also took up the frontal lobes as theme (Fulton, Aring, & Wortis, 1948). Part IV of these proceedings included eight chapters on frontal lobotomy, namely one by Rylander (1948) on personality changes before and after lobotomy, three on pain relief (Falconer, 1948; Koskoff, Dennis, Lazovik, & Wheeler, 1948; Watts & Freeman, 1948 a), three on the consequences of lobotomy for motor behavior (Chapman, Rose, & Solomon, 1948), cerebral blood flow and metabolism (Shenkin, Woodford, Freyhan, & Kety, 1948), gastro-intestinal hemorrhages and other changes (Sweet, Cotzias, Seed, & Yakovlev, 1948), and the last chapter gave the findings of a cooperative clinical study of lobotomy (B. E. Moore, Friedman, Simon, & Farmer, 1948).

In 1948 Ederle described a case with a history of about nine years of schizophrenia. After leucotomy the patient lost his spontaneity and was much less strange in behavior than prior to surgery. However, his disturbances in formal thinking remained, and Ederle also emphasized that surgeons should weigh all consequences of a "mutilation of the soul" and recommended leucotomy only in "the most severe cases" (cf. also Russell, 1948).

For a recent "review of the literature on post-operative evaluation" of psychosurgery see Valenstein (1980 b), for older ones Valenstein (1973) and Willett (1961). Patient-based evaluations (in part with substantial samples) were made by Barahona-Fernandes (1950, 1952), Berliner, Beveridge, Mayer-Gross, and Moore (1945), Birley (1964), Bridges, Goktepe, Maratos, Browne, and Young (1973), Dax, Cunningham, and Radley-Smith (1945/46), Frank (1946), Freeman (1953 a, 1954), Freeman and Watts (1946, 1947 a, 1948), Freyhan (1954), Greenblatt, Arnot, and Solomon (1952), Greenblatt, Robertson, and Solomon (1953), Greenblatt and Solomon (1953), Jones and Shanklin (1950), Joschko (1979), Michel (1948), Oltman, Brody, Friedman, and Green (1949), Petrie (1949, 1950), Pippard (1955), Risso, Poeck, and Creutzfeldt (1962), Rüsken (1950), Sands and Malamud (1949), Ström-Olsen and Tow (1949), Sykes and Tredgold (1964), Tomkins, 1948, W. W. Wilson, Pittman, Bennett and Garber (1953), among others.

In the study of Baeyer (1947) comparisons were made between the outcome of shock therapies and prefrontal lobotomy, in Bental's (1957) report the course of psychoses in lobotomized and non-lobotomized brothers and sisters was compared, Petrie (1952) assessed the psychological effects of different types of operations on the frontal lobes, and Dehnen (1961) compared the consequences of uni- and bilateral psychosurgical interventions.

W. W. Wilson et al. (1951), who had treated 100 patients, reported marked improvements in over one-half of the cases. They stated "We urge that this type of operation be considered for all chronically disturbed patients in whom other less strenuous forms of therapy have failed after one year. The economic advantages in the improvement of such a group of patients are stressed." (p. 448). An (even) less optimistic view was presented at the 1948 International Conference on Psychiatry in Lisbon by the Lisbon scientists (and therefore colleagues of E. Moniz) Furtado, Rodrigues, Marques, Alvim, and De Vasconcelos (1949). The diminution of affect and the changes in moral and ethical values in most of their patients led them to conclude: "The serious cerebral alteration which lobotomy produces and which is shown by the changes in the pneumoencephalogram, is also defined by serious changes of personality which today we still do not know if they will assume a progressive character. We conclude, therefore, that lobotomy, as a method of treatment, should only be authorized in special cases, when all the therapeutic means have been exhausted, and when hope has been lost of a spontaneous improvement, even at the end of a long time" (p. 74).

"Theoretical and critical remarks on prefrontal leucotomy" was the subtitle of Haddenbrock's (1949) paper. He first stated that with leucotomic surgery no ill or affected tissue was eliminated and that this meant that leucotomy was not a causal therapy. "Not the illness, but the experience of the illness defines the indication" (p. 70). This elimination of functioning tissue was done on an area which "constitutes a unique organic locus of disturbing the specific humane of the human" (p. 71).

According to Haddenbrock (1949) defrontalization constitutes "a definitive destruction of the self-consciousness and free human personality or of its rest which remains within the psychosis" (p. 73). He emphasized that leucotomized patients are no longer able to reflect their own nature and entity, they have no reflexive fear of death and are at the mercy of all external stimuli and of their own drives. In the worst case they are "intelligent creatures of drive" ("Triebwesen").

Spatz (1950) argued that while the frontal lobes may be important structures, they may be so only during certain times or stages. The frontal lobes could be an organizing apparatus which builds up capacities and makes them available to other areas of the brain (a manager function for the rest of the brain). When the frontal lobe has given up its creative performance, the individual could do without it.

Chronic schizophrenic patients with negative outcome after leucotomy were described by Stämpfli (1952; cf. also Stoll, 1954). Heimann (1951) pointed to the danger of post-operative defects of volition and affective responsiveness. Carscallen, Buck, and Hobbs (1951) ended their evaluation of 49 lobotomized patients with the words: "Although the operation frees the patient from his psychosis to the degree that he performs better along manual and practical lines, it also leaves him with the inability to concentrate sufficiently to utilize this asset" (p. 220).

Lastly, Bräutigam and Czernigewycz (1950) stressed the similar effects of a degenerative process affecting the frontal lobes and of prefrontal lobectomy on a compulsive disorder. Their case was a woman with a compulsive drive to wash her hands, whose abnormal behavior improved after multiple sclerosis-induced frontal atrophy.

Prospect

In the 1950's psychosurgery was still treated with optimism or even euphorically (Freeman, Davis, East, Tait, & Rogers, 1954; Gardner, 1957; R. E. Jones & Shanklin, 1950; B. E. Moore & Lutz, 1951; M. T. Moore & Winkelmann, 1951; Rylander, 1950; Simon, Margolis, Adams, & Bowman, 1951; W. W. Wilson, Pittman, Bennett, & Garber, 1951). Gardner, for example, reported results of 115 leucotomized patients, 44% of whom had remissions, 36% improved, and 20% failed. From this outcome he concluded that transorbital leucotomy "is an excellent technique for treatment of selected cases from private practice, as well as such institutionalized cases reported by others" (p. 142). Simon et al. (1951) emphasized several times the surgically caused "excellent adjustment as housewife" (e. g., p. 500). Similarly, Reihnert (1950) performed a leucotomy on a 29-year-old female patient with massive character deviations who then improved considerably. Within the next eight months of observation, she became much less hostile than before and was able to start working.

On the other hand psychosurgery may even result in the development of cystic lesions: Guthrie and McMullen (1978) reported the case of 62-year-old female who had received a bilateral transorbital leucotomy 21 years earlier and subsequently manifested bilateral frontal lobe cystic lesions.

Quite thorough discussions of the value as well as limits of psychosurgery appeared at the end of the 1950's (Busch, 1957; Greenblatt & Solomon, 1958; Häfner, 1957; Landis, Zubin, & Mettler, 1950), in the 1960's (Heimann, 1963) and later (e. g., Valenstein, 1980 c). But already before the 1950's McLardy and Davies (1949) gave the following conclusions in their summary (on p. 238):

1. Many of the symptoms and syndromes characteristic of affective and schizophrenic functional psychoses can recur after practically complete isolation of the prefrontal cortex from its long fibre connexions. Some schizophrenic symptoms, at least, cannot only persist but can disappear and then recur after full bilateral prefrontal lobectomy. Many neurotic symptoms can recur after disappearance following removal of more limited amounts of prefrontal cortex.
2. The illness which recurs is practically always of the same type as the pre-operative one.
3. There are indications that the power of environmental influences for both good and ill may be augmented after the operation.

Greenblatt and Solomon (1958) discussed lobotomy under three major headings:

1. What are the changes produced by frontal lobe operations on behavior, thinking and feeling?
2. What are the therapeutic implications of lobotomy?
3. What has twenty years of frontal surgery contributed to our understanding of the functions of the brain, especially the frontal lobes and mechanisms of human adaptation?

With respect to the first topic the kind of operation and the size and placement of the cuts are, of course, of important influence. "Early total bilateral operations, for example, evoked the fear that lobotomy produces a 'vegetable' personality ..." (Greenblatt & Solomon, 1958, p. 19). A reduced drive was considered the most likely result of lobotomy (Greenblatt, 1950). This reduced drive was sometimes termed apathy (A. Meyer, Beck, & McLardy, 1947; Ström-Olsen, 1946), laziness or lethargy (Golla, 1943, 1946), lack of initiative (A. Meyer, Beck, & McLardy, 1947), or loss of spontaneity (Ström-Olsen, Last, Brody, & Knight, 1943). Self-concern is a further personality trait which is reduced after prefrontal lobotomy (Hutton, 1943, 1947), as is affectivity and the patient's social sense (Hoch, 1949; Hoheisel, 1954; Reitman, 1947; Rylander, 1943, 1948). Though Greenblatt and Solomon (1958) acknowledged the likeliness of these consequences of psychosurgery, they still considered it a recommendable technique in view of the usual preoperative status of the patient and the gains obtained postsurgery.

The therapeutic implications of course derive from the consequences: thus, persons with "high tension" who are blocked in normal psychological functioning and social behavior might benefit most (and most likely) (Greenblatt & Solomon, 1953). Greenblatt and Solomon (1958) also summarized their own previously published data on the long-term outcome of prefrontal lobotomy (Greenblatt, Robertson, & Solomon, 1953; Greenblatt, Wingate, & Solomon, 1954; N. L. Paul, Fitzgerald, & Greenblatt, 1956), stating that the five year follow-up revealed results at least as posi-

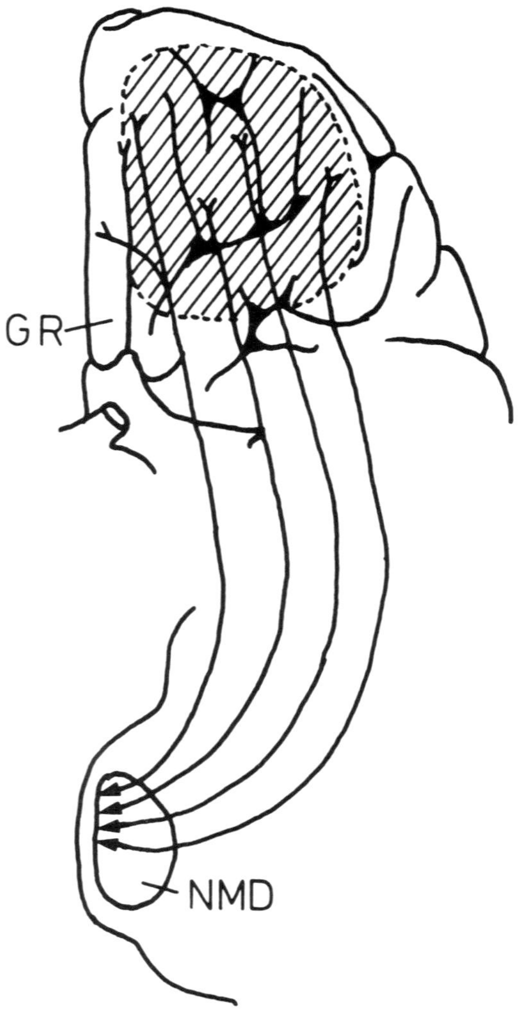

Figure 20. Anatomical relations between the medial portion of the thalamic mediodorsal nucleus and the orbitofrontal cortex of the human brain according to Pilleri; GR, gyrus proreus; NMD, nucleus mediodorsalis (after Fig. 10 of Pilleri, 1960).

tive or even improved compared to those observed after the first year postsurgery. In their table on page 24 Greenblatt and Solomon (1958) listed "good" work adjustment in 54%, "fair" in 12%, and "poor" work adjustment in 34% of their cases after five years.

With respect to the third heading – implications of lobotomy for redundancy in the brain – Greenblatt and Solomon (1958) described the main consequence of lobotomy as interfering with "long circuits": "The individual suffers 1) a reduction in drive, force or energy; 2) he is less affected by past experience and more bound to immediate stimuli; 3) he is less able to elaborate experience or to sustain experiences. One way of looking at this is that the mechanism of prolongation in time is impaired." (p. 27).

In discussing the contribution of Greenblatt and Solomon (1958) (which had been presented in 1956 on the Symposium on "The Brain and Human Behavior" of the Association for Research in Nervous and Mental Disease) S. Cobb criticized the lack of controls in psychosurgery (p. 29: "I think that we need about fifty volunteers, so-called normals, who would have lobotomy").

Psychological changes after prefrontal lobotomy were described in several publications by Scherer and coworkers (Scherer, Klett, & Winne, 1957; Scherer, Winne, & Baker, 1955; Scherer, Winne, Clancy, & Baker, 1953; Winne & Scherer, 1956). Rosvold and Mishkin (1950) also evaluated the effects of prefrontal lobotomy on intelligence, finding a deficit.

The pioneer of lobotomy, Walter Freeman, published a paper in 1971 on the long term follow-up of 415 lobotomized patients with the diagnosis of early schizophrenia. His statements were still quite enthusiastic, one of them being that "*the original hypothesis of Egas Moniz appears more probable than ever*" (p. 622), another that frontal lobotomy marked the turning point in effective therapy (cf. also Freeman, 1949a; M. F. Robinson & Freeman, 1954; Williams & Freeman, 1953). He also stated – what I find quite surprising, if not unlikely – that "I was unable to find any retrograde degeneration in the medial dorsal nucleus of the thalamus, or any other place at a distance from the incisions" (p. 622).

Aside from a more general review of Girgis (1971) I wish to mention some major recent publications: The proceedings of the Fourth World Congress of Psychiatric Surgery, held in 1975 in Madrid, that of the Third International Congress of Psychosurgery, held in 1972 in Cambridge, and that of the Second International Conference on Psychiatry, held in 1971 in Copenhagen (Hitchcock, Laitinen, & Vaernet, 1972; Laitinen & Livingston, 1973; Sweet, Obrador, & Martín-Rodríguez, 1977). (The first Congress on Psychosurgery had been held in Lisbon, where Moniz lived, in 1948). The volume of Sweet et al., however, contains less than half a dozen contributions on prefrontal psychosurgery (Hirose, 1977; Peraita & Lopes de Lerma, 1977; Saubidet, Lyonnet, & Brichetti, 1977; Scoville & Bettis, 1977; J. S. Smith, Kiloh, & Boots, 1977; K. W. Walsh, 1977). In these reports criteria are listed for performing operations (Scoville & Bettis, 1977; cf. also Scoville, 1954 b, 1960) and outcome evaluations are provided and technical standards are discussed. Taken together, however, neither this book nor any other recent one has provided any major new insights (but see Knight, 1972, and Ström-Olsen & Carlisle, 1972).

Implications for Anatomical Knowledge

Though some of the studies on psychosurgery made – more or less as a byproduct – remarks on anatomical connections, the overall outcome for this topic is – with few exceptions (e.g., K. Hartmann & Simma, 1952) – negligible in my eyes (Freeman, 1949 b, 1950; Freeman & Watts, 1947 a; Fulton, 1949; Glees, 1948 a, 1948 b; Hassler, 1950; McLardy & Davies, 1949; McLardy & Meyer, 1949; A. Meyer & McLardy, 1948; Pfuhl, 1954; Pilleri, 1960; Poeck, Pilleri, & Risso, 1962; Sperling, 1957; Yakovlev, 1954; Yakovlev, Hamlin, & Sweet, 1950), especially on the background of already existing old findings (e.g., Fukuda, 1919; Hirosawa & Kato, 1935; Monakow, 1895; Rutishauser, 1899). Nevertheless this judgement is primarily based on present-day possibilities and knowledge on the anatomy of the prefrontal cortex (ef., e.g., the review of Markowitsch, 1988 a). An example of anatomical relations between portions of the mediodorsal thalamus and the prefrontal (orbitofrontal) cortex is given in Figure 20.

A possible exception to the opinion given above may be seen in the fact that prefrontal psychosurgery reinforced the search for anatomical substrates of psychiatric illnesses (e.g., C. Vogt & Vogt, 1948; cf. also Fünfgeld, 1937, J. Schuster, 1930, and C. Vogt & Vogt, 1937), an attempt which is currently being followed quite vigorously (S. E. Arnold, Hyman, & Van Hoesen, 1989; Bench, Dolan, Friston, & Frackowiak, 1990; Benes, McSparren, Sangiovanni, & Vincent, 1989; Bogaerts, 1984; Fontaine, Breton, Dery, Fontaine, & Elie, 1990; Luchins, 1990; Mayberg, Starkstein, Robinson, & Wagner, 1989; Pearlson et al., 1989; Roberts, 1991; Rossi et al., 1990, 1991; Seidman, 1983; Young et al., 1991; Zibursky, Lim, & Pfefferbaum, 1991), but which has a long and controversial tradition (cf., e.g., Omorokow, 1914, and Heyck, 1954).

Conclusions

Psychosurgery, as mentioned at the beginning, is a relatively recent endeavor – compared to the time period covered in the rest of the book – and, furthermore, it can be compared to a comet: "quick rise – rather steep fall". However, a minority of authors in fact sees "the renaissance of psychosurgery" (Rylander, 1973). One of the focal problems for making inferences from the patients operated on is the fact that they have had a long-standing severe (psychic) illness.

Based on our knowledge of the anatomy of the brain and of the multi-faceted consequences of brain damage (e.g., Finger & Stein, 1982) which includes direct anterograde and retrograde degeneration, it is astonishing how well in principal the patients behaved post-surgery. This is all the more astonishing when considering just which area was damaged most frequently and most heavily – the orbitofrontal cortex – and still the patients behaved as positively and as "normally" as they did on the average.

This finding interferes with the view that in this area there is a major dopaminergic pathway which is interrupted, and – even more importantly – that the principal cholinergic neuron pools are separated from the rest of the brain – a theory which in recent times has been discussed as possibly being the principal cause for the severe mnemonic deteriorations observed in Alzheimer's disease (cf. the substantia innominata papers in Hitchcock et al., 1972).

As the degeneration of cholinergic neurons in three regions (the nucleus basalis of Meynert, medial septal area and diagonal band of Broca) is frequently considered the major cause of Alzheimer's disease (e.g., Markowitsch, 1987; Price, 1986; Wurtman, 1985), it is quite astonishing that the intellectual abilities of patients with frontal operations were so little affected on the average or even improved over postoperative time (e.g., Stuss et al., 1981, 1982, 1983, 1986). A conclusion I draw from this evidence is that there are indeed considerable interindividual differences between human brains and that these differences are obviously even more heterogenous in cases with a long history of behavioral deviations (cf. Markowitsch, 1988b, 1988c).

Chapter 5: Memory and Memory Disorders

Das Gedächtnis verbindet die zahllosen Einzelphänomene zu einem Ganzen, und wie unser Leib in unzählige Atome zerstieben müsste, wenn nicht die Attraktion der Materie ihn zusammenhielte, so zerfiele ohne die bindende Macht des Gedächtnisses unser Bewusstsein in so viele Splitter, als es Augenblicke zählt. [Memory connects innumerable single phenomena into a whole, and just as the body would be scattered like dust in countless atoms if the attraction of matter did not hold it together so consciousness – without the connecting power of memory – would fall apart in as many fragments as it contains moments.] (Hering, 1921, p. 12).

The action of reflexes, investigated for instance in the frog, has served as a model for understanding complex functions like mood and memory (e.g., Exner, 1881) (Figs. 21 and 22).

Pavlov's (1953) reflex theory – classical conditioning – was prominent in the days of Sherrington and other famous neurologists, as was the beginning of scientific memory research (Bergson, 1911; Charcot, 1892; Ebbinghaus, 1885, 1897; Forel, 1885; Häcker, 1914; Hering, 1895; Jaspers, 1910; Mabille & Pitres, 1913; G.E. Müller, 1911-1917; Semon, 1904), of psychology (James, 1890; Ebbinghaus, 1902; Jodl, 1903; Lipps, 1903; Losskij, 1904; Münsterberg, 1900; Pfänder, 1904; Watson, 1913) and of physiological psychology (C. Lange, 1887; Wundt, 1874; Ziehen, 1891, 1924). And the pros and contras of the possibilities of localizing memory functions in circumscribed entities within the nervous tissue had been discussed from Gall (1825) over Flourens (1842) to Broca (1861 a, 1981 b), Wernicke (1874), Hughlings-Jackson (1876, 1884, 1932; cf. Hitzig, 1900 a; E. H. Reynolds, 1988), Hitzig (Hitzig, 1903 c; cf. G. Anton, 1914), Freud (1900), Alzheimer (1897, 1904 a), Campbell (1905), Monakow (1909, 1914) and others (cf. H. S. Levin, Peters, & Hulkonen, 1983). In the last century, several books already appeared on possible relations between brain damage and memory disturbances (e.g., Forel, 1885; Hering, 1895; Meynert, 1878; Ribot, 1882/1881; Rittershain, 1871; Sollier, 1892). Ribot (1882) attributed three meanings to memory: "the conservation of certain conditions, their reproduction, and their localization in the past" (p. 10). Ribot subdivided amnesia into three variants as well: "1. Temporary amnesia; 2. Periodical amnesia; 3. Progressive amnesia ..." (p. 71). And in animals possible anatomical bases of mnestic functions were also studied (e.g., Edinger, 1899). Early reviews on the experimental investigation of memory appeared in 1885 (Ebbinghaus, Forel), 1889 (Burnham, 1889 a, 1889 b, 1889 c, 1889d), 1895 a (Titchener), and 1898 (Kennedy).

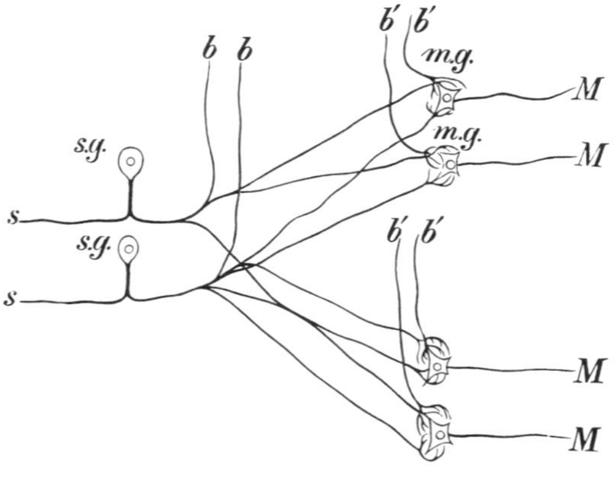

Figure 21. Schematic diagram (Exner's, 1881, Fig. 30) of theoretically existing connections between a sensory and two motor nuclei. *ss*, 2 sensory fibers which – after their connection with the spinal ganglion cell *sg* – divide in the gray substance and connect to the motor neuron *mg*. *b* and *b*' are fibers leading to the organ of consciousness. *M*, motoric fibers.

For a more recent definition of memory, I will cite that of Syz from 1937 (p. 355): "In its

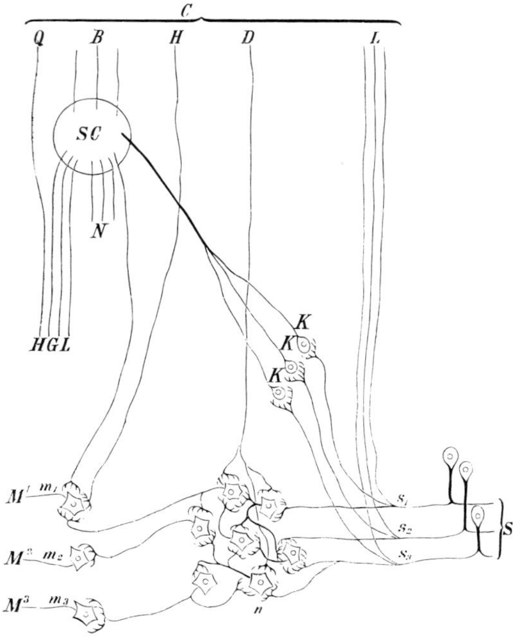

Figure 22. Schematic diagram (Exner's, 1881, Fig. 56) of a center of aversion. C., organ of consciousness; S, sensory; M, motoric spinal cord fibers; s, dividing points of the sensory fibers; m, motoric ganglion cells; n, center of spinal cord; K, centers of summation; SC, sum of the centers for the muscles performing the defense reaction; fibers 'N' lead to these muscles. Connected with these fibers are certain endings in the heart (H), the vessels (G), and the lungs (L). From these centers sensory fibers (Q) (which furthermore via the fibers B, H, D, and L receive information from the events occuring in the subcortical centers) lead to the organ of consciousness (after Exner, 1881, p. 209).

broadest sense memory may be defined as the capacity of the organism to retain, utilize and reactivate functional patterns which have been acquired through the organism's interaction with the environment. There is thus necessarily a close interrelation between memory and the problem of learning. The acquisition, retention and reproduction of action patterns may be observed in rudimentary form, as Jennings (1931) and others have pointed out, even in unicellular organisms" (cf. also McGeoch, 1928, 1930). Syz's definition is much more restricted than for instance that of Ziehen (1908, p. 29) who argued for similarities between human and animal memories, but also emphasized that it might be possible to attribute memory to any living matter. As examples he listed trees which are bent by recurring winds, and magnetic fields (the Chladni-sound figures; cf. the respective chapters in Delacour & Levy, 1988, for a modern treatment of memories in physics).

The field of memory and the brain is among the broadest – and not only because memory disorders belong to the most frequent symptoms after various kinds of brain damage or even only after brain concussion (e. g., Friedmann, 1906; Schneider, 1928). Anatomists such as Brodmann (1902, 1904) and Cajal (1895) contributed clinical work or hypotheses to the discussion of memory organization. (Korbinian Brodmann is principally known because of his development of a cytoarchitectonic atlas of the mammalian, including the human cortex, and Santiago Ramón y Cajal drew elegant depictions of neurons and conducted pioneering work in nerve degeneration and regeneration.)

On the psychological level, early approaches were strongly influenced by philosophy. Authors such as Volkmar (1875, 1876), who wrote a two-volume Lehrbuch [textbook] on psychology, quoted from the Greek and Latin, and included a good number of arguments from great philosophers such as Kant. Nevertheless, he had some insights which sound quite modern; for example his partitioning of memory, not only into memory as 'immediate reproduction' and as 'ability to remember', but also into as many kinds of memory as there are ways of imagining: For example, he subdivided verbal memory into memory for melodies, for rhythms, and for Gestalts (Volkmar, 1875, p. 461 ff; reference to a similar partition was later made by Marcus, 1926). Already at this early time there was apparently a vivid discussion of possible ways for improving memory, including memory techniques and mnemonic aids (e. g., Forel, 1885; Meumann, 1912). Again, the views of Greek and Latin authorities (Aristoteles, Cicero, Quintilian) and philosophers were major sources for Volkmar's argumentation (Volkmar, 1875, p. 465 ff) (cf. also Kühn, 1914, Semon, 1904, and Ziehen, 1908).

The fourth edition of Max Offner's book "*Das Gedächtnis*", published in 1924, included a large amount of factual material which had accumulated from experimental psychology during the first two decades of the present century. Subdivided into ten chapters, Offner commented on (1) memory within psychic experience, (2) sensation and imagination, (3) the term "disposition", (4) association, (5) strength of dispositions, (6)reinforcement and effectiveness of dispositions (reproduction), (7) emotions, will, and memory, (8) individual and gender differences in memory, (9) the memory which is independent of age of life, improvement, and the law of disintegration, and (10) on memory and intelligence and the merits of memory and forgetting.

Offner's section on "gender and memory" (pp. 181–183) is most interesting (he had been director of a high school). Starting with the common observation that women talk faster than men, and that the female sex is generally a little faster with learning, but a little less enduring in memorizing, he wrote the following (relying in part on the results of others) (p. 181 f):

Boys and girls differ with respect to the sensory modalities. Boys first have a better memory for words of visual content, then for memory for words of acoustic content, then for that of sounds and tones, numbers and abstract terms, and finally the memory for emotions develops. In girls, memory for words with visual content is best, followed by that for objects, then for sounds, numbers, abstract terms, then for words with acoustic content, then for imagining tactile events and movement, and finally for emotions ("Gemütsbewegungen").

Offner acknowledged that these observations needed further study. He then went on to discuss in detail learning aids and the use of mnemonic strategies.

Aall (1913) some years earlier had compared 15 and 16 year old boys and girls with respect to prose reproduction. He had found that for the first reproduction girls were superior to boys (largely independent of the time gap between presentation and reproduction), while for a second reproduction relations were reversed with boys being superior at an interval of both four and eight weeks.

Early Methods for Memory Assessment

As can be expected, around the year 1900 mnemonic assessment of brain damaged subjects was quite divergent and largely done by members of the medical profession. Standard psychological tests were non-existent, though, for example, Brodmann (1902, 1904), Gregor (1907, 1909; Gregor & Roemer, 1906), Jaspers (1910) and others used quite sophisticated and time-consuming test procedures. However, it was prevalent to rely on one's own inventions for memory assessment. One example is Strümpell's (1897) approach to test verbal memory. He just asked his patient personal data about his job, all four-legged animals he knew, the names of trees and birds he knew, or he told him to repeat sentences or names of cities (p. 407: "Stuttgart, Ulm, Friedrichshafen, Constanz"), or long words (p. 406: "Lotteriecommissionshausgesellschaft"). Bonhoeffer (1901, p. 125) gave a short description on how to test memory in Korsakoff's psychosis: "Mnemonic ability for the sensory modalities is tested, as is known, by presenting numbers, words, nonsense syllables, pictures, objects, and by repeatedly touching objects with the eyes closed. I have not investigated smell and taste. The older literature does not include anything on the ability of remembering within these sensory territories either."

Francis Galton, a cousin of Charles Darwin, is considered to be the father of modern statistics. In 1879, he published an article, entitled "Psychometric experiments" in the journal *Brain*. Some of his experiments are still referred to in present-day evaluations of old (retrograde) memories (e. g., Crovitz & Schiffman, 1974; Deisinger & Markowitsch, 1991; MacKinnon & Squire, 1989; Markowitsch, 1991 b; Zola-

Morgan, Cohen, & Squire, 1983; cf. Galton, 1883).

In 1888 Emil Kraepelin gave a talk (published in 1889) at the Dorpat Medical Faculty in Estonia in which he addressed effects of training on the duration of associations. He noted that even after $1^3/4$ years many previously acquired associations were reproduced in spite of the subjects' failure to realize that they had learned them – a phenomenon which was recently discussed in priming experiments with amnesics (Shimamura & Squire, 1988). I also wish to mention Talbot's (1897) attempt to train visual memory functions.

Determining the duration of associations was also the main aim of the investigation which Trautscholdt carried out in Wilhelm Wundt's "psychophysical laboratory" in 1880 and which was published in 1882 in the first volume of the "*Philosophische Studien*", edited by Wundt (cf. Meischner & Eschler's, 1979, biography of Wilhelm Wundt). Trautscholdt referred to Francis Galton's (1979) previous experiments and then described his own studies on reaction times, and the time needed to differentiate between words. An illustration of the equipment is given in Figure 23; it consisted mainly of two morse code printers and a chronoscope which was coupled to an electric magnet. Wundt, who was one of the three subjects tested, had the largest reaction times, but showed the fewest symptoms of fatigue. Trautscholdt concluded from these experiments that the shorter the reaction time had been from the beginning, the less it is influenced by training, and that on the other hand the shortest reaction time is influenced most by the process of fatigue (p. 235).

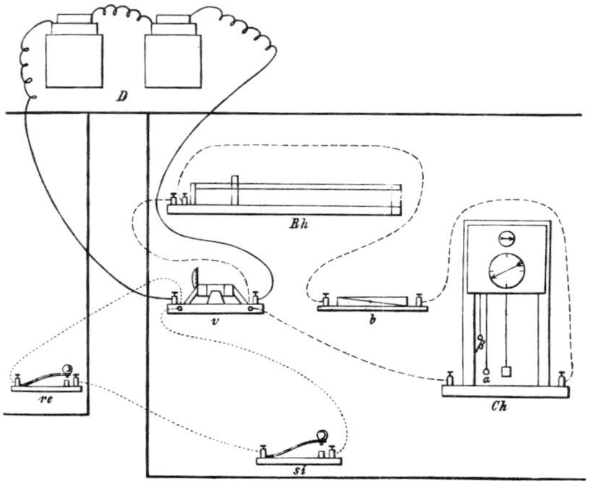

Figure 23. The equipment used by Trautschold (1882) for testing memory.

Korbinian Brodmann (1904) relied on procedures of Ebbinghaus (1885, 1897), G.E. Müller and Schumann (1894), G.E. Müller and Pilzecker (1900), and Steffens (1900). These included principally the acquisition of nonsense syllables, however in what he considered an improved form. He measured the influence of the number of syllables, the number of repetitions, and interval lengths. Comparable experiments were done by Ach (1901), who – similar to Kraepelin in 1882 and 1892 und Kürz and Kraepelin in 1901 – intended to study the effects of drugs (alcohol, bromine, paraldehyde, caffeine) on the acquisition of verbal material. Ach found the usual effects of alcohol on attention and speed of information processing, but concluded that – at least in the field he had investigated – alcohol did not impair memory performance. For caffeine he noted improved comprehension, and greater speed and accuracy in information processing; these effects were particularly evident under conditions of fatigue.

In the early experiments in which alcohol was used, wine and champagne were apparently favorite test substances, as reviewed by Kraepelin (1882). Small quantitites of champagne led to a reduced reaction time, while larger quantities resulted in slowing down. Kraepelin used Wilhelm Wundt's advice to try absolute alcohol, dissolved in water and with raspberry syrup added for taste improvement. His results were, however, not very different from those of the earlier experimenters, including Exner.

Intelligence and Association-psychology

Rieger, a professor of psychiatry at Würzburg, published two papers, in 1889 and in 1890, of altogether 126 pages on the description of intelligence defects after brain damage and included "the plan for a generally applicable method for testing intelligence". In the tradition of that time, he subdivided his plan into tests of (A) perception, (B) apperception, and (C) memory. Memory assessment he subdivided into (I) memory for early reminiscences in general, and (II) memory for fresh impressions. The (II) memory for fresh impressions was tested along the optic, haptic, and olfactory modalities. He refrained from testing memory for taste, on the one hand because he did not want to discomfit his patients too much, and on the other hand, as the so-called aftertaste would not have allowed maintaining pure test conditions. Finally, he tested (D) the ability to immediately initiate an activity, (E) the expression of intellectual actions which depend purely on inner associations ("speech expression"), (F) the ability for identifying recognition ("identificirendes Erkennen"), and (G) the ability to transform sensory impressions into verbal terms.

At the turn of the century, the use of associations to investigate memory increased markedly (Bleuler, 1905; Burnham, 1903; Diehl, 1902; Ephrussi, 1904; Heilbronner, 1904/05; Höffding, 1889, 1890; Isserlin, 1905; Jost, 1897; C. G. Jung, 1905 a, 1905 b, 1905 c, 1905 d; C. G. Jung & Riklin, 1904; Kraemer, 1912; Lipmann, 1911; Münsterberg, 1900; Netschajeff, 1902; Ranschburg, 1905, 1911; Reuther, 1905; Schneider, 1912; Talbot, 1897; Wahle, 1885; Wehrlin, 1904, 1905; Wreschner, 1900; Wundt, 1888; Ziehen, 1908; cf. the review of Stertz, 1928) . Quite exact time measurements were made and sophisticated apparatus for doing this were constructed (cf. Lipmann, 1908; Ranschburg, 1911). Kraepelin (1892), for instance, found that $^{43}/_{1000}$ seconds pass between starting to pronounce a word and the appearance of a measurable tone.

Aschaffenburg (1895) developed 15 different categories of possible associations (see his Table XIV); he also designed standard recording sheets (p. 298 f). Four years later Aschaffenburg (1899) described changes in the formation of associations under the influence of exhaustion (testing after a night without sleep and eating). Lottie Steffens (1900) trained verses of poems in English in different manners in order to develop conditions for economic learning. The persons tested included her sister Laura, E. G. Müller and A. Pilzecker (known up to today in experimental psychology for their work on retroactive and proactive interference: G. E. Müller & Pilzecker, 1900), and apparently a brother of Pilzecker.

A Swiss scientist – a university teacher with degrees in medicine and philosophy – wrote a long article "on associations in a case of idiocy" (Wreschner, 1900). The woman was 21 years old and showed some bodily abnormalities. What was striking in her memory abilities was the mechanical way of reproduction: She reproduced simple multiplication mechanically, knew "the main facts from the Bible", and was able to write. Wreschner emphasized the mechanical, automatic, or drilled way of reproductions. He used 46 adjectives which "represented nearly all areas of psychic life" (p. 244), allowing him to "investigate the influence of idiocy on the different steps of human intellect" (p. 245). The words used were related to concrete associations within the fields of all modalities, but also to such abstract ideas as consciousness and will. His main finding was that fixation on certain associations might be indicative of mental deterioration.

Comprehension, learning and retention were investigated by Finzi (1901). The selection of his 12 subjects is remarkable, the three females were described as "educated", seven of the nine men had an M.D.-degree, one a Ph.D., and one was a medical student. They were from Italy (1), Germany (4), the Netherlands (3), Belgium (1), North America (1), Norway (1), and Finland (1). Similarly Schneider (1901) tested comprehension and memory abilities in senile dementics. His investigation was based on Finzi's work.

At about the same time, the Russian psychiatrist Alexander Bernstein (1903) tested the ability to memorize in psychiatric patients, using two-dimensional pictures of geometrical figures. Recognition and reproduction were systematically studied by Eleanor Gamble and Mary Calkins (1903), using a large number of divergent odors.

Mention should also be made of the substantial contribution of Schneider (1912) on "clinical-psychological methods of investigation and their results". Schneider first broadly reviewed the available techniques and stated that at that time puzzles and related games were already in use (p.559; he wrote: "The presently again modern American 'puzzle game' also belongs in this list") (cf. the recent application of puzzles in procedural memory testing in amnesics: Grafman et al., 1990; Markowitsch, von Cramon, & Schuri, subm.).

He then applied his test battery, consisting of pictorial material (which had to be interpreted or in which details had to be identified), puzzles, and verbal learning tests, to 25 healthy subjects (mainly hospital staff) and to a large number of psychiatric and neurological patients (cases with multiple sclerosis, chorea Huntington, epilepsy, "hysteria", "psychopathy", obsessive-compulsive disorders, paranoia, progressive paralysis, senile dementia, and depression). He especially emphasized his repeated testing of three Korsakoff's patients. While Schneider emphasized the poor behavior of Korsakoff's patients which was worse for reading of words and for the omission of learned material than in patients with depression, schizophrenia ["dementia praecox"], and paralysis; his results on Korsakoff's cannot be generalized as the (only) three cases he had tested were quite special in their appearance.

Schneider himself was not quite satisfied with his test battery. He concluded his article with the words that "we have to acknowledge that our methods do not allow an exact determination of psychic disturbances in a satisfactory manner" (p.615).

Remembrance and Forgetting

Prominent psychoanalysts such as Sigmund Freud (1898, 1899, 1901a, 1901b) and C.G. Jung (1905a, 1905b, 1905c, 1905d; C.G. Jung & Riklin, 1904) published on remembrance and forgetting. They emphasized that especially the most important things (the repressed, aversive complex) are forgotten. Figure 24 gives an example on how Freud (1901) related word associations and how he included his main themes of death and sexuality in such a framework (cf. Sears, 1936, for a summary of work up to that time, written in English). C.G. Jung (1905a) furthermore pointed to the role of "systematic" forgetting which might provoke the development of the Ganser syndrome (cf. the section on "Psychogenic Amnesias").

The ability to memorize was analyzed, and discussed critically (e.g., Pick, 1905b) from psychological and neurological viewpoints as well. Diehl (1902) used numbers, colors, simple figures, and angles as stimuli and stressed the existence of individual differences. A lengthy textbook on "psychopathological methods of research" was written in 1899 by R. Sommer, including advice on how to study reflexes and direct expressions of affect. Furthermore, he gave instructions on the measurement and analysis of perception, orientation, memory, and calculation abilities. Boldt (1905) made three acoustic and four visual experiments on the ability to memorize: acoustic word memory (paired associate learning), picture memory (recognition of 5 out of 25 portraits), color memory, orientation, nonsense-words, memory for names (portraits with first and last names given), digit span. He used 35 patients as subjects, largely dementics, but also one case each with Korsakoff's psychosis and an hysterical psychosis. Boldt emphasized that

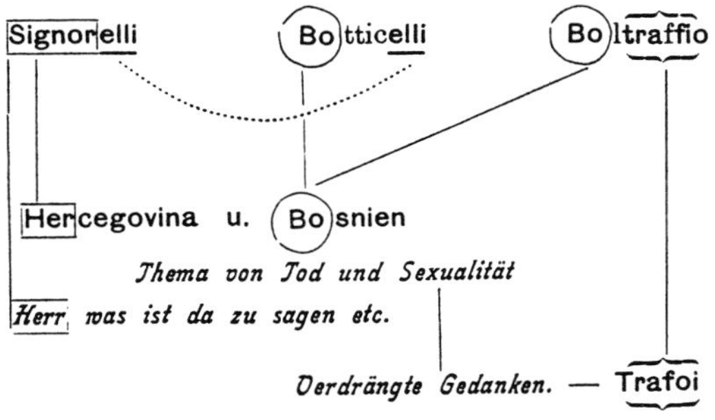

Figure 24. Scheme of relations between associated words and their possible underlying meaning. "Thema von Tod und Sexualität" = theme of death and sexuality; "Herr was ist da zu sagen" = Sir, what can be said here"; "Verdrängte Gedanken" = repressed thoughts. (Reproduced from the figure given on page 440 of Freud, 1901a.)

especially patients with Korsakoff's psychosis (he had data from additional Korsakoff subjects on record) manifested severe memory defects and retrograde amnesia. (However, one Korsakoff patient, a medical student, recovered completely.)

He gave vivid descriptions of special abilities or disabilities of patients with particular professional backgrounds: A female wool-ware trader with senile dementia had kept an extraordinary memory for colors, because – as she explained herself – she had dealt with wool colors life-long. An architect had kept special abilities for orientation. On the other hand, one patient, belonging to "the species of head waiters" ("zur Spezies der Oberkellner gehörig"; p. 108), had severe problems in name, person, and digit memories; however, he still had a good remembrance (or retrograde memory) of the regular guests (who were known to both the patient and the examiner "from his Berlin study period"; p. 109). Boldt's investigation is of interest, as he used tasks which in part are still considered to be useful in examining the patient's (everyday) memory (e.g., B.A. Wilson, Cockburn, & Baddeley, 1985; B.A. Wilson, Cockburn, Baddeley, & Hiorns, 1989), and as at that early time he already emphasized the selectivity of mnestic disturbances, their interindividual variability, and the existence of relations to premorbid preferences and specially trained abilities. A very detailed examination of the memory for figures in "paralytic" patients was written by Peters (1912) and Prager in the same year described in great detail the ability to memorize from a number of perspectives in patients with severe brain illnesses.

How acoustic-motoric and visual memories interact, was investigated by Cohn (1897) who used ten subjects, five with a doctoral degree and from the other five only one was female. He found that visual memory usually substituted when the acoustic-motoric one was disturbed. In 1894 Kirkpatrick already tested verbal memory by using 180 pupils from normal schools.

Kurt Goldstein (1906 b), who later became famous for his investigations and views on the organization of the brain in information processing, studied the ability to remember and the formation of associations. He used words, pictures, numbers, colors, and objects which had to be remembered, and tested memory for the alphabet, the months, days of the week, digits forward and backward, simple and compound multiplication, geographical and historical knowledge, the remembrance of prayers and other items.

Breukink (1907), a psychiatrist from Utrecht, described in detail his way of assessing memory (p. 115 ff). Memory for (I) earlier reminiscences in general was tested quite similar to the way it is done in present-day semi-structural autobiographical memory tests (e.g., Borrini, Dall'Ora, Della Sala, Marinelli, & Spinnler, 1989; Kapur, 1989; Kopelman, 1989; cf. also Potwins's, 1901, early analysis of childhood memories). Memory for (II) fresh impressions was subdivided into (a) optic impressions, (b) acoustic impressions, (c) passive movements, and (d) pain sensations. Than he tested (III) the "ability for immediate imitation", and (IV) "intellectual processes" .

At pretty much the same time Pappenheim (1907, 1908 a, 1908 b), working at the German Psychiatric Clinic in Prague, used quite a different way of assessing memory, namely what he termed "Assoziationsversuche". These were of the sort "What does the cat catch? – mice" or "bells – ring", "pencil – writing". Pappenheim also used meaningless syllables (after Ebbinghaus', 1885, suggestions and those of G.E. Müller and Schumann, 1894, which were presented in the trochaic rhythm), normal words, poems, numbers and names, prose texts, tests of optic memorizing, recognition, and intelligence. In fact, from the citations given in Pappenheim (1908) alone, it becomes evident that after the turn of the century experimental psychology was quite engaged and active in inventing and applying mnemonic tests (e.g., Aall, 1913; Bleuler, 1905; C.E. Browne, 1906; Ebert & Meumann, 1905; Gregor, 1909; Kogerer, 1920/21; Lipmann, 1903, 1904; G.E. Müller & Pilzecker, 1900; G.E. Müller & Schumann, 1894; Netschajeff, 1900, 1902; Ranschburg, 1901 b, 1905, 1911; Steffens, 1900; E. Stern, 1917; Stransky, 1905 a, 1905 b; 1905 c; Wehrlin, 1904, 1905).

Albert Gregor's Contribution

This engagement was found not only for investigating memory in unimpaired subjects, but also for testing the mnemonic abilities of Korsakoff patients (Brodmann, 1902, 1904; Gregor, 1907), senile dementics, depressives and schizophrenics (Gregor, 1909; Ranschburg, 1901 b, 1911). Adalbert Gregor, who worked in Flechsig's psychiatric-neurological clinic (cf. Busse, 1989) in Leipzig, explicitly stated that he intended to differentiate on the basis of applied tests between the stages of encoding and storage or retrieval. His subjects even had to learn poems and were retested between ten and 120 days after initial learning. Gregor's special interest lay in finding whether massed or distributed practice – or, as he formulated it – learning in toto and learning in parts, led to a better remembrance. He found that learning meaningless syllables profited better from more narrow spacing between learning sessions. For meaningless and meaningful words and stanzas spaced learning led to superior results compared to massed learning periods (cf. also Kühn, 1914; Lewin, 1922 a, 1922 b).

With respect to Korsakoff's patients, Gregor found that they were able to acquire new associations, especially under conditions where they could carefully pay attention to all impressions and were given the possibility to repeat them frequently. Daily events of relevance to the patients which they could observe repeatedly on their own free will had the highest likeliness of being remembered. Gregor (1907) estimated that about 8-10% of the normal every-day events met these conditions.

Gregor (1907) was apparently among the first scientists who tested experimentally something that the earliest students of Korsakoff's syndrome had observed repeatedly, namely that emotionally significant events have a higher probability of being remembered than more neutral ones (e.g., Bonhoeffer, 1901; Korsakow, 1890; cf. also Ziehen, 1908, p. 14). According to K. Gordon (1905), who was cited by Gregor (1907), the differential memorizing of more vs. less affective material is not found in normal subjects. Gregor furthermore argued that the strongly impaired time sense and ability to estimate time epochs hindered Korsakoff's subjects in acquiring information in a way similar to normals.

Attempts at Quantification

At Gregor's time it was already common to use lists of words and digits (cf. also Meumann, 1912; Ogden, 1903, 1904). Gregor furthermore pointed out that he quantified the remembrance of learned material on the basis of savings, and investigated the effects of temporal spacing on repeatedly presented material, of primacy and recency effects, and different error categories in the reproduction of learned material (e.g., semantic or phonemic errors). It was also common at that time to standardize the exposure time of material presented (words or pictures) by using apparatuses such as a "memory drum" (cf. Gregor, 1909, p. 226, and Figs. 1 and 2 in Ranschburg, 1901 a; Ebbinghaus, 1902, 1905; Wirth, 1902), or by providing detailed instructions (e.g., Pintner, 1915). The construction of learning curves was also common (Ogden, 1903, 1904) (Fig. 25).

Ranschburg (1901 b) wanted to determine the extent of memory and the certainty of mnemonic knowledge. He defined certainty as the percentage of incorrect remembrances, that is, of events when items were incorrectly recognized or reproduced, but the appropriate correction was given immediately after presentation. He used 50 items which were subdivided into seven groups: memory for words (2 groups; acoustic memory), persons, colors, names, numbers, and orientation memory. Twelve pupils of about 12 years of age were involved, 12 so-called non-educated adults (ward keepers at the psychiatric clinic), 13 adults with higher education and 12 so-called neurasthenic and 21 so-called paralytic patients. Ranschburg found that education enhanced the extent of memory but had an ambiguous influence on the certainty with which information was given. In his study, age had a positive influence on memory, especially for pair-associated and name memory. The patients were inferior throughout, but especially for words and word-pairs. Lastly, Ranschburg pointed out that the persons' oc-

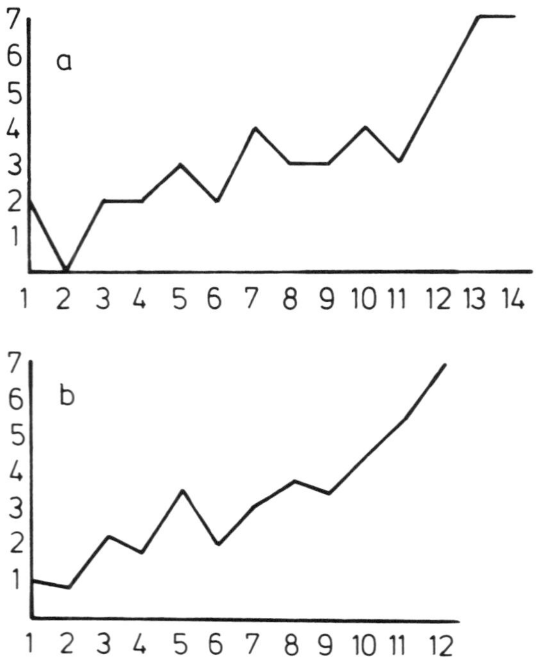

Figure 25. (a) Rate of word reproduction in 14 successive sessions in a patients with "progressive paralysis" (after Fig. 1 of Gregor, 1909); (b) Learning-to-learn phenomenon in a "progressive paralytic" patient. Gregor (1909) had trained the patient to learn 4 blocks of 7 digits in each of 12 sessions and then constructed this averaged curve, stating that the patient had improved over time from repeated testing (after Fig.3 of Gregor, 1909).

cupation was related to mnemonic abilities. Special memories were directly related to the job position: for example, waiters, teachers, or stock-brokers had retained special mnemonic abilities for numbers. In the following years, Ranschburg refined his assessment techniques and documented them in two extensive publications (Ranschburg, 1911, 1930; cf. below).

How far the memory deterioration in so-called paralytic states can go, was exemplified by G. Fischer (1904 a, 1904 b) with two case reports. The first, a 56-year-old physician, had extensive anterograde amnesia. When admitted to the clinic, he explained four times in half an hour that he suffered from extensive memory weakness and had had an infection (lues) in 1850. The second case, a 46-year-old merchant with good retrograde memory and apparently preserved memory for spatial relations and calculation, had at least moderate anterograde amnesia. During his stay in the clinic, his memory progressively deteriorated over a time of about seven months. He was discharged seven months after hospital admission and died after another five months after epileptic attacks.

An early review of techniques used for memory assessment stems from Lipmann (1903), and in 1911 and 1916 Ziehen and Terman published books on the measurement of intelligence. Ranschburg (1911, 1930) described results and methods of memory assessment in great detail. The development of memory was studied by Brunswik (1932). At the time border set for this book, in 1939, Rylander used a number of quite specific and original memory tests to investigate the consequences of prefrontal surgery. In order to study "reception, memorization and retention" (p. 61), he used series of digits, syllables and of figures, story repetitions, and paired-associate learning. Furthermore 60 nouns had to be named in three minutes, arithmetical tasks (such as 9 times 12 or 8 times 17), problems such as "If 4 apples cost 7 cents, what would 3 dozen cost?", geometrical forms, a picture story in color (from the "Münchener Bilderbogen"), 15 objects (pencil, fish knife, ashtray, book, etc.), distinctions between abstract words (e. g., "mistake – lie", "evolution – revolution"), proverbs and fables, comparison of nonsense figures, and a calculation test with interference, among others (cf. also Heine, 1914). These tests were in part taken or modified from other publications, but in part apparently created by the author. Isserlin's (1923) paper was more in Ebbinghaus' tradition, but already included tachistoscopic experiments on reading letters. Famous up to the present is the so-called Stroop test, originally created by Stroop (1935) as a measure of interference, but presently used as an index of aphasia.

Another careful set of experiments to test memory abilities was presented by Herta Seidemann (1926). For figural memory she used for example Bernstein's test, a multiple choice method which required from the patient

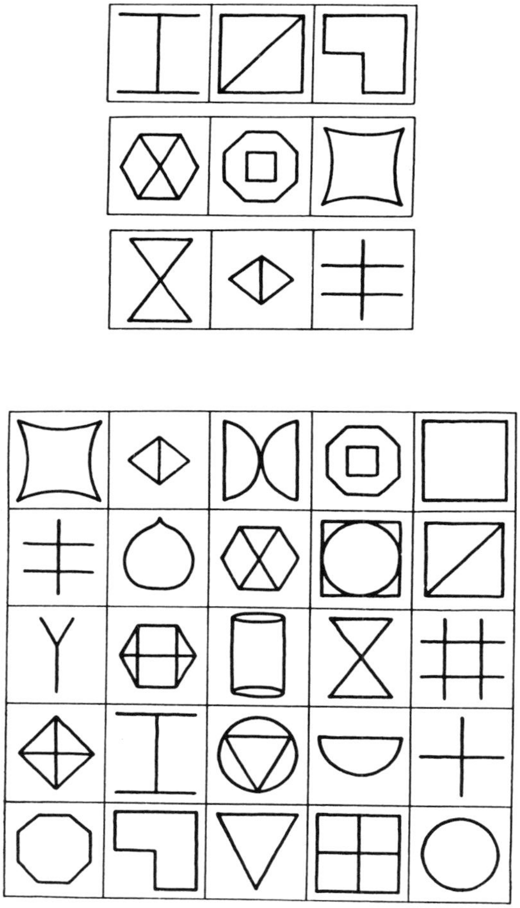

Figure 26. The geometric figures used as stimuli for learning (top) and for recognition (bottom) in Bernstein's (1903) and Seidemann's (1926) test batteries (after Figs. 1 and 2 of Seidemann, and Figs. 2 and 3 of Bernstein).

to reidentify nine out of 25 previously seen geometrical figures (Fig. 26). Bernstein (1903) had given the following performance measure (p. 261): if n being the number of presented figures, r that of correctly identified figures, f that of false responses, then performance should follow the formula $r/n+f$. At least two of the figures should be selected so similar, that they easily could be confounded.

Systematic experiments on particular problems such as card sorting were done in the 1920's (Weigl, 1927a, 1927b). For comparing the development of standardization in memory tests see for example Curran and Schilder (1937), Poppelreuter (1912), Hebb (1939, 1941, 1942, 1945), Nichols and Hunt (1940), or Hanfmann, Rickers-Ovsiankina, and Goldstein (1944). A short review and critique of the older methods for memory assessment was given by Zangwill (1943); he then suggested the use of verbal and performance tests which, when used in combination, might allow differentiation between memory disorders on an organic and on a functional basis.

In his book on "the diseased memory" Ranschburg (1911) first discussed the resemblance of memory research and what he called "pathological mnemology", with the head of Janus – there is anterograde and retrograde amnesia. He then described the kinds of memory loss which are most common in organic brain illnesses, including the memory for proper names. He explained this impairment with the frequently superfluous acquisition of names which are then associated with a number of old, similar sounding names, with the consequence that they are often reproduced only approximately.

He considered factors of attention and inhibition as playing a major role in the memory for names. He then gave a number of examples of memory span and memory duration for visually presented words in various samples of normals, psychotics, and patients with brain damage. In the second part of his book, he then described methods, techniques, and equipment for measuring memory abilities. An example is given in Figure 27.

Just within the historical setting for this book is the very interesting doctoral work of Ruth Clark Conkey (1938), who investigated the psychological changes which accompany head injury over time. For different recovery periods she made a number of psychological tests and quantitative records resulting in recovery curves. Her Figure 1 on page 26 (reproduced here as Fig. 28) demonstrates that there is a steep increase in recovery from weeks 2 to 8, a more flat one from weeks 8 to 20, and again a steeper one up to week 34. Conkey came to a number of remarkable results, including the

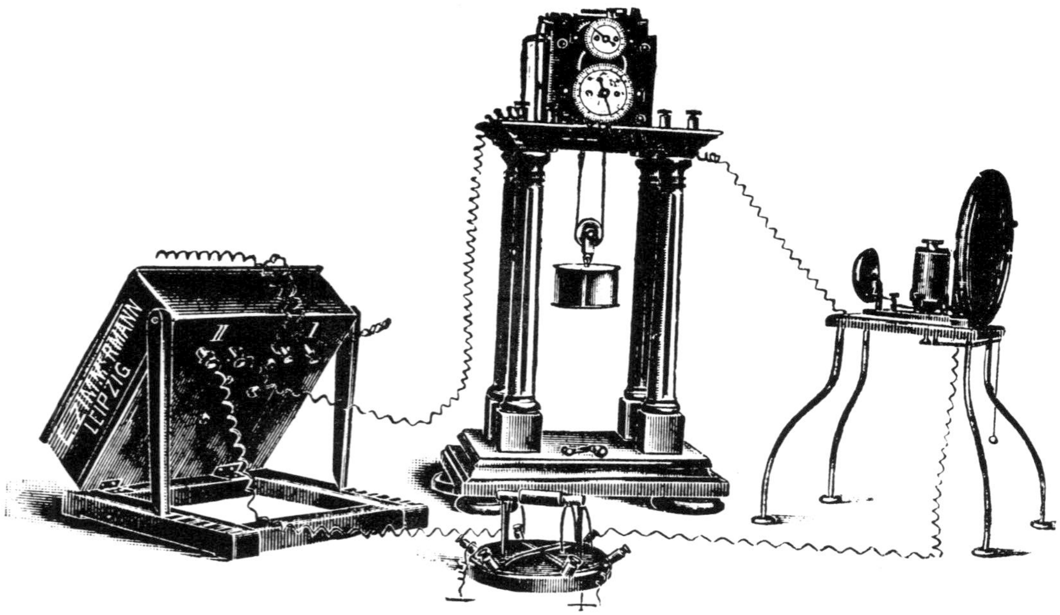

Figure 27. The Ranschburg-mnemometer connected to a Hipp-chronoscope and a Römer-sound measuring device ("Schallschlüssel") for the exact measurement of reproduction times (reproduced from Fig. 4 of Ranschburg, 1911).

ideas that hospitalization played little or no part in performance, that simple mental functions exhibited recovery earlier than more complex functions, that performance involving memory functions lagged behind other behavior, and that "the recovery of psychological processes lagged behind physical recovery and affected the performance of the patient after all apparent physical symptoms had disappeared" (p. 53). Her report also included a considerable number of references to the old literature. (For an early attempt to train visual memory functions see Talbot, 1897, and for an early discussion of possible mechanisms of cerebral recovery Monakow, 1914, and Niessl von Mayendorf, 1922.)

Psychogenic Amnesia

Simulating in general or feigning madness, has always been of special interest, reflected, for instance, in the dramatic literature (e.g., Shakespeare's "Hamlet" [Shakespeare, 1599–1601]; cf. the discussion in Maudsley, 1873) or in the classical psychoanalytic "Studien über Hysterie" of Freud and Breuer (Breuer & Freud, 1895; Freud & Breuer, 1970; cf. also Freud, 1910).

As described in Markowitsch (1990a), hysterical amnesia was apparently diagnosed much more frequently in earlier centuries than today (in part also related to war experiences: e.g., Bauer, 1917), and to a major extent it was only found in members of the female sex (cf., e.g., the case histories of Fräulein Anna O., Frau Emmy v. N., Miss Lucy R., Katharina, and Fräulein Elisabeth v. R., given in Freud & Breuer, 1970). This tradition may be traced back to "La possession de Jeanne Fèry, religieuse professe du convent des soeurs de la ville de Mons 1584", a description of possession in a nun summarized by Gilles de la Tourette in 1886 (cited after Donath, 1908). In the United States, Weir Mitchell (1889) described the existence of a case with some parallels to the medieval nun, namely of an 18-year-old girl who suddenly behaved like a new-born child ("... as being for the first time ushered into the world"). A closely related case was that of a Bavarian woman with a number of ecstatic, religiously motivated states (Hoche, 1933).

A detailed review on possible amnesic states – many of which were psychological in nature – was given by Heine (1911, p. 55 f). He listed

1. epileptic somnolence
2. hysterical somnolence
3. states of unconsciousness and of mnestic activity after traumatic damage of the brain
   a) commotio cerebri
   b) attempt to hang oneself
   c) reanimation after hanging
4. states of somnolence with a relation to physiological sleep
5. hypnotic states
6. migraine-based somnolence
7. affect-based somnolence
8. toxic somnolence, or disturbance of mind
   a) complicated states after intoxication
   b) disease of the mind after CO-inhalation
9. vasomotoric states of somnolence
   a) congestive (transitory mania)
   b) angiospastic (raptus melancholicus)
10. transitory disturbances of mind after infectious diseases
11. paralytic attacks
12. retrograde amnesia without previous disturbances of consciousness
13. Korsakoff's psychosis.

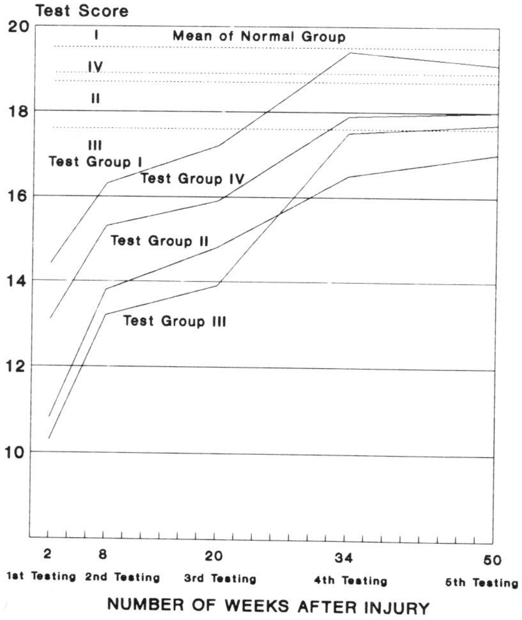

Figure 28. Recovery curves for the head-injury patients in the four test groups (Conkey, 1932).

There are numerous forms of psychogenic amnesic states and numerous attempts to test and therapy them (cf. e.g., Markowitsch, 1990 c). Of special interest are old studies in which these twilight states were manipulated experimentally (e.g., Bechterew, 1907; Brodmann, 1897; Kandinsky, 1885; Köhler, 1897; Prince, 1908 a; cf. also Jahrreis, 1928 a, Leavitt, 1932, Lundholm, 1932, and Sears, 1936).

A review on "sense and non-sense of the psychic-unconsciousness" was given at the time border of this book by Jancke (1953). He summarized his findings in the following sentences (p. 513): "One should not speak of a physiologically based unconscious, but of the background of consciousness. Illusions of motive in the healthy and the neurotic are not at all unconscious, but unknown, as one may see something in the absence of a sufficient level of anticipation, without being aware of it."

The Ganser Syndrome

The Ganser syndrome (originally named Ganser symptom; Ganser, 1898/1965, 1904; cf. Anderson & Mallinson, 1941) was a well-known (transient) amnesic state (e.g., Flatau, 1913; Hey, 1904; C.G. Jung, 1902; Lücke, 1903; Matthies, 1908; A. Meyer, 1904; Pick, 1905 b; Raecke, 1908; Stertz, 1910) and is also sometimes diagnosed today as well (e.g., Carney, Charty, Robotis, & Childs, 1987; Cocores, Santa, & Patel, 1984; Feinstein & Hattersley, 1988). According to Ganser (1898, 1904) it consisted of an hysterical semi-trance or twilight state and could be characterized by the tendency to give only approximate reactions, and to deny things under high pressure. Impairments of consciousness, amnesia, and the existence of hallucinations are prominent features.

Fugues

Fugue states (Bregman, 1899; Raecke, 1903, 1908; Schultze, 1903; Stier, 1912; Woltär, 1906) or poriomania (Donath, 1899, 1907; Heilbronner, 1903) were usually thought to be accompanied by amnesia (e.g., Burgl, 1900; Heilbronner, 1903, 1905 a, 1905 b), and were not uncommonly of "forensic relevance" (Zingerle, 1912 b). Fugue states were also preponderant in children and young adults (Bregman, 1899; Dana, 1894; Donath, 1908; Heilbronner, 1903, 1905 a, 1905 b; Hey, 1904). Franz (1933) gave a detailed description of a subject, named Jack, with a multiple personality who ostensibly traveled between Europe, Africa, and the United States and described being captured and held as a prisoner during World War I in East Africa.

Multiple Personalities

Other "dissociative reactions" (Janet, 1894, 1907) included cases with multiple personalities (and, as a defining criterion, amnesia for the respective other personality [state]) (Angell, 1906; Azam, 1876; Bregman, 1899; Burnett, 1925; Donath, 1908; Franz, 1933; A. Gordon, 1906; Pick, 1876; Prince, 1906 a, 1906 b, 1908 a, 1908 b, 1920, 1924; Read, 1923; Sears, 1936; Sidis & Goodhart, 1905; Viner, 1931; A. Wilson, 1903), somnambulism, "fausse reconnaissance", depersonalization, or a state of trance (cf., e.g., Abeles & Schilder, 1935; Gillespie, 1937; Heymans, 1904, 1906; Laughlin, 1956; McKendree & Feinier, 1927; Sears, 1936). A link with epilepsy was frequently assumed to exist (Bechterew, 1900 a; Cowles, 1900; Forel, 1885; A. Gordon, 1906; Kellner, 1898; Mörchen, 1904; cf. also Schilder, 1924).

Already in 1878, A. H. Bennett had published a "case of cerebral tumour-symptoms simulating hysteria" and had questioned the dichotomy between organic and psychic illnesses. He wrote (p. 120): "In conclusion, there appear to me to be at least two points of interest in this case: 1st, the anomalous symptoms of pressure caused by the tumour; and 2nd, that symptoms of what is called hysteria may coexist with organic disease of the brain – whether independent of it or the result, being in this patient doubtful. Under any circumstances it serves to indicate what caution should be exercised in diagnosing, and more especially in treating, as hysteria, any nervous affection in women which may appear indefinite or mysterious." (A case with related symptomatology after brain disease was reported by Savage in the same year and in the same journal.)

A. Gordon (1906) stated that "self-consciousness is a *conditio sine qua non* of normal life" (p. 480) and that amnesia is the most typical of all disturbances of consciousness. In persons with multiple personalities one personality, at least during the first stages of the illness, is unconscious (or totally amnesic) of the other(s). In rare cases, as in the patient K. J. W., described by A. Gordon, two egos might coexist at the same time. The most famous cases in scientific literature – Miss Christine Beauchamp, Reverend Mr. Henna, and Mary Reynolds – were among the earliest and most extensively described multiple personalities (Prince, 1906, 1920; Sidis & Goodhart, 1905; Weir Mitchell, 1889). Schultz (1924) later argued that recovery from amnesia constitutes an "experience of relief" and a "release from inner disorientation" (p. 129). For a recent, quite popular, description of a case with a multiple personality ("Sybil"), see Schreiber (1973).

Mainly based on the poetic works of Annette von Droste-Hülshoff (who lived from 1797 to 1848; cf. Droste-Hülshoff, 1925; Hüffer, 1911), Glaus (1953) gave numerous examples on depersonalization, double gangers, delusions, and related deviations, as they have been described in poetry. A short book on double gangers was written by Menninger-Lerchenthal (1946). Finally, I would like to mention Bechterew's (1898) old case of a man who heard his own thoughts, though this case reflects a different orientation compared to the above-mentioned symptomatologies.

Dana's Case

In 1894, Dana described "a case of amnesia or 'double consciousness'", and mentioned that 10 years earlier he had already collected and published 16 cases with 'double consciousness' or 'periodical amnesia', one of which had been published in 1822 in the *Transactions of the Royal Society of Edinburgh.*

Dana described a 24-year-old "active, intelligent, and healthy ... man" (p. 571). Due to carbon monoxide poisoning by domestic gas, his behavior changed. After being rescued, he was quite disturbed and "did not know who he was or where he was, and ... his conscious memory for everything connected with his past life was gone" (p. 572). His behavioral changes included the use and understanding of only the simplest words. After realizing where he was he "pronounced many of the new words with a German accent" (p. 572), similar to the way his German attendant spoke. He did not know what marriage meant and did not remember (previously) familiar persons though he seemed especially glad to see them. At first he was unable to read, but soon learned to read and write simple sentences. Old musical memories existed and so did habits connected with courtesy.

Interestingly, "in argument he showed considerable dialectic skill and logical power, [but] he evidently could not understand any conceptions at all abstract" (p. 573). "The moon, the stars, the animals, his friends, all were mysteries he impatiently hastered to solve" (p. 574). While at the beginning he did not recognize his parents or sisters, or his fiancee, from the beginning he said that he had always known her and subsequently his thoughts and feelings centered on her.

Exactly three months after his attack, his memory was completely restored. The recovery started during a visit in the evening at his fiancee's; she thought he was in a condition worse than during the previous months, and said "he felt as though one half of his head was prickling and numb, then the whole head, then he felt sleepy and was very quiet. ... At about 11 o'clock he woke up and found his memory restored. ... He knew all his family at once and was plainly just the same man as before. But the three months was an entire blank to him" (p. 575). So he did not know Professor Dana whom he had not seen before the accident.

While such an abrupt and nearly complete memory restoration, the total but time-limited loss of knowledge about his family and friends, and the age of the patient all favor psychogenic amnesia, the carbon monoxide poisoning provides a basis for an organic damage-based explanation. Possibly the poisoning but triggered the release or manifestation of an already existing tendency for psychogenic memory loss. (See Sibelius, 1905, for a detailed and extensive review on the consequences of carbon monoxide poisoning.)

Stevens' Case

A similarly "mixed" case was given by Stevens (1907), who described a woman, aged 44, coming "from a very refined, and intellectual family" (p. 447). At school she had been brilliant in certain subjects, but greatly deficient in others, particularly the exact sciences. She had never taken drugs or alcohol in any form. Her brother sent her to a sanatorium after she manifested "melancholia – painful emotional depression" (p. 448) and after suffering from somatic complaints, "an attack of severe pain in the head, face, and arms, lasting about 48 hours" (p. 448). However, no evidence of neurological abnormalities could be found.

While hospitalized, she had very severe anterograde and retrograde memory problems, was disoriented, and had a strong "feeling of unreality". Stevens described her abnormalities and the subsequent behavioral improvements in the following way: "... there is superimposed a condition of disorientation for time and place, an extreme amnesia for passing events, great disturbance of the time element in memory, fabrications, dreamy delusions, and hallucinations of hearing, ... This amnesia, disorientation, etc., continues for some six or seven weeks, and then rather rapidly disappears, her memory becomes excellent, fabrications cease, orientation becomes perfect, and hallucinations disappear, leaving her in the original state of severe emotional depression ..., and still later, nihilistic delusions" (p. 456).

While Stevens was convinced that "[c]ertainly we had here presented the Korsakoff's syndrome" (p. 458), he admitted having no evidence of the occurrence of a definite neuritic process, but I would rather see in this case a neurotic patient with major features of psychogenic amnesia.

Psychogenic memory loss is a fascinating subject (cf., e.g., Heine, 1911; Markowitsch, 1988d, 1988e, 1990b; Parwatikar, 1990; Schacter, 1986; Teahan, 1987), especially as we do not know any possible neuroanatomical and/or neurochemical or neurophysiological correlate of this altered state of consciousness. The memory dimensions affected in psychogenic amnesia differ considerably from those of amnesias with a known or likely organic basis (cf. Cramon & Markowitsch, 1992; Markowitsch, 1988a, 1988b, 1990b, 1990c; Markowitsch & Pritzel, 1985; Mayes, 1988; Squire, 1987).

Localization of Mnemonic Abilities

Emphasizing the Cerebral Cortex

As discussed in the chapter on the frontal lobes, the localization of intellectual functions and thus mnemonic abilities was vehemently discussed throughout the last century, but also during the first half of this century (cf., e.g., Bernhardt, 1874; Charcot, 1878; de Crinis, 1934; Exner, 1881; Ferrier, 1878b; Guder, 1886; Henschen, 1890-1908; Hitzig, 1901b, 1903c; Janzen, 1948; Jefferson, 1937; Kleist, 1934, 1936; Klingler, 1967; Kornmüller, 1937; J. Lange, 1937; Liepmann, 1913; Monakow, 1909, 1914; Solly, 1836; O. Vogt, 1951; A. Walker, 1834). Meynert (1884), borrowing from Munk, remarked: "Intelligence is not localized, its center is the whole cortex" (p. 137). With respect to memory ("Gedächtnis") he stated on the same page that no authors were looking for a special seat for memory anymore and he himself considered memory to be a general ability of the cortical neuron and fiber. Ziehen (1908, p. 27) argued that special fields of remembrance exist in the cerebral cortex.

Still interesting is the obvious fact that all authors adhered to the view that the cortex was the principal "memory structure", – while ignoring subcortical tissue such as the mammillary bodies of the medial thalamus, which only somewhat later attracted attention, at least for the passage of memories as in "diencephalic amnesia". (Cf. also the later discussion of Ewald, 1940, who emphasized that the mammillary bodies constituted the center of a memory system.)

The preference given to the cortex was most likely related to the dominance of psychiatry over neurology at those times and the prevalence of dementia as a diagnosis (Felmann, 1864; cited in Ribot, 1882). An example is Alzheimer's (1904a) paper on the anatomical bases of idiocy. "Dementia praecox, paralytic, epileptic, alcoholic dementia, states of weakness after certain other forms of mental illness" (Alzheimer, 1904a, p. 497) were the dominant clinical diagnoses – so-called secondary dementias. Seven years earlier, in 1897, Alzheimer published a manuscript which dealt principally with relations between amnesia and epilepsy. In this report he stated that he had no hint as to where in the cerebrum retrograde amnesia was localizable.

Aside from epilepsy (W. Sommer, 1880), common causes for dementic processes were seen in infections (syphilis: Köppen, 1896; Pick, 1893), various forms of encephalitis (Friedmann, 1890; Popoff, 1875; Rosenthal, 1881; Spatz, 1930; 1934; Stockert, 1932), and intoxications (e.g., Binswanger & Berger, 1901; Környey, 1931; Kraepelin, 1886b; Meggendorfer, 1928; Wechsler, 1933; Wernicke, 1881). Prevalent diagnoses were those of "progressive paralysis" (e.g., Gowers, 1878a; Gregor, 1909) or senile dementia (e.g., Freund, 1889a; Pick, 1906; Probst, 1903; A. Stern, 1914; Wernicke, 1881; cf. also Grünthal, 1930). But relations between multiple sclerosis and dementia were also traced quite early (Jolly, 1872; Raecke, 1906; Seiffer, 1905) and Meggendorfer (1923) thoroughly described mnestic disturbances in patients with Huntington's chorea.

Some of the best works on the localization of functions in the cerebral cortex stem from Goldstein (1927), Kleist (1934 a, 1934 b), and Monakow (1910 b, 1914). J. Lange (1938) commented on the consequences of extirpating total lobi or even hemispheres.

Semon (1920), who stated that his views generally were in close congruence with those of Monakow (1914), was of the opinion that engrams certainly are not laid down in accordance with cyto- or myeloarchitectonic maps of the brain. Nevertheless, he assumed that the storage of engrams would occur in the chromatic substance of the neuronal nuclei (p. 157).

Amnesia

A general weakness of the research done on memory disorders at that time is the lack of association between the observed psychological defects and their possible underlying brain pathology. The "amnesic symptoms' complex" was a favored term (e. g., A. Stern, 1914). As an example, in 1930 Bürger-Prinz and Kaila grouped four different cases with quite diverse etiologies all under the amnesic symptom's complex: one with carbon monoxide poisoning, one with arteriosclerosis, one with a skull fracture, and one with strangulation (cf. also Bürger, 1927).

While the authors acknowledged that not each case manifested all the same disturbances in full clarity, they stated that all demonstrated the identical basic elements. In spite of this, distinct, modality-specific amnesic disturbances had already been described in the last century. Bleuler (1893), for instance, provided a case with left insular degeneration, gray and white matter damage in the surrounding central gyri, and amnesic color blindness. And in the first decade of this century Goldstein (1906 a) described amnesic aphasia and Burr (1907) tactile amnesia. In addition the phenomenon of retrograde amnesia, which usually occurs in combination with anterograde amnesia (Markowitsch, 1984; Markowitsch & Pritzel, 1985; Ray, 1937; Russell & Nathan, 1946), was seen as a separate entity at the turn of the century (Konrád, 1907; M. Paul, 1899). And it should also be pointed out that Ziehen in 1908 already concluded that "only brain pathology has shown us that a general memory does not exist at all, but only subdivisions of memory or partial memories" ("Teilgedächtniss", p. 16, "Partialgedächtnisse", p. 17).

Retrograde Amnesia

While at that time retrograde amnesia was frequently related to hysterical amnesia (cf. Markowitsch, 1990 a, 1990 b), M. Paul (1899) also gave examples of cases with chronic alcohol, carbon monoxide intoxication, or with an amnesic status after hanging or after epileptic attacks which he had found, especially in the French literature between 1881 and 1898. He concluded that patients who had been saved from strangulation especially allowed a rather precise determination of the duration of retrograde amnesia and also of the effects of time-dependent improvements. He concluded that "the degree or extent of amnesia is to a certain degree proportional to the duration of coma" (p. 264).

The examples of retrograde amnesia mentioned by M. Paul, principally refer to episodes lasting at most hours or days (e. g., Lührmann, 1896). He did not discuss for instance Freund's (1889 a) case of a 52-year old woman who had had gross memory impairments for the last 20 years of her life.

Retrograde amnesia was sometimes investigated quite specifically and thoroughly (e. g., Burnham, 1903; Friedlaender, 1919/20; Konrád, 1907; Krafft-Ebing, 1898). Boedeker (1905) described the interesting case of an "ordentlicher Universitätsprofessor", 54 years of age, who developed Wernicke's encephalopathy (Wernicke, 1881). This case shows that remembrance frequently follows associations according to their sounds; the patient, for instance, answered that he lived in the "Fischborn" hospital, although in fact he lived in the "Fichtenhof". After three weeks of hospitalization there nearly was a complete recovery and after several further weeks he was giving lectures again.

Boedeker's second case was a "true chronic Korsakoff" (p. 314). When asked the same question as the patient mentioned above, he answered "Fichtenhöhe"; he also concluded that he could not be ill: "When you have appetite, you can't be ill, I say to myself, logically" (p. 316). However, some days later he repeatedly said that he had memory problems, especially with respect to the immediate past. While he remembered specific dates from history correctly (1648, 1756-1763, about 800), he thought that his two brothers had visited him in the hospital, though both had recently died. He attributed his memory problems to frequent masturbation in his youth ("... dass ich früher manustuprierte. Die Folgen bleiben ja nie aus."). He was quick and accurate with calculations (12 x 13, 220-21) and accurate with estimating numbers and in reporting four-figure numbers over time. But the discrepancy was striking between his ability to memorize "5679, 1235" over days and his inability to remember the deaths of several relatives and the fact that his daughter was 21, and not 7 years, as he estimated.

The stereotyped handling of numbers and dates, combined with the lack of confabulation, is an apparently specific feature of patients with distinct (episodic) amnesia. Bonhoeffer particularly remarked on the difficulty in examining retrograde amnesia. For his (second) patient he had been able to show that he had accurate recall for his childhood and military service up to the time of his marriage, but then he lost the time scale – for his daughter he consistently gave 7–9 years as her present age, that is, his retrograde amnesia had a duration of about 15 years.

Krafft-Ebing (1898) gave an early review of different forms of retrograde amnesia ("general", "localized", "retrograde destructive", "psychological", "organic"), and concluded that, in total retrograde amnesia the whole earlier performance as well as the consciousness for the personality were destroyed. He listed a number of earlier cases from the time period between 1880 and 1890, many of which had psychic (or in the terminology of that time "hysterical") origins and this is also reflected in Krafft-Ebing's conclusion that "general (hysterical) amnesia" (p. 224) usually diminished while the so-called commotio-caused psychosis could result in dementia (cf. also A. Gordon, 1927).

Bechterew (1900 b), who like many of the old neuroscientists, is known today for work done on the anatomical, physiological, and clinical levels, described the case of a patient who had a stroke and then periodically became amnesic, but never for more than 24 hours. Usually, the attacks followed hard, longlasting mental work. No specific cause could be made out.

Burnham at the turn of the century seems to have been the American specialist for memory and memory problems (cf. Burnham, 1889 a, 1889 b, 1889 c, 1889d); in 1903 he made an analysis of retrograde amnesia. His main thoughts were the following (p. 132):

a) In normal memory a process of organization is continually going on – a physical process of organization and a psychological process of repetition and association. In order for ideas to become a part of permanent memory, time must elapse for these processes of organization to be completed.
b) In cases of retrograde amnesia, the amnesia results from arrest of these processes of organization by shock or other causes. Memory is lost because it was never completely organized.
c) In normal memory these processes of organization are essential in order to fix impressions, and anything that interferes with them, fatigue, being in a hurry, distraction or excitement, hinders acquisition.

Burnham (1903), as well as others (Freud, 1899; Matthies, 1908; Naef, 1897; Read, 1923; Thyssen, 1988) discussed at length hysterical amnesic states and related amnesic conditions such as posteclamsic amnesia (Aschner, 1914; Heilbronner, 1905 c). Naef (1897) gave a very detailed case report of a 32-year-old well-educated man who at that time had already traveled all over the world, including the United States of America and Australia. Of interest is also Jung's (1905e) work on cryptomnesia which can also be found in his monograph on "psychiatric studies" (Jung, 1966). The book included occult phenomena, hysteria, cases simulating mnestic disturbances, and cryptomnesia (pp. 103–115). Cryptomnesia is a negative delusion of remembrance: facts (obtained from others) lose their mnestic associations and are, if recalled again, considered to be one's own thoughts.

Jung defined cryptomnesia as "hidden memories" (p. 110); he stated that most likely "no single, tiny impression is lost from memory, though consciousness works with innumerable losses of previous events" (p. 112). His further discussion of this matter included examples of a dying man who started to recite in Greek, and of an hysterical young woman who in an ecstatic state was able to cite a two-page long poem which she had just seen shortly before. All this resembles what we would presently subsume under priming, though the circumstances were indeed exceptional. A further case was given by Zahn (1903) about a 33-year-old epileptic with highly unusual memory abilities during his attacks.

Another example for retrograde amnesia with a psychic touch was given by Kohnstamm (1917) on a former soldier who had been buried alive, but had no somatic complaints. The patient's short-term memory was normal; however, he did not remember dates from history or geography, which he had learned at school. His musical repertoire, however, was still fully existent; while he was not aware of the musical titles, he was able to play them accurately. Similarly, he recognized his closest relatives, but not more distant friends, though he still was aware of the fact that he had known them. (A case with a closely related history and quite similar symptoms was given by Müller-Suur, 1949.)

Kohnstamm (p. 375) concluded that the "quality of familiarity" had survived in the patient (cf. also Claparede, 1911; Markowitsch, Kessler, Bast-Kessler, & Riess, 1984; Markowitsch, Kessler, & Denzler, 1986; Müller-Freienfels, 1915; Pick, 1903 b; Titchener, 1895 b). The patient, however, had a severe anterograde amnesia as well (but no trace of confabulation). Kohnstamm emphasized that the patient's remembering was greatly influenced (i.e., facilitated) by emotional stimuli and when he was interested and engaged in a topic (p. 378). He remarked that this observation might be used pedagogically and for memory training. Here again, as in other studies of this time, similarities are apparent to the presently discussed division of memory into episodic, semantic, and nondeclarative memories. When Kohnstamm stated that "knowledge of language, calculation, and requirements for daily living" (p. 380) were preserved, one is reminded of preserved semantic and procedural memory, and of grossly impaired episodic memory.

In more recent times, retrograde amnesia was found to accompany electroconvulsive therapy (e.g., Häfner, 1951), a phenomenon which in the last years was studied more extensively by Squire and coworkers (Squire, 1981; Squire, Cohen, & Zouzounis, 1984; Squire, Slater, & Chase, 1975; Taylor, Tomphins, Demers, & Anderson, 1982; Weiner, 1984) and others (e.g., Ringo & Guttmacher, 1988). Häfner gave a summary of the findings available until the beginning of the 1950's and included two cases of his own. Both of them showed quite severe retrograde amnesias; for the second patient these dated back for 32 years, three days after electroconvulsive thereapy (probably at least in part due to high dosages of shock and of drugs used). The patient then recovered, but had no knowledge of the last two to three decades with the consequence that he also had no memory of his psychosis. He died before a follow-up could be made. From summarizing and evaluating the results from a large number of cases treated with electroconvulsive therapy, Häfner concluded that more or less prominent symptoms of retrograde amnesia remained for nearly all cases even two years after the end of therapy.

Hanging

Unsuccessful attempts at hanging usually result in retrograde amnesia. This was described already by Boediker in 1986. Two of the first detailed reports of such cases were given by J. Wagner (1889, 1891) in southeastern Austria.

In his article from 1889 he referred to already 17 previous cases which had been described in the years between 1826 and 1887. Wagner (1891) also mentioned Leidesdorf (1865), who had given examples on hanging-related cases. Leidesdorf for example wrote (p. 123): "The rope which the Sibirian Shaman allows to be laid around his throat, until, shortly before choking, he goes into ecstasies ...". Of principal importance are Wagner's publications and a related report of Pick (which is cited in Wagner, 1891) as both emphasized the time point of the onset of retrograde amnesia before hanging.

Wagner (1891) noted that attempted hanging usually resulted in severe memory disturbances which he characterized as "dementia acuta" (p. 999), but that these amnesic states were usually only temporary; in a few cases he noted that the reverse pattern might even follow, namely an improvement of mnestic functions or the cure of a psychosis.

A few years later, Wollenberg (1897) described a 39-year-old carpenter, who hanged himself during a stay in a psychiatric clinic, to which he had been admitted as paranoid and because he had tried to hang himself eight days before. Wollenberg assumed that a preceding loss of consciousness was an important requirement for retrograde amnesia to occur, though unconsciousness did not necessarily lead to retrograde amnesia as a consequence (cf. the book of Bumke, 1922 on this matter, and Bleuler's, 1921, counter-arguments against Bumke's preceding article from 1920).

Some years later again, Wachsmuth (1907) reported the example of a 23-year-old merchant who had a shot-wound in his head of unclear origin; an attempted suicide was assumed to have occurred. The patient made a second attempt, this time by hanging himself during his hospitalization, and had a profound retrograde amnesia. At the time of Wagner and Wollenberg there was still a serious discussion on whether retrograde amnesia after hanging was organic or psychic in origin, and this was reviewed by Schneider (1928, p. 518).

The question was also central to M. Sommer's (1903) report on "the amnesic disturbances after attempts of hanging". On the basis of two cases of his own he confirmed the observation of other scientists that following strangulation there is a retrograde amnesia for a few days and usually also an anterograde one for one or two days.

In the ensuing debate over the views of Möbius (that the amnesia following strangulation is of hysterical nature), and of Wagner (that it is of organic nature), M. Sommer was strongly inclined to follow Wagner's opinion. (Likewise, M. Paul, 1899, had argued vehemently against Möbius opinion, and also E. Meyer in 1907 considered Wagner's view as the most plausible one.) M. Sommer assumed that the complete blockage of the carotids and the interruption of the venous discharge resulted in temporary but still severe nutritional disturbance of the nervous tissue with functional detriments of the neurons, without, however, damaging them permanently. (As a marginal note, the views of the just-mentioned scientist Möbius were discussed controversially already at the time of his most active research. "Famous" is still his book "On the physiological feeblemindedness of woman" which in 1922 was published in its 12th edition.)

E. Meyer (1910) combined a large number of psychological and neurological tests to determine the status of a 24-year old man. This patient had attempted to hang himself and was found and rescued early in the morning. Interestingly, he apparently had a preserved skill memory, knowing, for instance, how to salute, while his episodic memory was disturbed. E. Meyer compared the patient's behavior over several days, by asking every day the same questions and listing the respective answers in tabellary form. He concluded that the patient's behavior best is described by a Korsakoff's syndrom, and that strangulation typically will result in Korsakoff's symptomatology.

Fraenkel in 1911 reported the case of a 20-year-old woman who after strangulation had massive disturbances in anterograde and retrograde memory and was disoriented with respect to place and time. The patient remained in an amnesic condition even after four months, but had been somewhat abnormal in psychic condition already before the attempt of hanging. Fraenkel discussed this case as resembling the symptoms of Korsakoff's psychosis in many respects.

After the Second World War, Jacob and Pyrkosch (1951) made a detailed analysis of the consequences of hanging on the anatomy of the brain. They based their investigation on the painstaking investigation of 3 out of 20 brains from cases who died after hanging. It is interesting that here again, as in other cases with hypoxic or anoxic brain damage, the hippocampal formation was consistently affected. The subicular cortex and Ammon's horn especially showed degenerated neurons. Other areas of cell damage were in the claustrum, the pallidum, and the thalamus. It cannot be determined, however, whether the damage was primarily caused by the reduced oxygen consumption or by convulsions which may occur during hanging.

Retrograde Amnesia after Cerebral Concussion and after Shot Wounds

In 1894, Gussenbauer gave his introductory lecture as the new director of the Second Surgical Clinic of Vienna, centering on the consequences of cerebral concussion on behavior. He remarked that cerebral concussion might alter not only mnestic functions but intellectual behavior in general: "For the injured it is as if his brain had stopped its intellectual functions for some time" (p. 807). He wondered why some of the information lost might be recovered while other parts failed to do so. He described a patient whose concussion he could follow and investigate in detail from the very start, because he was an eyewitness: During a mountain hike a friend of his lost his balance and fell on his head in the ice which led to a short cardiac arrest, a cephalic hematoma and wounds. Gussenbauer noted the following (p. 808):

1. All memories for the last 24 hours, including imaginations, reflections, and affections were permanently lost. Even going over the same mountain route one year later failed to reinstate any remembrance.
2. Events from the previous two days were partially lost as well.
3. There was an anterograde amnesia for the next nine hours.
4. Some priming of emotionally significant memories from the last hours before the accident was possible.

Gussenbauer assumed that the effects of concussion were due to a partial ineffectivity of cortical neurons.

A case was published that had an interesting forensic sidelight (Härtl, 1916): A man was shot in the head, but in spite of massive bleeding, he took his instant and vehement headache for signs of a stroke; then another man gave him some help. It was not until later that he realized he must have been attacked by the other man when he read about an attempted murder in the same farm area where he had been, under identical circumstances as during his own visit there. Otherwise the patient was completely unaware of what actually had happened during the attack or of the shot which was only later discovered by x-rays.

The Case of Grünthal and Störring

Grünthal and Störring investigated (1930) and followed-up (Grünthal & Störring, 1933; Störring, 1931) a case of carbon monoxide intoxication with particular deficits in the anterograde memory range, but with massive retrograde amnesia as well. The patient's behavior with respect to memory performance, emotions, will, spontaneous activity, and abilities to think and reflect consciously was documented in more than 120 pages in Störring's publication from 1931.

The patient's retrograde amnesia followed typically Ribot's law (the more recent the information is, the more likely it is lost, while vice versa, the longer it had been stored, the more likely it is retained). He had a good remembrance of events from his youth, but practically no knowledge of his recent past. Grünthal and Störring (1930) speculated on the morphological substrate of his amnesia and negated the existence of diffuse brain damage, but acknowledged the possibility "that the more refined physical-chemical processes of large brain areas might have suffered so differently in their dynamics or quality that especially the correlates of mnestic functions are affected" (p. 368).

They preferred, however, to assume that distinct brain portions such as the mammillary bodies might have been damaged.

In 1933, the patient married his fiancée (which had been mentioned already in the 1930-report) and lived at home. He was still markedly amnesic and introduced his wife consistently as his fiancée. He was always happy to see her as if he had just fallen in love. He showed appropriate behavioral stereotypes, such as taking off his hat when entering the church or when being greeted, and was able to behave well during meals and to explain industrial drawings he made about 10 years previously. But he used external helps for memorizing. For instance, he once explained that it must be Sunday because he was wearing a suit or that he would not be traveling on a train, as he was not dressed appropriately. He also assisted his wife in climbing a mountain as he remembered from the time before his accident that she had difficulties on such occasions.

It is interesting that when asked about the present date he always said "the last day of May, 1926", and in fact his accident had occurred on the 31st of May in 1926. We recently made the same observation on an amnesic who had a stroke affecting the diencephalon. The patient always gave the year as 1981 – the year of his stroke – when asked (in 1990) (Markowitsch et al., subm.).

The various forms of retrograde amnesia (cf. Schneider, 1928, p. 516 ff) are still even less understood than anterograde amnesia, which is partly due to the diverse and inconsistent damage of brain tissue. While Grünthal and Störring's (1930, 1933) case is an old example, recent ones are those of Goldberg et al. (1981), Goldberg, Hughes, Mattis, and Antin (1982), Kapur, Young, Bateman, and Kennedy (1989), Kopelman (1989), and Roman-Campos, Poser, and Wood (1980) (cf. also the reviews of Dall'Ora, Della Sala, & Spinnler, 1989; Markowitsch, 1991 b; Markowitsch & Pritzel, 1985; and Tulving, 1989).

In the following memory disturbances will be subdivided principally on the basis of etiologies and/or loci of brain damage.

Chapter 6: Korsakoff's Syndrome

Alcohol-related Brain Damage

Korsakoff's psychosis can be characterized by focal intellectual deterioration which centers around problems in memory, and by brain damage which is found most prominently and reliably in diencephalic structures. Another form of ethanol-based brain damage, alcoholic dementia, leads to more widespread deteriorations of intellect, personality, and – possibly – brain damage than Korsakoff's disease. And, to complete this list, I mention the possibility that a Korsakoff syndrome can be associated with a vitamin deficiency-disease which can consequently occur independent of alcohol consumption: cf. Bowman, Goodhart, & Jolliffe, 1939; Campbell & Biggart, 1939; Cochrane, Collins-Williams, & Donohue, 1961; Cruickshank, 1950; De Wardener & Lennox, 1947; Ecker & Woltman, 1939; Ely, 1922; Goodhart & Jolliffe, 1938; Irle & Markowitsch, 1982, 1983; Jolliffe, Wortis, & Fein, 1941; Markowitsch, 1982; Markowitsch & Pritzel, 1985; Minski, 1936; Roemheld, 1906; Sittig, 1914; Wechsler, 1933).

Though a lot of pathological conditions have been subsumed under the heading "Korsakoff's disease" or "Korsakoff's syndrome" (e.g., Benedek & Porsche, 1921; Betlheim & Hartmann, 1924, 1951; Brie, 1892; A. Knapp, 1918a; Lückerath, 1900; Marx, 1921; E. Meyer, 1904; Schulz, 1908; Steinthal, 1921; Thiele, 1924; Weber, 1906), it might be worthwhile to call back to mind a differentiation made by Steinthal (1921). He pointed out that a clear distinction should be made between the "Korsakoff's symptom complex" and "Korsakoff's psychosis". Synonyms for the 'Korsakoff's symptom complex' would be 'Korsakoff's syndrome' and 'the amnesic symptom complex'. This symptom complex, according to Steinthal, could appear in "progressive paralyis, lues cerebri, brain tumors, after traumatic brain damage and strangulation, in the age-related illnesses of the brain, and after various infections and toxic illnesses" (p. 287) (cf., e.g., Giese, 1911; Meggendorfer, 1928). He reserved the term 'Korsakoff's psychosis' for cases in which the symptom complex appeared after year-long alcohol abuse, that is, he based this term on an etiological moment. An equally restrictive use of the term "Korsakoff's syndrome" was also suggested a few years later in the English-language literature: "If we are to use the term 'Korsakoff's syndrome' at all, it should be restricted to the condition which Korsakoff observed and not applied only to the psychical state which occurs in that condition" (Carmichael & Stern, 1931, p. 189).

An excellent monograph on the Wernicke-Korsakoff syndrome, including a chapter with an historical review, is the book of Victor, Adams, and Collins which appeared in 1989 in its second edition.

Korsakoff's papers on alcoholic polyneuritis, published at first in Russian (in 1887; cf. Victor & Yakovlev, 1955), and then in French and German, constituted the basis for sensitizing psychiatrists and neurologists to an illness which in previous times was apparently even more widespread than today (Korsakoff, 1889, 1890; Korsakow, 1890, 1891; Korsakow & Serbski, 1892).

Nevertheless, there were a number of articles and other contributions before Korsakoff's publications which dealt with alcohol-related multiple neuritis (Annan, 1840; Canton, 1860; Charcot, 1884; Dreschfeld, 1884; Fischer, 1882; Lawson, 1878; Moeli, 1883; C. H. Robinson, 1877; Strümpell, 1883; cf. also the reviews of Cambier, 1954; Moll, 1915; and Soukhanoff & Boutenko, 1903). Especially Wernicke's (1881) acute, haemorrhagic, superior poliencephalitis, described in paragraph 47 of the second volume of his "Lehrbuch der Gehirnkrankheiten für Aerzte und Studirende", was well-known (cf. e.g., Elzholz, 1900; Leichtenstern, 1892; Raimann, 1900; Salomonsohn, 1891; Sträussler, 1902). With his terminology Wernicke wanted to characterize a sudden, haemorrhagic infarct occurring at various loci of the gray matter dorsal to the medulla oblongata: "It is an independent, inflammatory, acute gray matter disease in the area of the eye muscle nerves, leading to death within 10–14 days" (p. 240: "Es handelt sich um eine selbständige, entzündliche, acute Kernerkrankung im Gebiete der Augenmuskelnerven, die in der Zeit von 10–14 Tagen zum Tode führt."; cf. Raimann, 1901, for a detailed discussion of eye muscle paralysis in alcoholics). While Wernicke's poliencephalitis is considered an acute form, Korsakoff's disease is considered the chronic form of the two usually alcohol-related, diseases (cf. Victor et al., 1989).

Moeli (1883) noted that already around 1880 about 1,000 "lunatic" patients were hospitalized per year in the Berlin Charité. While a large percentage of the patients he described were alcoholics, with delusions and other psychiatric symptoms, including dementia in many of them, he paid particular attention to the cases with alcohol-related illnesses and subdivided them into several subgroups mainly according to the observed symptomatology. Moeli also described some special cases with only sporadic, temporary loss of behavioral control, including a doctor of philosophy who because his drinking problems were known usually refused any offer of alcohol but soon lost control whenever he did start; both the quantities he drank and his subsequent behavior were excessive. The next day he was always totally amnestic of the foregoing day.

Moeli described another patient in detail, a man who had been hospitalized three times with delirium tremens and who died with all signs of peripheral nerve degeneration. His body and brain were examined post mortem, but the description of neural pathology concentrated principally on the peripheral nerves. Moeli concluded that alcoholic pathology can be restricted to the "peripheral nervous system" (p. 548). Orr and Rows (1901) and J. Turner (1903 a), a few years later, placed similar emphasis on the peripheral nervous system or – as J. Turner termed it – the "spinal ganglia". However, much of the literature then failed to mention possible alcohol-related disease etiologies. For example, on p. 46, J. Turner just wrote "This woman was stated to have had an alcoholic history". And still, in discussing his 33 cases, he mentioned S. J. Cole (1902) as an advocate of the position that alcohol has a direct poisoning action on the nerve cells (p. 61).

At the beginning of the present century, Chotzen (1902) already described in detail which functions of the Korsakoff's syndrome might recover in which sequence. First, orientation recovers, then the ability to memorize ("Merkfähigkeit"; short-term memory); thereafter, orientation for time recurs. However, some anterograde amnesia nearly always remains, together with a poor reaction towards the environment and lack of interests. Retrograde amnesia, on the other hand, usually shrinks considerably according to Chotzen's findings.

Spielmeyer (1904) emphasized that Korsakoff's psychosis is not an illness "sui generis", but more the outcome of a general disease, namely an alcohol-caused sickness.

Korsakoff's Descriptions

Sergei S. Korsakoff (1854–1900), a psychiatrist in Moscow, published the first case descriptions in several Russian journals (*Archiv Psychiatrii [Charkow], Westnik Psychiatrii, Medizinskoje Oboszenije,* and in the *Jeschenedelnaja klinitscheskaja gaseta*), and as a book "On alcoholic paralysis", which appeared in 1887 in Russian (cited after Korsakoff, 1890, and Korsakow, 1890).

Because the form of psychiatric disturbances which he was referring to in his articles was not dealt with by psychiatrists, but rather by general practicioners and gynecologists, he described it in the "*Allgemeine Zeitschrift für Psychiatrie*" in 1890 and 1891 (Korsakoff, 1890; Korsakow, 1891), in the "*Archiv für Psychiatrie und Nervenkrankheiten*" (Korsakow, 1890), and before that in French in the "*Revue philosophique*" (Korsakoff, 1889).

In this book I use the spelling "Korsakoff", though Korsakov might be the more appropriate one. The spelling with a double 'f' is most frequently found in Anglo-American literature, though sometimes 'w' (e.g., J. Turner, 1903b; Zangwill, 1941) or 'v' (e.g., Cutting, 1978) at the end can be found. In French literature (Delay & Brion, 1969; Korsakoff, 1889) the spelling with double 'f' is usual (though sometimes Korsakow may be seen as well: Lhermitte, Doussinet, & de Ajuriaguerra, 1937; Remy, 1942), and in German 'w', though sometimes (for instance in his first German-language publication) 'ff' can be found.

Korsakoff was of the opinion that in his cases memory for recent events usually diminished, while it was spared for far remote events (Korsakoff, 1890, p. 479). His description of a typical Korsakoff's patient can still be considered representative (Korsakoff, 1890, p. 479 f):

> At the beginning of a talk the mental disturbance is hardly noticeable; he gives the impression of a person with full mental powers – talking with full reflection, drawing correct deductions on the basis of given premises, playing chess, or a game of cards, in short – he behaves like a mentally healthy subject; only after longer conversation may one notice that he mixes facts quite substantially, and that he is unable to keep in mind anything of what takes place in his environment: he does not remember having eaten, or whether he got up from bed. Sometimes he immediately forgets what has happened to him. Patients of this kind may read for hours one and the same page, because they are unable to keep the contents in mind. They can repeat 20 times the same conversation without realizing the continuous repetition of their stereotyped talk. He does not know persons he met only during the time of his illness, such as the doctor or the nurse, though he sees them consistently; he is always convinced of meeting them for the first time.

It is interesting that Korsakoff emphasized that his so-called "Psychosis polyneuritica seu Cerebropathia psychica toxaemica" could occur quite often on a non-alcoholic basis. In 1890, he mentioned having published 14 cases with non-alcoholic etiology, and these included patients with a dead, decaying fetus in the uterus, septicemia, accumulation of feces, typhus, tuberculosis, diabetes mellitus, jaundice, a lymphadenome, and a disintegrated tumor. He further mentioned intoxication with alcohol, but also with arsenic, lead, carbon disulphite, carbon monoxide, and ergot (cf. also Jarho, 1973; recently, arap Mengech, 1983, described a case with Korsakoff's psychosis due to strangulation).

Korsakoff justified the label "toxaemic" with his experience that in all cases investigated "the composition of the blood is altered, toxic substances have accumulated, and it is most likely that these poison the nervous system, whereby in a few cases mostly the peripheral, in others the central nervous system, but frequently both are afflicted to the same degree" (Korsakoff, 1890, p. 484).

In his study "On a special form of a psychic disturbance, combined with multiple neuritis" (Korsakow, 1890), he gave detailed case reports, first of women (aged 28 and 22 years), then of six new cases which he had observed during a two-year-period (and on still a further case which he added in the proofs). He gave a careful and detailed summary of the psychological changes (p. 700 ff), emphasizing the irritability of the patients, their disturbed association of ideas, and their memory problems. He also mentioned again that conscious and rational thinking may be preserved, while the amnesia is still profound (p. 701 f: "not knowing 5 min past lunch that he had just eaten").

"Pseudoreminiscences" or "false memories" were the specific topic of a study which he published in 1891 (Kraepelin, 1887a, 1887b, had also published on 'false memories', as acknowledged by Korsakoff). Korsakoff mentioned that these pseudoreminiscences appear in two forms – as deja vu feeling and as the appearance of ideas or conceptions which had not occurred in reality – and that they could be found in a number of diseases (paranoia, progressive paralysis, senile dementia, polyneuritic psychosis). He had noted that most of these pseudoreminiscences had some relation to a true background, and so he hypothesized that they represent a rudimentary form of memory engrams ("The memory traces most likely correspond to the preservation of a function of neuronal elements, though in very minor intensity"; p. 410). He furthermore speculated that these rudimentary elements might then combine to "constant associative groups" which are first unconscious but at a later stage may come to consciousness and thereby simulate real memories.

In Korsakoff's last publication I have found on this matter (Korsakow & Serbski, 1892), a 27-year-old woman was described who had largely refrained from drinking alcohol and who developed the polyneuritic symptomatology due to a decaying fetus ("extrauterine pregnancy"). This case is described with great accuracy and at length; a detailed anatomical description is also given (which I assume is Serbski's contribution to the paper). However, the patient had no significant changes in the brain.

Bonhoeffer's (1901) Book on Alcoholics

Bonhoeffer (1901), a pupil of Wernicke (cf. Ackerknecht, 1985, p. 79, footnote 5, for a short description of Bonhoeffer's life, and Ziehen, 1905, for an obituary on Wernicke), wrote on "The acute mental diseases in chronic alcoholics" and gave a detailed description of the "Wernicke-Korsakoff-syndrome" (Victor et al., 1989; see Bonhoeffer's chapter II, and Nickel, 1990). The idea of four "cardinal elements" of the Korsakoff's syndrome – a memory defect for current events (*Merkunfähigkeit*), retrograde amnesia (*Erinnerungsdefekt*), disorientation, and confabulation – is traced back to his 226 paged-monograph (see p. 119, last paragraph). The memory defects are the most persistent and consistent of the four, as Korsakow (1890) had remarked earlier. (Bonhoeffer, however, criticized that Korsakoff had failed to make a sharp distinction between anterograde and retrograde amnesia.)

It is interesting that both Korsakow (1890) and Bonhoeffer (1901) emphasized that the amnesia is not complete, but that certain, usually emotionally significant, events can be memorized and that information which appeared to have been lost, may be regained even after years (cf. Markowitsch et al., 1984, 1986, for more recent experiments on this subject, which is also known as the "Claparede-phenomenon" [Claparede, 1911].) In Bonhoeffer's words: "The inability to memorize is complete only exceptionally. Usually it is possible, even in cases with apparent total amnesia, to determine some memory ability. For example, a patient was able to tell me a list of names of familiar distilleries even after a very long time, though he otherwise forgot nearly instanteously simple, indifferent words, names, or two- or three-figure numbers." (p. 126). (For very similar descriptions of Korsakoff's patients of more recent times see Zangwill, 1941; Zola-Morgan et al., 1983; Zola-Morgan & Öberg, 1980.)

Bonhoeffer further discussed the reduced apprehension of Korsakoff patients, which had been tested by Finzi (1901) in Emil Kraepelin's laboratory. He referred to a peculiar and interesting case of Liepmann (1898, 1910). In 1910 Liepmann admitted that his earlier short description of this case had appeared in a place which was inaccessible to the majority of other scientists (namely in the "Verhandlungen der Schlesischen Gesellschaft für Vaterländische Kultur"). In the earlier publication Liepmann (1898) had described this case as a 50-year-old journalist with an amnesic episode extending back about three decades, the border between preserved and lost remembrance dating to the year 1871. The patient, a philologian, had a good remembrance of his former school friends, knew Latin syntax and could name his University professors. Asked on his occupation, he told the physician "a student". The death of his parents (dating to the year 1874) was lost. All political answers dated 30 years back in time. But he was well educated on questions of political, historical, and moral nature.

Bonhoeffer criticized Liepmann's description of the patient's sharp border of memory loss; after all he had been able to calculate the age of Kaiser Wilhelm (I) correctly, though realizing that he would have to be 101 years old (in 1898). Bonhoeffer also argued that if the patient really only kept experiences up to the year 1871, he should have behaved like a 19-year-old adult (while in fact he behaved like a much older person considering his available background of knowledge). Bonhoeffer concluded that there is no case with a total loss of that individuality which had accumulated over time; instead, the total character and degree of the mental maturity is preserved.

In 1910 Liepmann stated that he had followed his case in detail for another five years and, in the proofs added to his article, he had even provided some additional material he had on another case which gave an up-date to the present time (i. e., to about 1909).

The case was that of a well-educated student who had worked as a reporter until shortly before hospitalization. Liepmann noted a marked dissociation between his optic and acoustic memory abilities. The student immediately forgot pictures and objects just seen, but could remember words he had heard such as "Omnipotnekatmehum" (which is not German) for 3 or 4 minutes. While his memory ability was largely reduced, he had what Liepmann called a "phenomenal ability" for mental arithmetic (e. g., multiplying four-figure by two-figure numbers).

It is of interest to note that the patient could play chess quite well (winning against all other occupants of the hospital), but minutes later, he had no knowledge of having played a game. A similar description of a patient, who in spite of dense amnesia, played a particular game well, but immediately forgot the game, was recently given for Damasio's patient Boswell (e. g., Damasio, 1989; Damasio & Tranel, 1989) and is also known from other present-day amnesics, described in the current literature.

Later in time, after another five years, the patient gained partial knowledge of his present situation (i. e., that Bismarck was no longer chancellor, that Kaiser Wilhelm II reigned, etc.). In the note added in proof, Liepmann noted that the patient still had a gross Korsakoff-like symptomatology, but some islands of knowledge of the more recent past. For instance, he stated that he had been brought to the hospital by the "Wernicke'sche Kanaille" (p. 1161).

Coming back to Bonhoeffer: After discussing the psychological consequences of Korsakoff's psychosis, he gave a detailed analysis of possible or likely neuropathological changes associated with Korsakoff's psychosis (pp. 136–168). He started out by pointing to peripheral nerve damage, cerebellar damage, and likely damage of the vagal nerve. Then he discussed the picture of the so-called "Polioencephalitis haemarrhagica superior" (p. 146 ff), described first by Wernicke, which is characterizable above all by eye muscular disturbances (cf. also Salomonsohn, 1891). With respect to the Korsakoff syndrome, Bonhoeffer considered the existence of cortical damage as likely, though he stated that this had as yet not been investigated in sufficient detail. (Creutzfeldt in 1928 emphasized that he had seen much more severe cortical damage in nine Korsakoff's patients than was found in Gamper's publications from 1928, 1929 and 1931.) Haemorrhagic processes were seen consistently and in high numbers and had a tendency to occur symmetrically (a statement which was confirmed by Creutzfeldt, 1928, and has recently been corroborated by the detailed neuroanatomical evaluations of Mair, Warrington, & Weiskrantz, 1979). Furthermore, likewise in accordance with more recent results (Victor et al., 1989; cf. also Markowitsch, 1982), periventricular damage was noted by Bonhoeffer.

Lastly, Bonhoeffer made some remarks on possible functional restitution. He stated that some degree of recovery may be possible, though not the full restitution of all personality dimensions. As therapy he suggested refraining from memory training at the beginning; he also prefered practical work over memory training at a later stage of recovery. The main emphasis, he thought, should be placed on improved nutrition (a factor which is also emphasized in recent work; see, e. g., Victor et al., 1989).

Korsakoff's Psychosis at the Time of Queen Victoria and King Edward VII

Serbsky, a Pupil of Korsakoff

After Korsakoff's papers (and book), results on a number of cases were published in the two decades around the turn of the century (e.g., Hurd, 1905; Jelliffe, 1908; A. Knapp, 1906; Moeli, 1883; Murawieff, 1897; Raimann, 1900, 1901, 1902; Stanley, 1909/10; J. Turner, 1903a, 1903b). In 1907, Serbsky (written this time with a 'y' as last letter) summarized the state of the art on "Die Korsakowsche Krankheit", starting with the observation that Korsakoff's disease represented the biggest success of the last decades in the field of psychiatry (in these words: "Die Korsakowsche Krankheit stellt die grösste Errungenschaft der letzten Dezennien im Gebiete der Psychiatrie dar"; p. 389). The term "Korsakoff's disease" had been suggested by P. Jolly at the International Medical Congress in Moscow in 1897 (cf. also Jolly, 1897).

In Serbsky's publication the case of a 30-year-old woman with septicemia due to a decaying fetus was described in extenso; as Serbsky remarked, the case had a number of parallels to the one previously published (Korsakow & Serbski, 1892). Based on this description he then discussed all possible varieties of "psycho-polyneuropathies" (p. 408) and referred to a close relation between beri-beri and Korsakoff's disease which had been suggested by a South American professor of forensic medicine (Rodrigues, 1906; cf. also the later report of a South American neurology professor on beri-beri: Austregesilo, 1927). (Serbsky wrote that Rodrigues' observation contradicted that of English physicians who had been in the Far East; today we know that the link in fact does exist: cf., e.g., references in Irle & Markowitsch, 1982.) He then presented – in almost as much detail as for the first case – the case of an alcohol-based Korsakoff psychotic (aged 42 years), who had had severe memory problems, but was still able to think logically, could make jokes, and won games, and of a third case, a female patient, aged 33 years, who drank large amounts of alcohol: every day, though usually only in the night, she had 1 to $1^1/_2$ bottles of brandy, the same amount of schnaps, up to 10 bottles of beer, liqueurs, rowan-berry wine and other alcoholic beverages. The woman survived, but suffered feelings of jealousy for her husband. Serbsky ended his description by elaborating on a dilemma: The woman wanted frequent intercourse with her husband, but was not physically fit enough to become pregnant or have an abortion. Serbsky was of the opinion that coitus interruptus or reservatus might lead to epilepsy (in women), so he suggested as an alternative bringing the woman to a "special sanatorium".

Other Early Authors and Single Case Descriptions

"Multiple alcoholic neuritis", as a defined illness, existed in the literature long before Korsakoff. In 1887 Witkowski referred to works of about a dozen authors; for the first of his own cases (a 48-year-old shoemaker), he remarked his "very short memory" (p. 810). For his second case, Witkowski noted an imbalance in the widening of the pupils and ("the usual") peripheral muscular atrophies or paralyses. Thomsen (1888, 1890) was another psychiatrist who described the anatomical changes in cases with Wernicke's "acute haemorrhagische Poliencephalitis superior" (Wernicke, 1881, p. 229), or, more simply, the multiple alcoholic neuritis (polyneuritis) (cf. also Strümpell, 1891).

While Witkowski's and Thomsen's cases were principally on the acute ("Wernicke") side, with Freund's (1889a) article a "true" Korsakoff's case appeared (as Korsakoff acknowledged himself; cf. Korsakow, 1890, p. 691). Prior to publication Freund gave the contents of his paper in a talk held at the "Verein der Ostdeutschen Irrenärzte zu Breslau" in 1887. His first case was a 52-year-old woman with memory disturbance as the most prominent symptom. As in other cases, she had a cut-off point between retrograde amnesia and preserved memory (at age 30), though she was able to answer being about 50 years old (but stating that her parents were "already in the fifties"). His second case was a 65-year-old woman whose retrograde amnesia went back to the age of 20. In spite of her old age, she thought she was 18, or, at most, 30 years old. She thought she was just married and had a child of at most half a year of age. Freund gave a number of examples of recent memory disturbances in this case ("musical memory, auditory memory, simple multiplication, writing, spelling").

A gastro-intestinal origin for Korsakoff's psychosis was found in the case given by Raimann (1902) (for a recent case, developing into Korsakoff's syndrome after intravenous feeding and intestinal surgery, see Parkin, Blunden, Rees, & Hunkin, 1991). From his patient, Raimann concluded that the polioencephalitis superior acuta and the Korsakoff psychosis were only different manifestations of the same process of illness. The same opinion had been published by Elzholz in 1900 who already included 56 citations of the relevant literature on Korsakoff's disease.

A course similar to Raimann's patient from 1902 can be seen in a diabetic acidosis case published a dozen years later by Sittig (1914); the psychosis retrogressed hand-in-hand with the retrogression of the acidosis. (For a recent example of the Wernicke-Korsakoff syndrome without alcoholism see J.T. Becker, Furman, Panisset, & Smith, 1990; an old description on gastric influences on the brain was given by Neubürger, 1937.)

The term "Korsakoff's psychosis" was already used around and before 1900 (e.g., Brodmann, 1902, p. 227; Elzholz, 1900; Mönkemöller & Kaplan, 1899; Raimann, 1900). Brodmann's (1902, 1904) psychological experiments with Korsakoff's patients were mentioned above (cf. the section on "*Early Methods for Memory Assessments*"). With Kalberlah's (1904) article from Hitzig's clinic in Halle, a relation was established between commotio, brain damage, and Korsakoff's psychosis.

Kalberlah (1904) also described in detail two individual cases, the first one being that of a 42-year-old bricklayer who had an accident with commotio during work. Kalberlah noted all errors his patient made during the period of his recovery, especially the memory disturbances which were quite marked and followed (as in other cases) Ribot's law. This "law of regression" meant that the most recent things learned prior to an injury are largely lost; memory recovers starting from older events moving up to more recent ones. Kalberlah's main concern was to trace parallels between his two cases with commotio, and Korsakoff's psychosis. He cited the work of others (Kraepelin, 1896; Tiling, 1892; Wernicke, 1900) which according to him seemed in high congruence to his own cases (cf. also Tiling, 1890).

His principal statement was: "The immediate and in time nonseparable appearing mental disturbances after commotio or coma constitute etiologically and clinically a congruent group, which is characterizable by quantitatively and qualitatively manifold disturbances of the memory and their extensity and intensity may come to expression quite variably" (p. 437).

A. Knapp's (1906) book on "The polyneuritic psychoses" was not quite as voluminous as Bonhoeffer's; nevertheless, on 141 pages he gave detailed descriptions on six female and two male cases with a Korsakoff symptomatology. He included comments on changes caused by peripheral nerve damage, but also by telencephalic damage, and gave a detailed analysis of psychic disturbances.

Already within the first decade of the present century, Baumgarten (1907) made experiments on animals, namely on dogs, rabbits, and guinea pigs in an attempt to corroborate the role of gastro-intestinal origins for Korsakoff's psychosis, but failed to find evidence for liver damage and concluded that in the species tested the toxic substances found in human subjects might not be present in the stomach-gut system of the animals.

Wehrung's Survey

Gaston Wehrung (1905) from Strasbourg contributed a further case, stressing especially the "pathological anatomy". (It is interesting to note that although Strasbourg was German at that time, he used the French writing "Korsakoff".) He gave a very thorough review of the history of Korsakoff's psychosis, stating, for instance, that Magnus Huss (1852) was (according to Korsakoff) the first who dealt with the consequences of alcohol on the psyche. As he demonstrated, between 1860 and 1885 a large number of papers were published in which the likeliness of the coexistence of multiple neurosis and heavy drinking was emphasized. For those who wish to follow the history of papers on alcohol-related neuropathology, his article is a very rewarding choice. He gave not only long case descriptions, but also a long table on 34 cases published up to that time (including many French publications). For the case he examined himself (an innkeeper's wife of 28 years of age who had been drinking heavily since 8 years), he particularly emphasized anatomical deviations. As in Serbsky's (1907) case, the woman had been quite sophisticated in simple math, in spite of her otherwise deteriorated memory. A neuroanatomical examination revealed a number of pathological changes, as in the frontal lobes.

Boedeker's Cases

Boedeker (1905) then, again, related Wernicke's acute with Korsakoff's chronic states of alcoholic memory disturbances. He described an acute case of a 54-year-old university professor who had drunken beer excessively but had not been considered an alcoholic. He showed a weakness of his extremities, double sightedness and confabulated. His anterograde memory was poor: He did not know the name of the doctor in charge, or that of the clinic, or the correct day of his admission. After three weeks he was already considered to be cured and within less than another three months he was able to continue his lectures.

He also described a chronic case of a 57-year-old merchant who was a chronic alcoholic and had had repeated episodes of delirium tremens prior to his admission. He had anterograde and retrograde amnesia, but was oriented with respect to his hospitalization and behaved quite appropriately. He had been in the hospital for examinations for three years. However, he was able to give approximate answers with respect to specific episodic events (dates of poets, historical dates). The ability to calculate was good (e.g., "What is 12 times 13?"). It is interesting that when given the task to reproduce the number 3579, he said 5679 after five minutes, but this and another (invented) number (1235) he kept in his mind throughout the time of testing (that is, for weeks). When asked after weeks why he remembered these two numbers, he answered that the difference is 23 for both (between 56 and 79 and between 12 and 35).

Boedeker tested the extent of his anterograde amnesia and found that the patient could remember events from his school and military service up to his marriage, but apparently had lost memory for roughly the next 15 years of his life, including the deaths of his parents and his brother and his first admission to the psychiatric hospital. Whenever he gave wrong answers and these were questioned, he remarked that it might have been a hallucination.

Very detailed case descriptions of altogether eight cases were given by E. Meyer and Raecke (1903). The patients were between 34 and 67 years old with a median of 51.5 years. The authors concluded that the Korsakoff syndrome constitutes an irreparable lesion of the central nervous system, although the actual locus or loci of the lesions were unknown at that time. Three years later, Kutner (1906) pointed to focal cortical lesions in "polyneuritic psychosis". However, his arguments, based on four cases, were largely speculative in nature.

Mathematical Abilities Versus Episodic Memory

There are striking differences in the descriptions given in the above-mentioned reports for episodic verbal memory on the one hand and the ability to calculate and even that to remember numbers on the other. Offner (1924) reported the ability to memorize numbers as a "peculiar speciality". On pages 172ff of his book, he gave a number of examples of phenomenal mathematical abilities in individuals.

While most of these "jugglers with figures" used visual imaginations, one subject who only learned to write numbers at an age of 20 years, worked on an acoustic-motoric basis, hearing the numbers and speaking them voiceless. Offner remarked that usually there is even a discrepancy between intelligence and an extraordinary ability to calculate.

For musical ability, he mentioned astonishing abilities of W.A. Mozart and of the daughter of the composer Anton Dvorak who already sang difficult compositions of her father's at an age of one and a half years.

Forel (1885) wrote a short section on hypermnesias and stated that certain, special memory abilities may exist even in idiots and that some subjects "store all sensory impressions as if they were photographed" (p. 43). From his survey, he concluded that "human unconscious ('unbewusstes') memory is indeed developed colossally" (p. 44).

Theissen's case. Theissen (1924) described in detail the case of a 20-year-old imbecile who was able to give the exact dates for Easter from the year 1583 up to the year 2000, and already at an age of 4–5 years had been able to give the Latin names of all flowers which grew in the garden of the charity he lived in. Asked about 318 Easter dates, he made only 14 errors (4.4%), reacting on the average in 1.76 s! At the age of 12 years, the pupil had received the Gregorian calendar from a priest and from that time learned its contents by heart, by reading it daily for three or four times, on some days for ten times. Later, he developed a system to relate all other days of the year to the date of Easter . The subject was then tested on a large number of dates, and thereafter he was required to learn new data such as geometrical figures and time tables. The patient had supranormal spans for learning and remembering non-associated facts, but was inferior whenever the data were embedded in a system, or followed logical or spatial sequences and relations. Most recently a similar talent of calendar calculation ability was described in an 18-year-old subject whose left hemisphere had been removed at age eight, and who had a full IQ of 84 points (Dorman, 1991); earlier so-called idiot savant-cases with this phenomenon were documented by Hill (1975) and Horwitz, Kestenbaum, Person, and Jarvik (1965) (cf. also Luria's "mind of a mnemonist": Luria, 1968).

The peculiarity of numbers and number symbols (as opposed to words) was summarized in the volume of Menninger (1969); an early review on the psychopathology of calculating was given by Peritz (1918). In the article of Peritz a good deal of information was given on the old history of calculating, on calculating in children, and on patients with different pathology and calculation disturbances (mostly hemianopics). He concluded that the center for calculating is situated in the left angular gyrus.

Wizel's Case

Wizel (1904) ascribed "a phenomenal talent in calculating" to his case. The patient was a 22 year-old woman, from an "intelligent family" (p. 122). Her development had been normal until the age of seven years when she suffered from severe epidemic typhus. Thereafter she had epileptic attacks and lost her intelligence almost completely. Wizel wrote that at the age of eleven years her intelligence was that of a child of only a few years and she preferred to play with children aged two or three years. Her sense of time was grossly impaired.

The patient's speciality had been to collect buttons and small coins and she soon developed an astonishing ability to calculate: She could immediately tell what the result of 27 times 16 is, or of 900 divided by 16. A further speciality was her ability to always answer in rhymes, sometimes even with humor.

After she had been hospitalized for four years, her answers to the question of how long she might have been in the hospital, were "a few weeks", "two years", "900 days", "17 years". She had at most a very crude conception of her surroundings, including persons, and had been unable to read figures. In spite of these deficits, her ability to deal with figures was extraordinary, with multiplication being her speciality. For example, she immediately knew the answer to 56^2, 85^2, or 78^2; on the other hand she made errors and was quite unsure when asked to add or to subtract (examples: 57 + 63 = 141 [instead of 120]; 48 + 53 = 163 [instead of 101]). Another exceptional ability was apparent when she was asked what 23 x 23 is; here she answered 529, but also remarked in addition that this is the same as 33 x 16 + 1. For 729 (27 x 27) she added that this equals 24 x 30 + 9. The number 16 played a special role in her calculations which apparently was related to the fact that as a child she had collected coins and that the Polish and Russian coins are specially related (Wizel worked at the Israelitian Hospital in Warsaw): 1 rouble = 100 copecks = 200 polish pennies. Given this relation, her answer to the question as to how many pennies are in a rouble, was 16 x 12 + 8.

In discussing his case, Wizel referred to some older reports on imbeciles with extraordinary mathematical abilities: Among them was a person who knew the day of death of all persons who had lived nearby and their first and last names (case of Forbes Winslow), a person who knew the birthday and day of death and the most important life events of numerous important personalities (case of Falret), or that of a person who could immediately transform the age of a person into minutes (case of Heim). He also mentioned the cases of Inaudi and Diamandi, who had been tested by Binet, Charcot, and several mathematicians.

Wizel's explanation for the calculation abilities of these cases was that they rely on a method of dividing numbers into smaller ones (e.g., 83^2 into [80 x 80] + [80 x 3] + [83 x 3]) and that they have a phenomenal memory for figures and know all products up to 100 x 100. He remarked that most of the jugglers with figures started to work with figures very early in their life, frequently at the age of 3 years.

Other Cases with Unusual Mathematical Abilities

Liepmann (1910) mentioned the phenomenal ability for mental arithmetic (multiplying four-numbered figures by two-digit numbers) in his patient and Boedeker's (1905) case showed the long-term remembrance of two four-figure numbers. Cases with alcohol-related memory disturbances or Korsakoff's syndrome, described by Ransohoff (1897), Wehrung (1905), Bonhoeffer (1901), Boedeker (1905), and Serbsky (1907), had been quite sophisticated with tests for calculating. Chotzen's (1902) case was much better on the mathematical than on the verbal memory level. Likewise, Grünthal's (1932) patient was told to remember "Schwalbennest" [swallow nest], and the number 151; after three minutes of talking he only remembered 151; and Krauss's (1904, 1930) patients apparently had no difficulties with simple multiplication and remembrance of numbers. Also, a further patient of Grünthal (1939) gave, I think, one of the last published examples at all on the mathematical performance of a Korsakoff's patient, a 40-year-old stoker, who died within less than six months after hospital admission. After a few examples of the patient's calculating abilities, Grünthal summarized: "Calculating in all species quick and without errors ..." (p. 83).

On the other hand, rational conclusions and reflections, in particular when they revolve around the patient's own daily living, have been much less reported on (Pick, 1915; Sittig, 1914). The frequent discrepancy between the very poor episodic memory of Korsakoff's subjects and their preserved abilities in the mathematical field suggests a profound difference between memory for numbers and for applying mathematical rules on the one side and memory for episodes on the other, whether autobiographical ones or from more general knowledge.

This distinction may in part be in accordance with the episodic-semantic memory distinction (Tulving, 1985, 1987); however, it cannot apparently be fully explained on this level in as much as Korsakoff's patients, for instance, sometimes manifested a subnormal digit memory span but were still able to multiply two two-digit numbers, or remembered other numbers for an extensive period of time though they failed to remember the doctor's name over much shorter periods.

While it might be overstating to extrapolate from these findings in Korsakoff's patients and to conclude that Bartlett's (1932) distinction between "knowing that" (episodic) versus "knowing how" (procedural, or in part semantic) (reviewed for instance by Squire, 1987) is unjustified, this finding is nevertheless in line with recent findings in experimental and clinical memory research which also question the efficiency of a distinction into episodic, semantic, and procedural memory systems (e.g., Humphreys, Bain, & Pike, 1989; Jacoby, Baker, & Brooks, 1989; Wilson, Baddeley, & Cockburn, 1989; Wood, Brown, & Felton, 1989).

Though in the recent literature on Korsakoff subjects (e.g., Mair et al., 1979; Mayes, Meudell, Mann, & Pickering, 1988; Squire, 1982; Winocur, Kinsbourne, & Moscovitch, 1981) the mathematical abilities usually remained untested, it would seem worthwhile to perform just such an investigation with present-day methodology. Support for this view also comes from experiments on non-Korsakoff patients and normal subjects (e.g., Berger, 1926; Bischoff, 1912; Henschen, 1919; Lewandowsky & Stadelmann, 1908; Singer & Low, 1933; Sittig, 1921; Vieregge, 1908). The frequently found dissociation between general intelligence and ability to keep numbers in mind and/or to retrieve them has fascinated scientists as well as the interested layman (e.g., Jaensch & Mehmel, 1928; van der Kolk & Jansens, 1905).

The Search for the Anatomical Bases of Chronic Alcoholism and Korsakoff's Syndrome

While Stevens in 1907 still assumed "that the occurrence of a neuritis" is not necessary in Korsakoff's syndrome, "so that the only symptoms produced are in the psychic field" (p. 458), other neuroscientists were eager to obtain evidence for neuropathological changes associated with the symptomatology.

Most of these investigations were done in the time period during and after the First World War (e.g., Bender, Curran, & Schilder, 1938; Bogaert & Helsmoortel, 1928; Gamper, 1928a, 1928b, 1929, 1931; Kant, 1932; Stertz, 1933; Tsiminakis, 1931; Tuwim, 1914), though, for example, Wernicke had already provided some hints in 1881 (hemorrhages surrounding the third and fourth ventricle), and Flechsig (1896b) was of the opinion that changes are most prominent within the somatosensory and prefrontal cortex (p. 103). Ewald Grimm (1868) stated that in some drinkers pathology of the frontal lobes is certain. Early studies sometimes appear naive, such as Baumgarten's (1907) injections and oral applications of different concentrations of alcohol to dogs, rabbits, and guinea pigs.

Probably the first article to give a clear statement on diencephalic damage in Korsakoff's syndrome was from Gudden in 1896; however, his results were not generally acknowledged or referred to in the papers which appeared around the turn of the century. The same was true for Bonhoeffer's (1901) findings on the neuropathology of Korsakoff's disease. This is regretable, as both authors had made very careful and detailed observations and furthermore had provided thorough reviews on previous cases. (Gudden's reference list included 110 entries.)

Gamper's Findings

A major contribution then came from Gamper (1928a, 1928b, 1929), an Austrian scientist who in 1930 became professor of psychiatry and neurology at the German University in Prague.

Gamper performed histological investigations on 16 brains of chronic alcoholics who had died as Korsakoff's psychotics. The average age of the nine men was 53.6 years and that of the seven women 47.7 years. Most patients died within 8–14 days after disease onset, while in three cases the illness lasted two months, and in one nine months. Brain sections were Nissl-stained, complemented by eosine-hematoxyline stains and Spatz' iron-sensitive technique.

Gamper emphasized that he failed to find any characteristic, specific changes in the cortical mantle of any of the patients' brains. On the other hand, marked changes were observed from the onset of the medulla oblongata up to the level of the anterior commissure. The affected regions included the dorsal motor nucleus of the vagus, sometimes the descending vestibular nucleus, the central gray, the inferior, but not the superior colliculi, sometimes medial portions of the oculomotor nucleus, the mesodiencephalic transition zone, and the nuclei Darkschewitsch and interstitialis. In all cases the mammillary bodies were regularly affected. Gamper stated that they apparently constituted the nodal points of the disease process and that they were also degenerated in cases in which no other areas were involved.

Furthermore, changes in the diencephalon were found in the nuclei along the medial wall of the third ventricle. The medial portions of the mediodorsal thalamic nuclei were affected, that is, areas which partly overlap with the nucleus reuniens. The nuclei parafascicularis, submedius, and reuniens were frequently damaged. Generally, however, destruction within the diencephalon was diminished in regions close to the dorsal and anterior thalamic boundaries, while lateral and anterior nuclei were not affected. In the subependymal area a glia proliferation was observed. This same, somewhat unexpected finding was documented in the cases reported on by Mair et al. (1979; cf. their Figs. 8 and 15, or Figs. 15 and 17 of Markowitsch & Pritzel, 1985). In these cases also the mammillary nuclei and the most medial portions of the mediodorsal thalamic level were also degenerated (cf. their Figs. 4 and 12, or Figs. 14 and 16 of Markowitsch & Pritzel, 1985).

Gamper mentioned that Gudden first found atrophic mammillary bodies in the brains of Korsakoff's patients with a longer disease process, and he furthermore remarked a strong proliferation of the vascular system and of glia cells and a restriction of the degenerative changes to nerve cells without invading the passing fiber systems.

It is important to note here that Gamper's findings are frequently mentioned only in a curtailed form as if he had only mentioned the mammillary nuclei as the essential affected brain structures in Korsakoff's psychosis, while in fact (with the exception of cortical areas) his minute descriptions include principally all the structures – if not more – which today have been found to be damaged in Korsakoff's alcoholics (e.g., Colmant, 1965; Mair et al., 1979; Torvik, 1987; Victor et al., 1989).

Gamper's findings changed the view on the importance of the cortical areas for higher cognitive processes (though he did face some opposition: see e.g., Carmichael & Stern, 1931). He noted this change in appraisal when concluding for instance in his article from 1929 that "doubting the absolute supremacy of the cerebral cortex is no longer a sin against the Holy Ghost" (p. 239).

Tsiminakis' Neuropathological Study

While Gamper emphasized the importance of the mammillary bodies and the negligible role of the cerebral cortex, Tsiminakis nearly at the same time tried to reverse these relations by arguing that the mammillary nuclei have "on the basis of their connections relevance only for the osmic sphere" (p. 25), and that the cortical changes in Korsakoff's syndrome are more severe than assumed by Gamper" (p. 26) (cf. Carmichael & Stern, 1931). ['Osmic sphere', translated from 'osmische Sphäre', most likely meant 'odorous sphere'.]

Tsiminakis' detailed and long article was based on only three cases, two of which were non-typical Korsakoff's patients. The first one died at the age of 58 and was characterized as "a Korsakoff's syndrome of perhaps unclear provenance" (p. 26). This case, a waiter, had had a CO-poisoning at age 45 and at age 46 skull damage occurred due to an explosion in an ammunition factory. Chronic alcoholism and Korsakoff's psychosis were given as diagnosis, though nothing at all was said about the patient's drinking habits. His psychic status was characterized by anterograde and retrograde amnesia, and also by a general diminuation of intellectual functions. A postmortem inspection of his brain revealed a number of changes in brain stem regions, severe degeneration in the locus coeruleus, and focal stripe-like softening in the thalamus next to the third ventricle, but terminating immediately before the periventricular nuclei. Spots of glia infiltration were found in this region as well. On the other hand "in the area of the mammillary bodies and the hypothalamus no obvious changes" (p.32f) were noted, while focal neuron-free or neuron-sparse areas were found in the hippocampus, especially in Sommer's sector. (My interpretation of these changes is that they are due to the severe carbon monoxide poisoning.) In the cortex only some diffuse changes without regional concentration were noted.

Tsiminakis' second case was a clerk who died at 39, after consuming about a quarter of a liter of rum per day and other alcoholic beverages; he was incontinent and in quite a poor physical condition. The post-mortem brain examination revealed again a number of affected brain stem loci, especially in the region surrounding the fourth ventricle, damage in the locus coeruleus and the raphe nuclei. The corpora mammillaria were drastically atrophied. The mediodorsal thalamus also showed neuronal degeneration, glia infiltrations and widened blood vessels, though the damage here was not as prominent as in the periventricular sectors. Specific cortical damage was not found.

The third case, a coachman, had had repeated alcohol-based hospital stays (21 times) and died at the age of 69. His physical condition was accompanied by epileptic attacks, hallucinations, and dementia. In spite of the alcoholic background of the patient's physical status, Tsiminakis considered it as proven that this patient had not been a Korsakoff's psychotic, but a simple (alcoholic) dementic. As in the other two cases, a number of brain stem loci were altered, and the periventricular nucleus was affected (with capillary and glia proliferation, bleedings, and ependymal changes). Blood vessels in the cortex had been widened but the cytoarchitecture was not altered.

In comparing the neuropathology of the three cases, Tsiminakis attributed a wider, more diffuse distribution of brain stem alterations to the first as opposed to the second one. For the second case, he found vascular and glia reactions were most prominent with the main focus of the hemorrhages being in the neighborhood of the dorsal portion of the third ventricle. He judged brain damage in the third case to be quite similar to that observed in the second one, but possibly even more restricted.

Tsiminakis' discussion of the comparability of his findings with those of Gamper is highly interesting. He stated that his second case – the (young) clerk – was a typical Korsakoff's patient. Comparing the findings in the brain of this patient with Gamper's results, Tsiminakis remarked that in his case more widespread and more diffuse nuclear damage was existent in the regions surrounding the fourth ventricle, including the nucleus Bechterew and fibers terminating in and arising from the cerebellum.

As to the mammillary bodies – Gamper's nodal points of the damaged zones in Korsakoff's subjects' brains – Tsiminakis emphasized that he confirmed the existence of the damage, but questioned its consistency and severity in Korsakoff's subjects. (I would like to note here that while Tsiminakis based his inferences on only three brains of subjects differing in a wide number of respects, Gamper had had 16 subjects, all of whom were typical Korsakoff's patients according to him.)

Tsiminakis furthermore stressed the likely difference between brain pathology in severe alcoholics (his case 3) and Korsakoffs' (his case 2). For the former he pointed to the severe mammillary body damage, while for the latter he remarked only mild changes in this nucleus. (It seems appropriate at this place to point to the early remark of Gudden that atrophy of the mammillary bodies is frequently associated with complex alcohol neuritis, possibly with any kind of alcoholism.) For Tsiminakis, "the disease process in the region of the elongated nuclear column of the nucleus paraventricularis" (p.55) constitutes the core area of damage in Korsakoff's psychosis.

He concluded from his findings "that the toxic component of diverse processes in the central nervous system may result in a qualitatively and quantitatively similar, if not identical change. On the other hand, neither its character nor its topical focus allow making firm conclusions on the clinical consequences, as the same psychic syndromes may have different anatomical biases, while deviant clinical pictures may follow identical processes in the central nervous system" (p.62).

Carmichael and Stern on the Neuropathological Changes in Korsakoff's Patients

In 1931 Carmichael and Stern gave a very balanced review on the Korsakoff syndrome – in particular on its neuropathology. The authors surveyed a considerbale amount from the international literature – French, German, Swedish, British, and American. They mentioned the findings of a Swedish worker (Marcus) who had published his findings in 1920 on the pathology of the brains of five Korsakoff's patients and had found "lesions ... confined mainly to the frontal region and to the deeper layers of the cortex (p. 194) in acute cases and much brain atrophy in chronic ones". He concluded therefore (according to Carmichael and Stern) "that the outstanding lesion in Korsakoff's syndrome was a parenchymatous degeneration in the cerebral cortex. The changes were greatest in the deepest layer of the cortex, only slight in the superficial layers, whilst the predilection of the process was for the anterior part of the frontal lobes" (p. 194).

Carmichael and Stern's own findings were based on the examination of five cases. In spite of the very careful examination (with the use of, however, stains largely different from those taken by Gamper) the authors failed to detect diencephalic damage (except for a slight change on the thalamic level in one case), but stressed the existence of cerebral cortical changes, most consistently and intensively in the prefrontal and motor areas.

The authors did not try much to integrate their observations into those of others, except for the fact that they assumed a similarity between the brain damage following the alcoholic Korsakoff's syndrome and pellagra, a condition of vitamin malnutrition (cf. Irle & Markowitsch, 1982). One might speculate that the differences between their cases and those of, for example, Gamper (1928 a, 1928 b, 1929), Remy (1942), or Mair et al. (1979) in more recent times could lie in the drinking and eating habits of Carmichael and Stern's cases: Case 1 (a 40-year-old man) "for three to four weeks past ... had had practically no food, but had been drinking large quantities of whisky" (p. 195); case 2 (a 48-year-old man) had lost his appetite and "had drunk 1 to $1^1/_2$ bottles of whisky a day" (p. 199); case 3, a 43-year-old woman who died three days after hospital admission, was described as "a heavy whisky drinker at times ...[with] chronic gastritis" (p. 202 f); similarly, case 4, a woman of 41 years, had been "a regular spirit drinker 'for some time'" (p. 204) and had had eight children; case 5, a 43-year-old woman, was described as "first drinking brandy, then bitters and ale" (p. 206). While the descriptions given were not very detailed, they still indicate that these cases had multiple nutritional problems which might have resulted in cortical neuron damage. Still the failure to detect diencephalic abnormalities remains unexplained.

Kant's Review of the State of the Art in 1932

Under the headline "The pseudoencephalitis Wernicke of the acloholics", Kant (1932) gave a detailed, thorough review of the available material. He first pointed out that Wernicke had given a rather narrow definition of the "alcohol psychoses" and that he had emphasized (Wernicke, 1881) the appearance of symmetrical hemorrhages in the surroundings of the third and fourth ventricle. He then referred to the findings of Gamper (1928 a), Spatz (1929) and Neubürger (1929), all of whom emphasized the atrophy of the mammillary bodies (Neubürger, 1931, p. 192 f. emphasized that softening of the mammillary bodies occurs more frequently than atrophy). Somewhat different from the observations of these authors were the findings of Bonhoeffer (1901), Creutzfeldt (1928), and Troemner (1899), who had detected a large number of small cortical zones of hemorrhage in addition to the mammillary body damage.

Concerning the etiology of Wernicke's pseudoencephalitis, Kant briefly mentioned that it was much more likely to occur in consumers of schnaps than in beer drinkers, where neither he nor Bonhoeffer ever found typical delirious states.

Kant had the opportunity to study 17 cases himself, some of whom were from Gamper's material. He gave a number of thoroughly selected photographs of brain sections which showed the principal loci of damage, especially in the brain stem and on the diencephalic level. Also the description of the neuropsychological results was quite detailed, including for example findings on memory disorders.

Kant emphasized that in all 17 of his cases, the mammillary bodies had been affected, usually showing the most severe damage of all changed loci. Principally, the inner regions were deteriorated most, while the border zones were free of damage. In two cases the mammillary body damage was the only one found. The hypothalamic regions next to the ventricle, the central gray, and the inferior colliculi were the other most commonly degenerated regions. Contrary to Gamper, Kant found the superior colliculi affected in three of the seventeen cases affected as well. Dot- and ring-shaped bleedings were not uncommon; they occurred in 11 of the 17 cases. Liquor changes were not detected.

One of the core sentences within the conclusions of Kant's paper was that "Wernicke's disease and Korsakoff's psychosis are one and the same, only the more severe expression of the focal neurological symptoms of the brain stem gave the impetus to discriminate pseudoencephalitis from Korsakoff's disease" (p. 760). Another core idea was that (in accordance with Stertz', 1931, findings) Korsakoff's syndrome may occur with and without involvement of the cerebral cortex (p. 762). Lastly, Kant emphasized that women in comparison to men have a higher likeliness of developing Korsakoff's syndrome as the strength of resistance of their tissue is lower than in the male sex. While infiltration via the liquor seems intriguing and has been commented on (Markowitsch & Pritzel, 1985) in the light of the results of Shashua and Schmidt (Shashoua, 1982; Schmidt & Shashoua, 1981, 1983), Kant argued against such a possibility by pointing out that central regions are more likely changed than peripheral ones in Wernicke's and Korsakoff's disease.

In my eyes the early results of Gamper, Kant, Neubürger, and the many colleagues cited in Kant's paper taken together, principally contain the same information which was later given in the thorough monograph of Victor et al. (1989) and the paper of Mair et al. (1979), to list just two examples. Particularly, the symmetry in the degeneration of the mammillary nuclei and the thalamic structures has been emphasized repeatedly as in the studies of Neubürger (1931), Colmant (1965) and Mair et al. (1979).

Korsakoff's Syndrome in the Time before the Second World War

A number of further articles appeared on the alcoholic Korsakoff syndrome in the decades between 1910 and 1940. In many of these the authors tried to further characterize the syndrome and to find out why memory disorders were so prominent in this complex. In other articles the combination of Korsakoff's psychosis with delirious states (progressive paralysis) was investigated (Pfeifer, 1928), or psychoanalytic interpretations of emotional and mnestic behavioral changes in Korsakoff's psychosis were given (Betlheim & Hartmann, 1924, 1951).

Gamper (1928 a, 1928 b, 1929) supposed that the principal deficit of Korsakoff's patients lies in their inability to form a spatial-temporal background, "... which in normals comprehends in passive attentiveness the basis of the temporal-spatial integration of a distinct event complex in the mnestic continuum" (Gamper, 1929, p. 238). In referring to the finding that Korsakoff's subjects frequently still possess the ability to perform the most complicated combinatory processes (calculating ability; see above: *Mathematical abilities versus episodic memory*), he argued that in experimental examination the ability to remember (short term) was hardly altered; what was altered in Gamper's eyes is the ability to embed an event into its proper context which therefore results in its loss.

The contribution of Grünthal (1932) has the same line of arguments. Like Pick (1915), Grünthal protocolled his talks with Korsakoff's patients (and published them word by word, which alone resulted in roughly 28 pages). In addition to analyzing the protocols, Grünthal gave a number of psychological tests to one of his own cases, a 22-year old medical student, who, for instance, admitted that he once drank "prophylactically 28 glasses of schnaps against influenza" (p. 117).

From the discussion between Grünthal and the patient it became evident several times that the patient had some knowledge of time and place but "hung in the air with his dates" so that for instance he switched back and forth between Munich (correct), Rome and Ravenna (both incorrect) and between saying that today was the 18th and yesterday had been the 9th. Corrections with respect to time and place he accepted apathetically.

The same phenomenon was described and discussed at length by Pick (1915). His patient thought he was 17 years old, but in fact he was married and already had four children. Pick stated that his patient "under full consciousness" (p. 346) kept to both statements, that is, Pick excluded the possibility that the patient just might have lost remembrance of his first sentence. Nevertheless, additional answers of the patient revealed that he had some feeling that his argumentation was not logical.

Grünthal assumed that the memory disorder of his patient (who later recovered) was due to an incorrect adjustment or mental attitude to the material remembered. He concluded: "A closer look through the publications reveals for nearly every case ... a clue to the fact that the ability to memorize has not been lost completely, and that instead surprisingly traces of remembrance can be found now and then. Korsakoff already mentioned that events from the time of the illness can emerge in patients after years. Kalberlah as well emphasized that the ability to memorize is never completely lost. Similarly, Boedeker (1905) stated "that the degree of the memory disorder is not always on the same level but fluctuates within certain limits without making it possible to say why this occurs ... beyond doubt, the ability of attentiveness is a changing one" (p. 129f).

Before Grünthal, Steinthal (1921) had given an extensive description of a former officer with Korsakoff's psychosis. Steinthal discussed in detail the psychic defects of his patient and explained why on the basis of the observed abilities and disabilities the diagnosis 'Korsakoff's psychosis' was justified, while labeling the patient as 'dementic' or 'schizophrenic' was not.

Hartmann (1930) reviewed results of others in which some savings for learned material could be demonstrated (Brodmann, 1902, 1904; Gregor, 1907, 1909). He referred to one of the publications of van der Horst (see below) who had stated that the principal disturbance of Korsakoff's patients lies within their ego, "the relation of the contents to its place in personal time experience" (p. 497) being disturbed. Hartmann then asked the reverse question: What is preserved in Korsakoff's psychosis? He gave his six patients six short stories of one or two sentences length which had to be reproduced at later times. Parts of the stories were of emotional content, others were emotionally indifferent. He found that the patients were able to better reproduce the more emotional stories. Frequently, the content appeared, however, somewhat distorted; for example, human sexual organs and coitus were given different, less obvious names. Hartmann concluded from these results that the ability to reproduce material is affected by its emotional content, a finding which has been made repeatedly since then (see, e.g., Markowitsch et al., 1984, 1986; Ziehen, 1908, p. 14). Another report on recovery from Korsakoff's syndrome was given by Siebert (1933).

Case descriptions were made in 1904 and 1930 by the psychologist Stephan Krauss which became rather influential (at least within Germany) in the discussion of the phenomenon of Korsakoff's psychosis. Krauss was of the opinion that Korsakoff's psychotics had a reduced apprehension so that they recognized given stimuli or events slower and with greater difficulty than normals. Furthermore Krauss (1904) assumed that the (engram) traces disappeared at a much faster rate than they did in normals (cf. the present-day discussions of this context by Huppert & Piercy, 1979, 1982).

As a final point, I would like to mention the articles of Remy (1942) and Riggs and Boles (1942). The last mentioned authors found the mammillary bodies to be damaged in all 42 of their examined cases with – what they termed – Wernicke's disease. Of interest are especially their Tables 6 and 7. In Table 6 the location of brain lesions was given for 29 cases, subdivided into five loci within the cerebral hemispheres, four within the hypothalamus, three within the thalamus, four within the midbrain, seven within the brain stem, and the cerebellum; in Table 7 the clinical and neuropathological findings were given individually for the 29 cases for which this information was available.

Remy (1942), working in Grünthal's laboratory, had done a painstaking analysis of the brain pathology of a Korsakoff's case who had remained stationary for ten years and who had been free of any delirious signs. The brain damage was found exclusively confined to the mammillary bodies "without any other metamorphosis in the diencephalon, mesencephalon and telencephalon" (p. 144).

Chronognosia

In line with frequent descriptions of others (e.g., Grünthal, 1932, 1939; Grünthal & Störring, 1930, 1933; Pick, 1915; Steinthal, 1921) Krauss (1930) pointed to the discrepancy between an undisturbed intelligence and a changed nature of drives and will. While Korsakoff's patients lack insight into their illness, they still manifest a number of uncertainties which indicate that they know that something is wrong with them (p. 651). 'Time consciousness' was a key expression of Krauss (1930) for describing the cognitive problems of Korsakoff's patients. The patient (a butcher) whom Krauss presented in 1930 was totally stoic in behavior, had no desires, no interests, no anxiety, restlessness, or doubts.

According to Krauss (1930) van der Horst (1928) was the first to define the central symptom of Korsakoff's patients, namely the fact that these patients had lost "the temporal signs of the events", showing an "amorphism of the time sense". Krauss furthermore cited the paper of Bouman and Gruenbaum (1929) who differentiated between three levels of time consciousness: "chronognosia" (unreflected, immanent experience of time), "chronologia" (comparing the inner history with the external), and "chronometria" (total objectivity and measurement of time). In the patient of Bouman and Gruenbaum time consciousness had shrunk from 30 years to three years with every event still in the correct chronological order but reduced ten times in time compared to the actual time period. The patient for example remarked: "Between picking blackberries and picking blackberries there is one whole year. Suddenly, however, I realized that between the last and the present picking only two months had passed." When asked whether hours were equal in time he responded: "That's the way one has to think. This is assumed by those who understand the time. I do not understand the time ...". And Grünthal's (1932) patient stated "I have lost all feeling for time" and "I can determine my time only by the clock and I assume it [the clock] works wrong" (p. 108). Two further cases with left-hemispheric thalamic infarcts and disturbances of the sense of time were given by A. M. Becker and Sternbach (1953), and another, early report on disturbances of time comprehension was given by Ehrenwald (1931). In Becker and Sternbach's (1953) first case, time seemed to run compromised so that years shrank to months. In their second case, the contrary phenomenon occurred, time seemed to extend indefinite so that a day would never pass. This patient could, however, be cured pharmacologically.

Scheid (1935) interpreted the memory behavior of a Korsakoff's patient as being much less time-bound than in normals. Furthermore, his patient said he dreamed what he in fact had experienced. The author had the special opportunity to see his patient, a 48-year-old American teacher, under what he called "experimental" or "natural" conditions, namely by accompanying him during a trip from Munich to New York. For a more recent discussion of disorientation (and therefore a disturbance in time) in Korsakoff's syndrome see Scheller (1961) and Liebaldt and Scheller (1971).

I wish to comment briefly on this fascinating phenomenon which can, at least in related forms ("speeded-up motion") also be found in other abnormal states of minds such as in a mescaline-delirium (Beringer, 1927; R. Fischer,

1946) and after right parietal lobe damage (Hoff & Pötzl, 1938). This phenomenon is also documented in the reviews of Häfner (1953, 1954) and Pötzl (1939) and in the more recent articles on this subject written by Gloning, Gloning, and Hoff (1955), Pötzl (1951, 1958), and by J. Brown (1990).

In a series of studies with mediodorsal stereotaxic thalamotomy, Spiegel and coworkers (Spiegel & Wycis, 1949, 1955; Spiegel, Wycis, Freed, & Orchinik, 1953; Spiegel, Wycis, Orchinik, & Freed, 1956; Wycis, 1972) found that what they termed "chronotaraxis" constitutes the major symptom following surgery. "Chronotaraxis is characterized by an inability to identify the date; the patient may not know the time of the day, may make incorrect statements regarding the season of the year though this is obvious if he looks through the window" (Spiegel et al., 1956, p. 97). Therefore it seems likely that the change in the dorsal thalamus is responsible for changes in the ability to estimate time or for controlling the dimension of time altogether. Thus the findings of Spiegel and coworkers (cf. also Markowitsch, 1982) confirm the view that a true Korsakoff's symptomatology is neuropathologically accompanied by damage to the mediodorsal thalamic zone. Related findings on disturbances of the time sense in diencephalic damaged patients were made by Häfner (1954).

Coming back to Krauss' (1930) article: Krauss argued that "Korsakoff's syndrome consists of a characteristic interplay of performance- ("Handlungs-"), time- and memory-disorders, in the course of which we see the lack of psychic activity in the change to inner performance or action, which impedes the formation of constructed entities" (p. 689).

Three years later van der Horst (1932) wrote a German-language publication "Über die Psychologie des Korsakowsyndroms". He gave a number of examples on the disturbance of the sense of time in Korsakoff's subjects, both from other sources and from his own observations. Some patients, for example, stated 15 minutes after having had a cigar: "Yes, I have had a cigar, but that was last week" (p. 70) or when an assistent entered and then left the room: "Yes, he was here yesterday."

Recently, investigators who prolonged the exposure time to stimuli in Korsakoff's patients (Huppert & Piercy, 1977, 1978, 1979), were able to confirm van der Horst's conclusion: "As the temporal factor is very important in remembering, we can state a priori with respect to the existence of amnesia that in Korsakoff's patients occasionally few or no memory defects will be observed, as when encoding occurred in a way in which the temporalization played no role" (p. 71). As Korsakoff's subjects have no consciousness of time contiguity, they work with "pieces of time" and "points of time" (p. 74). In van der Horst's argumentation they are able to work with weeks and days, but they have lost the ability to experience their duration. (Consequently, they may also deteriorate in their ability to attend with the effect of further memory deterioration: cf. W. G. Smith, 1895.)

'Disorientation in time' constitutes one of the first symptoms and the inability to estimate time epochs takes longest for recovery, van der Horst stated. One could mention here the frequent findings in animal experimentation and human case analyses on prefrontal cortex damaged subjects which indicate a function of this cortical region in time analysis (e.g., Fuster, 1989; Markowitsch & Pritzel, 1977, 1987). The prefrontal cortex is the principal projection area of the thalamic mediodorsal nucleus (Markowitsch & Pritzel, 1979; Markowitsch, Pritzel, Wilson, & Divac, 1980; Van Buren & Borke, 1972).

Van der Horst summarized: "The actual comprehension of time and time as a principle of order are disturbed. This is most likely the basic defect of the Korsakoff's syndrome" (p. 83). In his last paragraph he mentioned that Wernicke had already assumed that the defect in Korsakoff's lies in "allopsychic orientation" and not in the field of memory.

Taking up the tradition of van der Horst (1928, 1932) and Krauss (1930), Kleist (1934 a) assumed the anterograde memory defects of Korsakoff's patients were attributable to an unclear and erroneous determination of time and of the temporal or chronological integration of recently experienced events. For Kleist true memory defects were caused by cortical damage while the time-related or time-dependent amnesia was caused by mammillary body damage (the same view was somewhat later expressed by Benedek & Juba, 1940, 1941; cf. also Morsier, 1929, and Marchan & Courtois, 1934).

In 1939 Grünthal discussed the hypotheses of Gamper, Kleist, van der Horst, and others. He disagreed with their assumptions and conclusions. Based on his anatomical studies in animals and man, particularly on the study of the one case of a 40-year-old stoker (cf. above under the heading: *Mathematical abilities versus episodic memory*), who had a tumor-based complete, isolated atrophy of the mammillary bodies, Grünthal argued that in Korsakoff's patients "disturbances in adjustment and re-adjustment of thinking" (p. 89) are prevalent. "The principal defect appears to lie in the inability to relate an actual experience to the total experience of the personality. The patient is fully engaged in the momentaneously experienced situation ... The ability of 'circumspection' in the most direct sense of the word, ... is lost" (p. 90). Reasons for this deficit lie, according to Grünthal, in the passive, aspontaneous personality, living in a suspensed manner (cf. also Grünthal, 1936 b).

Though Grünthal was apparently unaware of Papez's influential paper (Papez, 1937), he argued along somewhat similar lines when relating the mammillary bodies to the anterior thalamus and the anterior thalamus then "with the dorsal portions of the agranular frontal cortex" (p. 92). The lack of mammillary impulses to the prefrontal cortex resulted, he said, in diminishing or losing the activity for relating experiences and events.

Chapter 7: Diencephalic Amnesia

"The role of the thalamus is one of the most interesting and most important problems" (Dercum, 1925, p. 289). With this sentence Dercum started his talk on the occassion of the fortieth anniversary of the foundation of the Philadelphia Neurological Society in 1924. Then he gave a description of the phylogenetic development of the thalamus and of its relation to the cortex. Under the normal conditions of the brain, the cortex would inhibit the thalamus, while in the damaged brain this inhibition would be strongly altered.

Dercum assumed that "consciousness is the property of the neurons actually engaged in the train of transmission through the cortex. This is the 'conscious field'. Further, all consciousness is attended by 'feeling' ..." (p. 293). Dercum went on by stating that the basic importance of the thalamus lies in the fact that it is the seat of all sensations, feelings, and emotions so that under normal conditions the interactions of cortex and thalamus" favor and lead to the safety, the success, the comfort, the pleasure and the happiness of the organism" (p. 294).

Tumors and Degenerations

About one percent of cerebral tumors are primarily thalamic (Cheek & Taveras, 1966; McKissock & Paine, 1958). While this number is most likely smaller than that of thalamic damage following chronic alcohol abuse, mention should be made of some tumor-based cases and of some of the even much rarer degenerative lesion-based cases on the thalamic level. One of the first major reports on neural tumors, Bruns' (1897) book on "Die Geschwülste des Nervensystems", did not contain the description of a thalamic tumor-case. Probably among the first thalamic cases described was that of Schüle (1899): The patient, a 16-year-old girl, died within two months after the first appearance of symptoms. The gliosarcoma was situated in the medial portion of the left thalamus and was massive (Fig. 29). Unfortunately the neurological and psychological examinations did not relate anything on the girl's cognitive performance. Vision was reduced, walking movements and body balance disturbed. Soon after this time, the "thalamic syndrome" became prominent (Dejerine & Roussy, 1906; Roussy, 1907; cf. also the review of Langworthy & Fox, 1937).

In 1922 Dandy described the "diagnosis, localization and removal of tumors of the third ventricle". In spite of the ambitious title the report was quite short – less than 200 words in length – and consisted of only one case. No mention was made of psychological or neurological changes pre- or postoperatively.

A larger series of thalamic and third ventricle tumors was included in the 368-page long book of P. Schuster (1902). He began his introduction on thalamic tumors with the statement that these are "diversified" (p. 163). He referred to several cases which had been published in German- and non-German-language journals at the end of the nineteenth century and then gave a detailed description of one of his own cases, which was characterized on the psychological level by a strong inclination towards crying. The patient had been 18-years old and had had heavy headaches since $2^1/_2$ years. Post-mortem examination of her brain revealed a tumor which may have originated in the pulvinar area of both hemispheres, but had infiltrated the total thalamic substance.

P. Schuster then listed in tabellary form 16 further cases in which mental deterioration was a prominent symptom. In three of these cases pure memory disorder with intact intelligence was remarked.

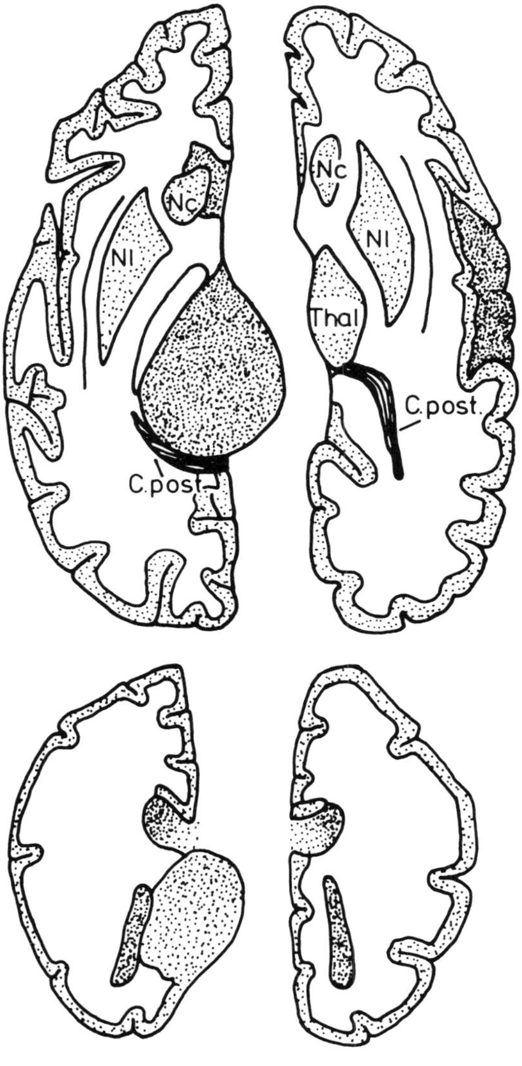

Figure 29. Appearance of the thalamic tumor in the left hemisphere of the brain of the 16-year-old maid observed by Schüle (1899). The extent and locus of the tumor are shown in a horizontal (top) and a coronal (bottom) section. In the horizontal section the length of the tumor is 5.4 cm, the width 4 cm; in the coronal section the height is 4 cm. Abbreviations: C. post., commissura posterior; Nc, nucleus caudatus; Nl, nucleus lentiformis; Thal., thalamus.

It is astonishing that at this time memory disturbances were already reported after thalamic damage (cf. Martin, Yap, Nei, & Tan, 1983 for a recent publication on selective thalamic degeneration). Much later, for instance in 1933, Stertz still emphasized thalamic involvement in mainly vegetative functions, especially the regulation of sleep (which, however, is not without justification either: cf., e.g., Beyerman, 1912; Bushnell & Duncan, 1989). (In 1937, however, Lhermitte et al. described the occurrence of Korsakoff's symptomatology in a case with a tumor of the third ventricle.)

A substantial survey of the consequences of damage in the areas surrounding the third ventricle was given by Högner (1927); his report contains 119 references. He listed cases with vegetative disturbances, including pupillary reactions, disturbances of vasomotilation, sweat secretation, sphincter control, and temperature, glucosuria, a disturbed salt and water conservation, adiposity, sleep disturbances, and sudden death. In addition, he mentioned the occurrence of disturbed consciousness and epileptic attacks.

Ependymal cysts are rather frequently found in the third ventricle, as described by Bruns (1897), (cf. Bailey & Auvrey, 1928; Beal, Kleinman, Ojemann, & Hochberg, 1981; Bassoe, 1916; Burkle & Lipowski, 1978; Cairns & Mosberg, 1951; Carmel, 1985; Dandy, 1933; Drennan, 1929; Geffen, Walsh, Simpson, & Jeeves, 1980; Horrax & Bailey, 1928; Lhermitte, 1922; Lobosky, Van Gilder, & Damasio, 1984; E. Meyer, 1899; Nitta & Symon, 1985; Piazza, 1909; Rabinowitsch, 1925; Riddoch, 1936; Sachs, Avman, & Fisher, 1962; Sprofkin & Sciarra, 1952; Trescher & Ford, 1937; Weisenburg, 1910; S. A. K. Wilson, 1906).

In 1934 Foerster and Gagel already mentioned 31 cases from various sources in the literature between 1858 and 1932. Though this number sounds impressive, exactly the same number of cases had been documented in 1910 in Weisenburg's table, given on pages 238-243. Foerster and Gagel themselves first reported the case of a 54-year-old patient who after removal of an ependymal cyst in the third ventricle recovered completely from his amnesic and other disturbances. Before removal of the cyst he had been disoriented with respect to time and place and had a very poor anterograde and retrograde memory. Even his ability to calculate had been quite deficient (5 x 7 = 40, 5 x 17 = 32). In 1932 he regarded Emperor Wilhelm II as the present ruler of Germany.

Following removal of the cyst the patient regained orientation in time and place and the ability to remember new events, learned a new game of cards, and was able to calculate accurately. However, he had a complete retrograde amnesia of about one-and-a-half months duration (the time prior to his surgery and for a few days thereafter).

The authors then described the cases of six further patients who died in spite of surgical interventions. In these patients the tumor was generally more basal (and sometimes more posterior), originating in the hypothalamic or hypophyseal area. The patients were characterized as maniacal. Foerster and Gagel closed their report with the comment that up to then they had had experience with altogether 70 cases with tumors of the hypothalamus or of the quadrigeminal plate. Manic-depressive psychoses in cases with diencephalic tumors were also described by Pötzl (1938).

Da Fano's Analysis of Neuronal Changes in Paralytic and Senile Dementia and Three Related Reports

One of the early papers which tried to relate psychological changes to abnormalities in the thalamus was Da Fano's contribution from 1909. For his analysis the author had "five cases with dementia paralytica, three with dementia arterio-sclerotica, and two of dementia senilis" (p. 4). Interestingly, though one would not expect it, Da Fano, similar to numerous old studies, cited some dozen articles which noted investigations on possible relations between dementic states and dorsal diencephalic changes, and an even larger number of reports on relations between dementia and other regional brain changes.

What he found were alterations similar to those which Alzheimer (1907) for example had described, namely as Da Fano described it "an abnormal increase of pigments in the cell body" (p. 17). As is emphasized in present-day research, these cell changes need not have pathological consequences as long as their number remains low. This fact had already been known to Da Fano, as he wrote on page 17.

Da Fano concluded (p. 23) that in paralytic dementia the neuronal changes in the thalamus show no major differences from those in other regions of the central nervous system. The changes include demyelination, fiber degeneration, blood vessel and glia proliferation, pigment sedation in the neurons and neuronal atrophy extending up to a total loss of the chromatic and fibrillary substance. Da Fano also noted fibrillary disintegration with "their metamorphosis into irregular pieces and particles" (p. 24).

As Da Fano documented in a number of figures, he found the fibrillary changes (bundles) which are seen today as characteristic for Alzheimer's dementia in his brains of senile dementics and in what he termed the brain of subjects with "dementia arteriosclerotica" (p. 24 ff). He pointed out differences between the cell and fiber changes he had found in paralytic dementic cases on the one hand, and those he had found in cases with arteriosclerotic and senile dementia on the other, and thought that these differences might be important for differentiating the primarily age-related "organic psychoses" from the other ones. Da Fano commented in great detail on plaques and tangles and noted that his descriptions were directly comparable with the observations O. Fischer (1907) had made.

While this article is of importance as one of the early documents on neuronal changes in the brains of senile dementics, Da Fano's last speculation on interpreting the fibrillary changes as regenerative processes turned out to be wrong.

It is interesting that Pfeifer (1910) after reviewing the literature stated that "we do not know whether any psychic functions may be attributed to the thalamus ["Sehhügel"] (p. 653). His own two cases (Nos. 61 and 62) with thalamic tumors demonstrated Korsakoff's psychosis in a clear manner, as he remarked. In case No. 61 both thalami had changed into a gray-red tumorous mass. In case No. 62 the posterior two thirds of the thalamus were encapsulated by a small walnut-sized tumor with softened surroundings; in the basal part of the posterior half of the right thalamus a second pea-sized tumor was found, again with softened surroundings. While for the first case moderate drinking was acknowledged, no mention was made of alcohol dependence for the second one. However, Pfeifer gave a particularly clear and detailed description of the latter patient's condition which mirrored Korsakoff's syndrome.

Before Da Fano, three German-language papers dealt with thalamic changes induced by progressive paralysis: Heinrich L. Lissauer is known for the description of Lissauer's tract (tractus dorsolateralis) and of Lissauer's marginal zone (zona terminalis of the spinal cord), and for defining what later became known as Lissauer's paralysis or the Lissauer-type of general paresis (Lissauer, 1890 b) – despite the fact that he only reached an age of 30 years.

While working in Wernicke's clinic, Lissauer (1890 a) noted thalamic changes in nine cases of progressive paralysis. The degeneration was most marked in the posterior thalamus, in particular the nucleus pulvinaris and appeared to progress from posterior to anterior. According to his observations, the degeneration in the thalamus was secondary, that is, it resulted from primary degeneration in the cortical mantle (p. 564). Zagari (1893) principally confirmed Lissauer's observations, though he stated that he had failed to confirm the close relations between thalamic damage and progressive paralysis as they had been stated by Lissauer (p. 106).

Lastly, Schultze (1898) made a major contribution on possible relations between thalamic pathology and progressive paralysis. As Lissauer before him, he emphasized the involvement of the pulvinar. He also stressed the similarity of his and Lissauer's results by writing that the thalamus is an index which provides in a condensed and synoptic way information on degenerated cortical foci. Schultze commented on the differences between Lissauer's and Zagari's interpretations of observed thalamic changes and concluded that Zagari was in higher concordance with Lissauer than he himself had supposed.

P. Schuster's Contributions to the Pathology of the Optical Thalamus

Aside from his early monograph (P. Schuster, 1902), Paul Schuster later published four articles in 1936 and in 1937 of altogether more than 200 pages (Schuster, 1936 a, 1936 b, 1937 a, 1937 b). He reported the case histories of 26 patients who were supposed to have pathological changes in the thalamus and classified his cases according to disruption of particular arteries invading the thalamus. These would be the regions of invasion of two arteriae: *thalamo-perforata*, invading ventral parts of the posterior mediodorsal nucleus; and the *tubero-thalamica*, invading the anterior ventral part of the mediodorsal thalamic nucleus (cf. George, Raybaud, Salamon, & Kircheff, 1975, for a description of the anatomy of the thalamo-perforating arteries).

The cases in which mediodorsal thalamic changes were observed (cases 8–11, 21, 26; median age of the patients at onset of hospitalization: 69 years; range: 49–75 years) were of limited value for an assignment of specific functions to the mediodorsal nucleus, as the damaged regions were mostly asymmetrical and infiltrated a multitude of other regions in addition. It should, however, be emphasized that, in spite of substantial damage to thalamic regions, memory impairment was not among the characteristic symptoms registered in the six patients. This was also true for case 26, a patient whose left thalamus had almost disappeared, together with the adjacent hypothalamus and internal capsule (P. Schuster, 1936 b, p. 588). The one patient (case 25) in whom P. Schuster noted considerable dementia had had a tumor which included among other areas the whole caudate nucleus and putamen on the right side, the whole lateral border of the right thalamus, and further parts from the anterior two-thirds of the right thalamus. Destruction of the mediodorsal nucleus was not mentioned.

A Cyst, Tumors, Infarcts, and the Degeneration of the Thalamus: Contributions in the Fourth Decade of this Century

As I mentioned in the description of Da Fano's (1909) paper, it is astonishing how many earlier articles the old authors could refer to. Foerster and Gagel (1934) listed 28 earlier papers (with altogether 31 cases) with cysts within the third ventricle.

Foerster and Gagel's case nevertheless is an exception in the authors' eyes "not only because of its special symptomatology, but also ..., because it is the first case in which the tumor was removed operatively and the case could not only survive due to this, but was also freed from its symptoms" (p. 313). (The authors may not be correct with this statement since, as I mentioned above, Dandy in 1922 had already briefly described the removal of a cyst and noted that their patient recovered from the operation.)

Clarifying the role of the mediodorsal thalamus in memory related mechanisms is confounded by the reports of Kleist and Gonzalo (1938) and Grünthal (1942). Only in the second of Kleist and Gonzalo's two cases (patient Mandel) was considerable destruction of the right mediodorsal thalamus noted. This infarct-caused destruction was considered to have resulted in affective disorders, whereas changes in memory were not reported. In his article "Über thalamische Demenz" Grünthal described a female patient whose most prominent brain damage was a symmetrical degeneration of the mediodorsal thalamus. Small parts of additional thalamic nuclei and the red nucleus were also degenerated. The damage had probably been caused by thrombosis in the arteria thalamo-perforata (Fig. 30). Grünthal considered damage of the mediodorsal nucleus to be the most likely cause of the patient's progressive dementia appearing during the last ten years of her stay in a psychiatric hospital. The patient, however, cannot be considered a typical case as her mother and all three children and she herself were described by Grünthal as having always been feebleminded too.

Speculations on a direct relationship between impaired memory functions and damage of the mediodorsal thalamic nucleus arose particularly from cases described by Smyth and K. Stern (1938) and by K. Stern (1939) (cf. for example, Horel, 1978, p. 428, and Schulman, 1956, 1957). Of the six case histories presented by Smyth and K. Stern (1938) it is most likely that three of them died from tumors which originated and spread outwards from the midline nuclei of the thalamus. In four patients, mental deterioration, particularly various forms of amnesia, were prominent. In case 3, tumorous tissue "appeared to involve almost the whole of the left optic thalamus [although] a very small rim of the thalamus along the medial (ventricular) surface seemed to be preserved" (p. 350). Microscopic examination of the thalamus revealed that while nerve cells could still be seen in the mediodorsal nucleus, the pulvinar had been replaced entirely by tumorous tissue. White matter, surrounding the hippocampus, was infiltrated by the tumor as well. Case 4 could be characterized by a tumor in the left thalamus, reaching from the anterior nucleus to the posterior tip of the pulvinar. Furthermore, "almost the entire white matter of the temporal lobe lateral to the inferior horn" (p. 353) and parts of the Wernicke field were infiltrated.

In case 5 the left thalamus was almost completely destroyed, once again including the nucleus pulvinaris. Further, medial thalamic regions of the right hemisphere and portions of tissue around the left hippocampal area had also been infiltrated. Lastly, in case 6, the posterior part of the left thalamus, the mediodorsal nucleus on both sides, Forel's fields, the zona incerta, and the Wernicke region were the main centers which had shown tumorous destruction.

The patients were 64, 67, 63, and 44 years old at the beginning of hospitalization. All four died within about one month thereafter. As "the tumours were large and had led to abnormally high intracranial pressure and ventricular dilatation" (p. 369) in cases 3 and 4, Smyth and K. Stern (1938) considered a critical evaluation of their mental state as worthless. For cases 5 and 6, the authors suggested a connection between the occurrence of dementia and the bilateral invasion of the mediodorsal thalamus,

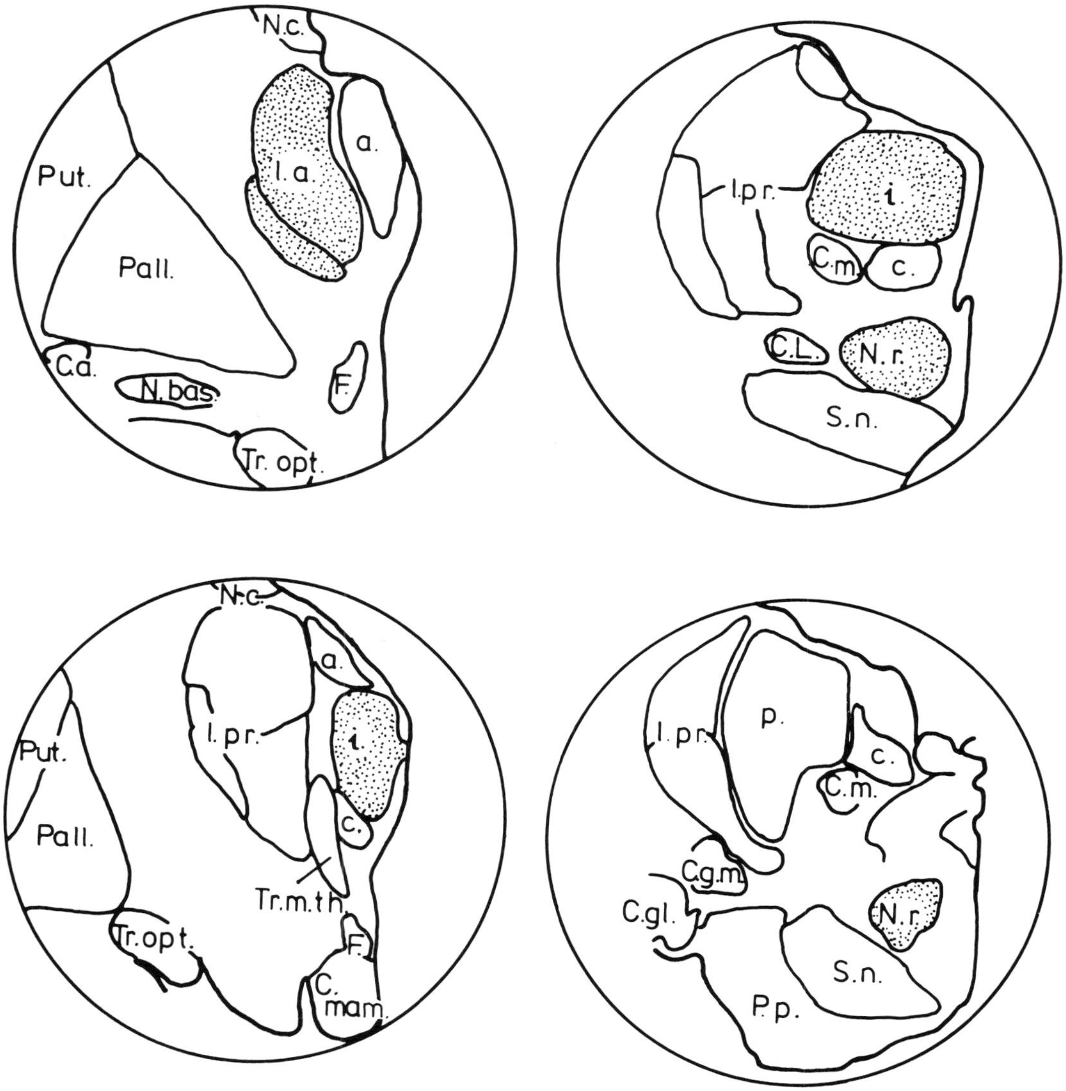

Figure 30. The extent and locus of the thalamic lesion described by Grünthal (1942). The atrophic areas are stippled. The figure part on the top left is at level 20, top right at level 40, bottom left at level 190, and bottom right at level 210, according to the atlas included in Grünthal (1934). Abbreviations: a., nucleus anterior; C., nucleus circularis ; C. a., commissura anterior; C. gl., corpus geniculatum laterale; G. g. m., Corpus geniculatum mediale; C. L., corpus Luysi; C. m., centrum medianum (Luys); F., fornix; i, nucleus internus; l. p. r., nucleus lateralis principalis; N. bas., nucleus basalis; N. c., nucleus caudatus; p., nucleus pulvinaris; Pall., pallidum; P. p., pes pedunculi; Put., putamen; S. n., substantia nigra; Tr. m. th., tractus mammillo-thalamicus; Tr. opt., tractus opticus. (After Fig. 1 of Grünthal, 1942.)

though they considered such a relation to be "admittedly conjectural" (p. 370). A. E. Walker (1940), in reviewing this report (as well as that of P. Schuster, 1936a, mentioned above), doubted the significance of Smyth and K. Stern's findings for an interpretation of the function of the mediodorsal nucleus, owing to the diffuseness of the thalamic damage observed.

In an evaluation of these cases, and of the case reported by K. Stern (1939), the involvement of regions next to the hippocampus and the temporal cortex should not be neglected. In addition to diffuse changes in the temporal cortex, the posterior parietal, small parts of the prefrontal cortex, and the posterior limbic region were affected in the patient of K. Stern. This 41-year-old man furthermore had an almost symmetrical degeneration of most of the thalamic nuclei. Similarities to both the Korsakoff and the Klüver-Bucy syndrome (Klüver, 1958; Klüver & Bucy, 1937, 1939; Marlowe, Mancall, & Thomas, 1975; Shraberg & Weisberg, 1978) were apparent. Figure 6 from K. Stern's report reveals that attributing the cause of dementia to damage of the mediodorsal thalamic nucleus goes beyond the data. In this figure the approximate extent of cortical areas which correspond to degenerated thalamic nuclei is visualized. These areas include, in addition to the dorsalateral prefrontal cortex, the motor cortex, the parietal and partly the occipital cortex, and most of the cingulate regions.

Chapter 8: The Corpus Callosum

To include the corpus callosum in a survey on the intellectual functions, in particular memory, may appear somewhat odd and unjustified. However, the situation was different at earlier times. This is best documented in Schuster's (1902) monograph. Aside from discussing his own cases (p. 141 ff), at the end of his book in chapter 15 he analyzed the frequency of psychic disturbances following tumors in different brain regions by comparing cases with similar localized tumors with and without psychic disturbances. He took the results of Gianelli (1897) as supporting his findings. Altogether Gianelli had collected data on 588 cases – 265 tumor cases without and 323 with psychic involvement. Figure 31 reproduces the results which Schuster presented and illustrated in his Table f. Lemke (1937, p. 66) stated that "the complete loss of memory for a long time was considered to be a callosal syndrome" and Mayer-Gross, Slater, and Roth (1969) much later noted that "[t]umours involving the anterior two-thirds of the *corpus callosum* produce a mental picture that is indistinguishable from the frontal lobe syndrome" (p. 494).

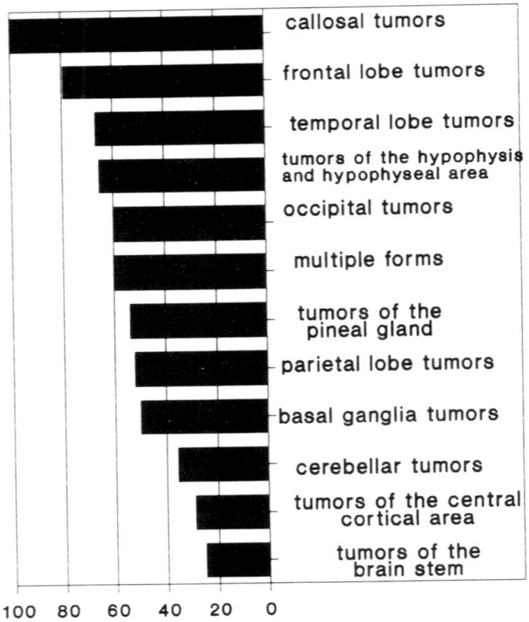

Figure 31. The percentage of tumors in different regions of the brain (bottom, 0–100%), resulting in psychic disturbances. Data from Schuster (1902, Table f), who had based them on the findings of Gianelli (1897).

Reference should also be made to P.C. Knapp (1906) who made similar surveys and tabulations as had been done by Bruns and Gianelli, and who had the same view as these authors. His argumentation for the importance of the callosal fibers was, however, based on a largely incorrect assumption of their course, as when he stated (P.C. Knapp, 1906, p. 47 ff):

> It is readily conceivable, assuming that a given association tract with a definite function runs from the occipital lobe, that a lesion in any one of the three regions might break the conduction and give rise to the same phenomena of deficit, just as a lesion anywhere from the cuneus to the chiasma may give rise to the same symptom of deficit – hemianopsia. It is not unlikely that disturbances in the higher visual centres in the occipital region in Flechsig's posterior association centre, may be responsible for much of the disorientation of confusional states, for example, and that the special phenomena of attention, and many of the ideas of personality, are dependent upon associated processes in the frontal lobes; but this is still undetermined, and the cases at present under consideration unfortunately give no definite information upon the subject.

In 1875 Pick already referred to a contribution which Wigan had written in 1844 ("*Duality of mind*") explaining the phenomenon of "double consciousness" as caused by an independent action of the two hemispheres. Artom (1923,

p. 119) strongly emphasized that Korsakoff-like amnesic states more likely follow callosal than temporal lobe damage, and Donath (1923) was of the opinion that the effects of callosal lesions correspond to those of the prefrontal cortex (and for the prefrontal cortex he reserved the highest psychic functions). A few years later then, the contribution from cortical somata and from callosal fibers was differentiated (e.g., Niessl von Mayendorf, 1930).

The corpus callosum and especially cases in which it was missing in the human brain had long fascinated authors (cf. e.g. Arndt & Sklarek, 1903; Kaufmann, 1887, 1888; Mingazzini, 1922; Onufrowicz, 1887; Probst, 1901 b; H. Vogt, 1905), as the corpus callosum constitutes the largest interhemispheric fiber system in the primate brain, but is non-existent in the most primitive forms of mammalian species. An old paper on the non-existence of the corpus callosum was Sander's (1868 b). He referred to an earlier survey of Griesinger (1867/1964) and then mentioned ten cases with sufficient information which had been described earlier, starting in the year 1812. He (1868 b) concluded that there were two principal functions attributed to the callosal fiber system: "it either should transmit coordination, or should be the substrate of higher mental functions" (p. 138) and "that the task of the corpus callosum would then be important enough if it controlled ordered thinking and hindered ideas and thoughts created on each individual side from intermingling in a confusing way" (p. 139). Lack of a corpus callosum was usually associated with feeblemindedness (e.g., Arndt & Sklarek, 1903).

Zingerle in 1900 described a "50-year-old Catholic, married construction worker from the Steiermark" (p. 367) who died 15 days after hospital admission and had shown a major deterioration of memory. He was disoriented in time, unable to make simple calculations spontaneously (i.e., he only could do so in a sequence like 2 x 2, 2 x 3, 2 x 4, ...), and behaved rather motion- and emotionless.

Post mortem examination of the brain revealed a tumor which was confined to the corpus callosum; it "at no place invaded the white matter, ... and is largest at the level of the third ventricle" (p. 369). Zingerle assumed that the tumor had originated on the right thalamic surface and then infiltrated the corpus callosum. The patient had been fully able to work and had shown no psychic disturbances seven weeks prior to hospital admission. Soon after the first appearance of behavioral abnormalities, memory defects were among the most striking symptoms. In accordance with other scientists of this time, Zingerle assumed "that the highest and most complex associative performance, which allows the cooperation of the two hemispheres as an integrated, harmonic whole, is abolished" (p. 373) in cases with callosal tumors.

In addition to this coordinative activity with respect to the highest functions, Zingerle at this time already acknowledged that the corpus callosum is not only related to the higher psychic and sensory functions, but is also involved in the innervation of bodily muscles and in the coordination of common activities of both body halves (p. 373).

Liepmann (1907 b), a psychiatrist with a strong background in psychology and philosophy, emphasized that a dissection of the corpus callosum would influence the relation between apraxia and intelligence (cf. also Liepmann & Maas, 1907). Ascenzi (1908) pointed to the well-known memory disturbances which follow callosal degeneration and are known up to the present as the Marchiafava-Bignami disease (Marchiafava & Bignami, 1903), a syndrome which neuropathologically consists of a callosal degeneration with laminar cortical sclerosis; excessive drinking of specific sorts of red wine are assumed to trigger the degeneration. The condition leads to depravation and dementia.

Seletzky and Gilula (1928) gave a thorough review of old assumptions for the functions of the corpus callosum. They furthermore reviewed research on animals and conducted their own study on rabbits and dogs. Though they mentioned a number of reports in which psychic detriments, including mnestic disturbances, were observed after callosal damage, they failed to find lasting alterations in the animals they treated. According to them, conditions of shock and temporary anaemia occur after callosal transections and are responsible for the behavioral deteriorations, but diminish with time.

A different view was given by Bruns (1897) at the end of the last century. Bruns wrote that the tumors of the corpus callosum lead to interpretable symptoms only when they affect neighboring cortical regions and even then the symptoms are usually not very characteristic (p. 121). Nevertheless, Bruns assumed that callosal tumors disrupt the important association fibers between the hemispheres and thereby lead to intelligence defects. He also pointed out that the deficits depend on the location of the callosal damage: "Anterior callosal damage may lead to frontal symptoms – frontal ataxia ... – quite posterior damage may result in ... hemianopia or amaurosis" (p. 122).

Five years later, P. Schuster (1902) concluded from the "lack of somatic functions of the corpus callosum" that "with a certain likeliness the corpus callosum will be all the more important for psychic functions" (p. 141). In support for this idea he cited old sources (Lapayronie from the beginning of the 18th century, and Saucerotte [1805–1884]) who considered the corpus callosum to be the seat of the soul). Other authors, according to Bruns, considered the corpus callosum to be necessary for the unity of intellectual processes, or hypothesized that consciousness is lost after illnesses affecting the corpus callosum (p. 142).

Bruns (1902) then reviewed case reports of altogether 31 patients with callosal tumors. He grouped them into patients in whom the anterior, the central, or the posterior portion of the callosum had been affected. From his survey he concluded that states of simple mental weakness are correlated with anterior and delirious states with posterior callosal damage; but as a cautious note, he remarked that for many of the cases reviewed surrounding tissue was affected in addition and that in the six cases with anatomically pure callosal damage quite diverse mental disturbances had been found (p. 159).

The importance of the corpus callosum in integrating mental activity is nevertheless evident from today's analyses of split brain subjects (e. g., Gazzaniga, 1970; Gazzaniga, Kutas, Van Petten, & Fendrich, 1989) and can also be seen in patients with callosal agenesis (e. g., Chiarello, 1980; Eichler, 1878; Ferriss & Dorsen, 1975; Gott & Saul, 1978; Jeeves, 1990; Kessler, Huber, Markowitsch, Pawlik, & Heiss, 1991). Recent memory disturbances have, however, to be attributed to extracallosal damage, particularly of the fornix and its connections (Clark & Geffen, 1989).

Chapter 9: Medial Temporal Lobe Amnesia

Examples of early studies on the temporal lobes

While Korsakoff's syndrome and other forms of diencephalic amnesia were intensively studied at the turn of the century (e. g., A. Knapp, 1906), there was much less investigation on the role of specific cortical areas in the processing of intellectual behavior (though modality-specific functions were analyzed frequently: cf., e. g., Cushing, 1922; Horrax, 1923). For the parietal cortex, for example, there were (aside from the books already mentioned of Bruns, 1897, and P. Schuster, 1902, on tumors, the monograph of Allers, 1916, on shot-based brain wounds and Monakow's, 1910 b, 1914, books on cortical localization) only a few sporadic articles (e. g., D. G. Anton, 1899; Kleist, 1923; Saelan, 1886; Wernicke, 1889).

The temporal lobe area received somewhat more attention. Bruns (1897) emphasized laterality effects, namely "sensory aphasia" as a "characteristic and very certain local symptom" (p. 117) after left temporal lobe damage. He referred to observations of others who had also found this left temporal lobe symptom in left-handers.

Aside from symptoms related to audition, Bruns mentioned observations of Ferrier, Hughlings-Jackson, and Oppenheim, who had found that the hippocampal area constitutes a center for taste and especially for smell. Bruns also pointed to the connection of epileptic attacks and temporal lobe changes, a connection which W. Sommer had already studied intensely in 1880 (cf. also Kühlmann, 1908; Zingerle, 1912 a; and, for a recent overview on this relationship, Gloor, 1990).

Paul Schuster (1902) began the fifth chapter of his book with the remark that the temporal lobe is the seat of one, perhaps of several, cortical sensory centers and that it consequently has to play a role in psychic functions. In addition to being an auditory center, the temporal lobe would most likely be a center for smell and taste. though there was no firm basis for this view according to P. Schuster. Otherwise, and especially for the right temporal lobe, scientists were still in absolute darkness (p. 105). P. Schuster then referred to Holländer's (1900) interpretation that the seat of the "folie furieuse" – raving madness – would be in the basal part of the temporal lobe.

A few of P. Schuster's cases make it clear that already at that time amnesic disturbances were diagnosed in cases with temporal lobe damage. This especially holds true for his own case number 9 (p. 108 f): A 52-year-old woman who shared a combination of amnesic and Klüver-Bucy-syndrome signs: She had severe amnesic disturbances "and her mood suddenly changed to a happy, gay state, she felt completely healthy, ..., and laughed unmotivatedly" (p. 108). After an epileptic attack she suddenly died. P. Schuster found a hemorrhagic focus in her left posterior temporal lobe which was surrounded by a tumor covering most of the temporal lobe.

A number of the other cases reviewed by P. Schuster had "memory weaknesses", "amnesic disturbances", "Korsakoff's psychosis" and the like, as a consequence of temporal lobe damage. Consequently, he concluded that "with high likeliness the intellectual disturbances after temporal lobe tumors are not bound to the existence of a language disturbance" (p. 117). In two cases even "isolated memory weakness" was the diagnosis (p. 121). Smell on the other hand was affected in only four out of 44 patients.

Among the first reported lesions of the temporal lobe is probably the case of Harvey (1846), who described a 30-year-old agricultural laborer who had been kicked by a horse.

First, there was not much of an injury visible (in fact he "Slept pretty well, answers questions readily, ..."; p. 503) and the wound was treated conservatively. Then there was a waxing and waning in his condition which was documented from the first visit of the surgeon on June 30th until his death on October 9th. There were repeated attempts to bring the protruding brain tissue under control, but the patient finally died, as it turned out, due to a piece of bone which had been driven so deeply into the brain on the occurrence of the accident, "as not to be discernible when the depressed portions were removed after the application of the trephine" (p. 506). There was not much precision in the description of the psychological consequences and of the exact anatomical damage. With respect to the neuropathology "the temporal region had entirely disappared" (p. 506); with respect to behavioral changes, he sometimes had naming disturbances (for the words knife and spoon, for example), a defective memory, but no systematic attempt to measure his behavior was attempted.

More than 40 years later, in 1888, S. Brown and Schäfer made their studies on the "functions of the ... temporal lobes of the monkey's brain". The authors' aim was to decide, if possible, between the conflicting results of preceding experimental observers, and especially those of Ferrier, Munk, and Luciani and Tamburini" (p. 320). However, this aim was restricted principally to determining how far the senses of hearing, taste, and smell had been affected by the, with one exception, bilateral lesions.

Several years earlier Yeo (1878) (who worked with Ferrier, studying the consequences of lesions in monkeys: cf. Ferrier & Yeo, 1884) provided the case of a patient with a large tumor in the left cerebral cortex. This patient's "memory was greatly impaired, and although she would attend to and take interest in what was read to her, she would almost immediately forget it, and take the same interest in its repetition" (p. 273). Her tumor was described as a glioma which was situated chiefly in the white matter of the central posterior lobe. One year later a related case was given by J. W. Hunt in the same journal (J. W. Hunt, 1879); the memory disturbances were described as very considerable, though there had been no deeper investigation of them. Contrary to Yeo's case, this patient had had a tumor at the outer surface of the left brain near the Sylvian fissure.

Another approach was to study epileptics (cf. Gloor, 1990, for a recent review). In addition to the mile-stone article of W. Sommer mentioned above, I would like to mention here Bratz' (1898) contribution, who noted that 25 out of 50 patients with epilepsy had hippocampal changes, 11 times on the right, 13 times on the left, and once on both sides.

Albert Knapp's contributions

A. Knapp wrote several works on the psychic consequences of tumors of the temporal lobes (e.g., 1905, 1918b; further citations can be found in his book from 1905), but also on Korsakoff's syndrome ("polyneuritic psychoses") (A. Knapp, 1906). In 1898 he gave the case of a 32-year-old woman who died within less than two years after her first hospitalization. The behavioral description corresponded to her somatic deterioration so that specific changes due to the involvement of the temporal lobe can only be guessed. Among them were an increased emotionality and a reduced mental capacity. The somewhat imprecise nature of the behavioral description may, however, correspond to Kaplan's view of brain-behavior relationships: He stated that he explained all "purely organic" and "purely functional" disturbances from a common viewpoint, "namely from the viewpoint that the symptoms of a brain tumor always are due to the influence of the tumor on the respective central nervous system, and that consequently the development of a tumor in an a priori abnormal brain will not only lead to changes, which are primarily due to the kind and locus of the tumor, but also to such which predominantly have their cause in the special circumstances of that respective brain" (p. 978).

In his book from 1905, he described ten temporal lobe cases and provided a thorough theoretical background of the state of the art at that time. He started with the observation of others

(Bruns, 1897; Oppenheim, 1902) of whom Oppenheim (in the first edition of his book which appeared originally in 1896) had stated "We are never allowed to make the local diagnosis ('Lokaldiagnose') of the right temporal lobe" (A. Knapp, 1905, p. 7) as there are no observable local symptoms to be found following damage in this area. A few years later, Lücken (1909) wrote a dissertation on this topic, while Kolodny still cited Oppenheim's statement in 1928 (on p. 385); Schwab on the other hand in 1925 had entitled his contribution "On diagnosing tumors of the temporal lobe".

As other authors before him, A. Knapp referred to the changes in audition, taste, and smell which frequently accompany temporal lobe damage. The auditory changes may include aphasic disturbances and often do so, as was shown in a number of contributions of that time (Goldstein, 1911; Heilbronner, 1901, 1908, 1910; Kehrer, 1913; Knauer, 1909; Lewy, 1908; Moranska-Oscherovitsch, 1910; cf. Stafiniak et al., 1990, for a recent analysis). Though A. Knapp's section on "amnesic aphasia after temporal lobe tumors" (p. 15 f) is interesting, here again (as in his publication from 1898) he argued against the localization of amnesic aphasia in the left temporal lobe. His principal argument was that amnesic disturbances and amnesic aphasia may occur even after cerebellar damage, and in patients with diffuse organic brain damage such as in "senile, polyneuritic, and paralytic conditions" (p. 16).

The last contribution of Albert Knapp on this subject was once again substantial, accumulating to over 60 pages (A. Knapp, 1918 b). In this article he saw a continuation and supplement to his monograph from 1905. Again, as in the earlier reports, he emphasized individual differences: "There is no illness which does not sometimes occur without symptoms, and especially in brain tumors – even if they are located in the known and generally acknowledged centers – there are always surprises and exceptions to be found" (p. 227).

After describing two cases in detail, A. Knapp classified the symptoms into (a) focal symptoms of the left temporal lobe, (b) focal symptoms of the right and left temporal lobe, (c) disturbances in consciousness, (d) disturbances in balance, and (e) local and distant symptoms. With respect to psychic disturbances (pp. 253–255) he again emphasized that "Korsakoff's syndrome has a special liking for temporal lobe tumors ("... mit besonderer Vorliebe"; p. 254). Futhermore, he remarked the occurrence of "character changes" ("rude, stubborn, inclined to use abusive words and violence"; p. 255), that is, changes which have some resemblance to the later described Klüver-Bucy syndrome (Bucy & Klüver, 1940; Klüver, 1958; Klüver & Bucy, 1937, 1939).

The chapter on "temporal lobe tumors and Korsakoff's symptom complex" (pp. 22–25) is also interesting. It starts with a definite statement: "I do not want to fail mentioning that in all temporal lobe tumors I have observed, which were accompanied by asymbolic, apraxic, perseverating, amnesic-aphasic and echolalic symptoms, coincidently the typical amnesic mental deterioration, the Korsakoff symptom complex, existed. Anterograde and retrograde amnesia, confabulations, disorientation in space and time were found markedly in several of his cases. A. Knapp deemphasized these findings, however, by stating that E. Meyer had described a case with a sarcoma in the third ventricle who had a Korsakoff's syndrome and that he himself presently had several cases under his observation with tumors in the cerebellum or the quadrigeminal plate with Korsakoff's symptomatology.

Bechterew's case

A frequently cited case of Bechterew (1900 a) demonstrated "a brain with destruction of the anterior and medial parts of the cerebral cortex of both temporal lobes". The bilateral destruction of the uncinate and hippocampal gyri was accompanied by an "extra-ordinary anterograde amnesia, and a partial retrograde amnesia".

As the patient during his lifetime had appeared in the sessions of the Russian Society of Psychiatrists and Neurologists in Moscow, as a Korsakoff's case ("with polyneuritic psychoses"), Bechterew concluded that this symptomatology could occur after temporal lobe damage as well; and with respect to functional localization he questioned the view of Munk and Ferrier that the respective brain area is primarily involved in taste and smell sensations. (Taste had been well preserved, while no data are available for smell.) Bechterew then gave a quite correct location of the cortical taste center by assuming that this is situated on the outer surface of the cerebral hemispheres, in the outer sectors of the motor region, in those parts which correspond to the opercular area of the human brain (p. 990 f).

The Temporal Lobes and Memory

In the first decade of the present century, the importance of the temporal lobes for mnestic information processing was reinforced considerably, as was discussed by Knauer (1909), though the picture was still blurred by diverse, individual-specific outcomes. For instance, Pfeifer (1910) described a number of cases with different unilateral temporal lobe tumors. The majority of the right-hemispheric tumors manifested no or only minor changes in intellect (p. 597 ff). For left-sided temporal lobe tumors, intellectual changes generally were more marked, but sometimes covered by signs of the Klüver-Bucy syndrome. Here, the thirty-second case of Pfeifer was especially characteristic: This 18-year-old girl was rather agitated, and apparently had the hyperorality and grasping reflexes described later in such patients (Aichner, 1984; Dahlmann & Schaefer, 1979; Gascon & Gilles, 1973; Lilly, Cummings, Benson, & Fraenkel, 1983; Marlowe, Mancall, & Thomas, 1975; Shraberg & Weisberg, 1978; Terzian & Dalle Ore, 1955). Pfeifer most likely misdiagnosed her condition as chorea Huntington. Bechterew's old case, published in 1894, may have had both signs of the Klüver-Bucy syndrome and damage of the brain confined to the temporal lobe region.

Of particular interest is the case description of Ludwig Edinger, who, like many neurologists of that time, was an all-round capacity. (In neuroanatomy, e.g., his name stands for the Edinger-tract and the Edinger-Westphal nucleus; cf. also his papers on brain ontogenesis, on the functions of the cerebellum, and on the relations of the fornix and the mammillary bodies: Edinger, 1905, 1913, 1914; Edinger & Wallenberg, 1902.) In 1902 Edinger pointed out how difficult it was at that time to diagnose a tumor which was not situated in the motor or in the occipital zones of the cerebral cortex. He wrote that nevertheless he had been able to diagnose a temporal lobe tumor with such accuracy "that the surgeon considered it justified to interfere" (p. 305). Indeed, a large melanosarcoma was removed involving most of the right temporal lobe. As the patient died later due to multiple small brain tumors, Edinger was able to give a detailed description of anatomico-behavioral relationships in this 19-year-old patient. The surgery had been performed by Heidenhain (1901) who described the case in extenso from page 864 to page 876 of his article (case 3).

The extent of the removal in the temporal lobe was quite similar to that dissected in Zingerle's case, described below (cf. Fig. 33). The extirpation probably invaded sectors of the temporal lobe situated a little more anterior and medially, compared to Zingerle's case, but the posterior border was a little more ventral

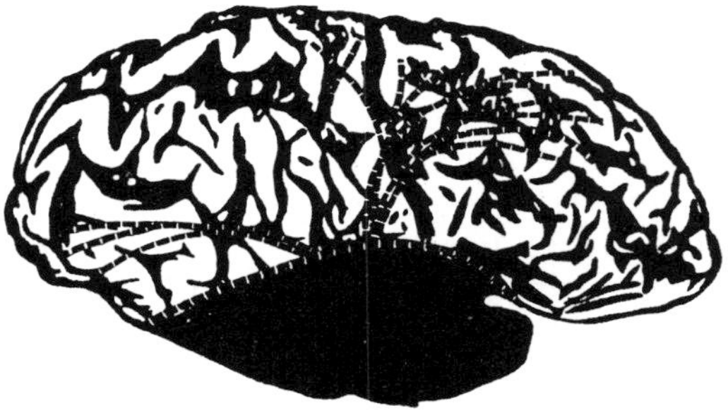

Figure 32. Schematic view of the extent of brain damage in the patient described by Edinger (1902); the broken lines demonstrate the course of degenerating fiber bundles. (After Fig. 1 of Edinger, 1902.)

and anterior than the removal in Zingerle's case (Fig. 32).

Unfortunately, not much information was given on the status of the patient's intellectual functions, neither before nor after surgery; at both times his language expression was retarded, but he was oriented in space and time and no memory disturbances were reported. With respect to his postoperative intellect the following description was given: "The assistant physician tested his intelligence repeatedly by using the pictures of a weekly journal, and always remarked that he had an appropriate comprehension."

The neuroanatomical evaluation revealed that the anterior two thirds of the right temporal lobe were missing, while the region of the uncus and of the hippocampal gyrus or subiculum were partly preserved. The large cortical association fibers connecting the temporal lobe with the frontal, parietal, and occipital cortex (cf. Fig. 32) were partly degenerated.

Edinger concluded that "the complete and smooth resection of the right temporal lobe and of the insula in a right-handed man failed to show any symptom of deficiency. All that was found of such symptoms can with certainty be attributed to other secondary softened or surgically insulted parts of the brain" (p. 320 f).

While Edinger had "dared" to diagnose a tumor of the right temporal lobe and proved to be right, Ulrich (1910) again stressed the view of a number of authorities from the turn of the century (Bramwell, Bruns, Monakow, Oppenheim; cf. also A. Knapp above) that a tumor of the right temporal lobe could never be diagnosed with certainty. (For left-sided temporal lobe tumors, the most frequently diagnosed symptom was that of a "sensory-amnesic aphasia"; cf. also Biro, 1910).

For Ulrich's case there was, as he wrote, no comparable counterpart in the literature, as the tumor was restricted to the right dorsal temporal lobe. The patient had been less than 22 years of age and was described as mentally very alert, having graduated from all schools with exceptional success. Since the occurrence of her menses, she had had minor epileptic attacks. Her memory deteriorated successively. Apparently seven physicians had misdiagnosed the case as "hystero-epilepsy". In 1903 she was hospitalized in the Swiss sanatorium for epileptics in Zurich where Monakow gave the tentative diagnosis of a cerebellar tumor. "After larger correspondence the patient's parents agreed with trepanation, after the intelligent patient had also so decided" (p. 4).

Surgery was performed one year after hospitalization. However, based on the misdiagnosis, the left hemipshere of the cerebellum was removed instead of the right temporal lobe! Consequently, other symptoms appeared (problems with space orientation and balance) and the patient frequently had symptoms of an internal hydrocephalus and consequently cerebro-spinal fluid had to be removed several times per week. The examination of the brain revealed the true cause of her symptoms, namely a tumor in the posterior part of the dorsal temporal gyrus.

Contrary to Edinger's anatomical diagnosis, Ulrich's therefore proved unsuccessful; however, in both cases, surgery brought little benefits anyway.

A case with an exceptionally detailed and thorough anatomical documentation was given by Zingerle (1912 b). Grossly viewed, the main portion of the right temporal lobe was absent along its total breadth and length, "as if it had been cut horizontally by a sharp knife" (Fig. 33). Behaviorally, the 40-year-old patient was characterized by an inappropriate orienta-

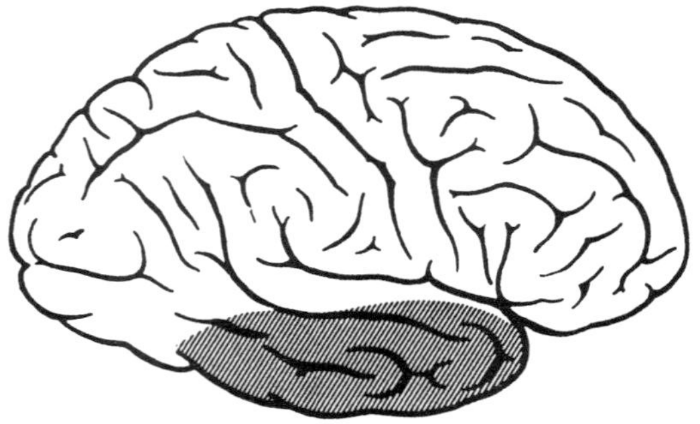

Figure 33. Schematic view of the extent of brain damage in the patient described by Zingerle (1912). (After Fig. 1 of Zingerle, 1912.) The defects enclosed the whole ventral part of the right temporal lobe from lateral to medial.

tion with respect to space and time, and by marked memory disturbances with reduced intelligence. Zingerle's case is remarkable as the tumor was unilateral, right-sided, and it isolated the amygdala and the hippocampal area from the rest of the brain, though marked damage was not detectable (the right hippocampal gyrus was, however, smaller than the left one).

Interestingly, at the University of Kiel, Germany, at least four dissertations were written between 1909 and 1919 which had the analysis of behavioral consequences of temporal lobe tumors as subject (Gast, 1912; Janus, 1911; Lücken, 1909; Singelmann, 1919).

In 1928 Kolodny wrote on "the symptomatology of tumours of the temporal lobe". He emphasized that writers before him had tried "to establish too rigid and too definite symptom-complexes. The temporo-sphenioidal lobe is too large an area of brain for it to be possible for lesions of it, variable in type and extent, to produce any definite train of symptoms and signs. For these reasons I shall not attempt to formulate here a definite temporal lobe syndrome, but shall merely enumerate the various symptoms and signs in the order of their frequency in this series of thirty-eight tumours of this lobe" (p. 413).

He observed memory disturbances in half of them, but -as he remarked – they were equally frequent in cases with frontal lobe tumors, though he concluded that frontal lobe tumors affected only recent memories, while temporal lobe tumors affected both anterograde and retrograde memories (p. 414). His final sentence on psychic disturbances is quite surprising: "The tendency to attribute psychic disturbances to lesions of the left hemisphere in right-handed people is not supported by clinical facts and, therefore, they have no lateralizing value" (p. 414).

Artom's Documentation

A monumental article was written by Gustavo Artom (1923) who worked in Rome's university clinic under the directorship of Mingazzini. Of special interest is the first of his eight cases – a patient with an intratemporal, isolated sarcoma in the right hemisphere which affected the anterior half of the second and the third temporal gyrus and the fusiform gyrus. The patient had been only 15 years of age. It is quite astonishing that in this patient with such massive temporal lobe damage (cf. Fig. 34) the psychic functions had been largely intact: The patient was described as generally apathetic, but as having had a preserved memory and a preserved ability of association. Likewise, he had been well oriented with respect to time, locus, and persons, and had had neither illusions, hallucinations, or delusions.

For Artom the question of whether temporal lobe damage results in psychic disturbances was a difficult one. Though he discussed psychic symptoms at length, and also mentioned the existence of Korsakoff's symptomatology, he was (in accordance with A. Knapp, 1905, but not with Stern, 1914), of the opinion that callosal more than temporal lobe damage would result in amnesic disturbances. As additional argument he refered to individual factors such as heredity and intoxication which may lead to different kinds of psychic outcomes.

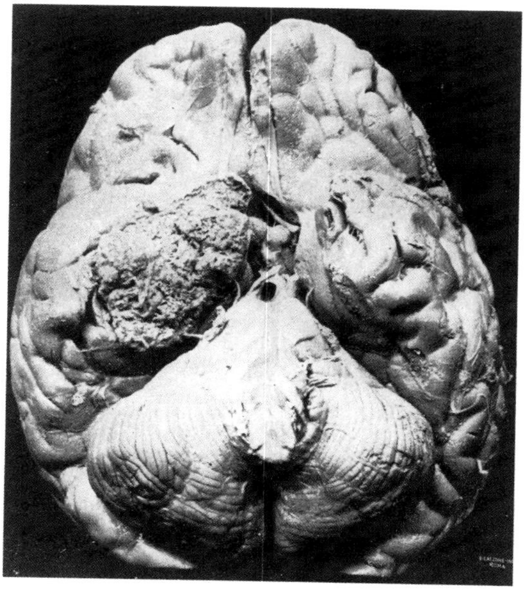

Figure 34. Basal view of the brain of Artom's (1923) first case, demonstrating the large extent of the right temporal tumor (probably a sarcoma).

The Hippocampal Formation

To flood the darkness, behind which the function of the hippocampal formation is presently still hidden, at least with a little twilight, the following rare, extraordinary case seems appropriate to us, and thus we will give its clinical-pathological description in the following (Grünthal, 1947, p. 3).

The importance of the hippocampal area within the temporal lobe was only recognized after the Second World War. Grünthal (1947) was among the first who complemented the detailed anatomical descriptions of, for example, Altschul (1935), Lorente de Nó (1933, 1934), M. Rose (1926, 1927), Schaffer (1892), and Uchimura (1928) with material on the behavioral level. Kleist (1934 a, p. 1270) had already mentioned that the sense of smell might not be directly associated with Ammon's horn, but with the surrounding tissue of the periamygdaloid cortex and of the amygdala itself.

Grünthal's case is that of a woman with mild diabetes who was hospitalized at the age of 67 due to an infection. After successful treatment she was released, but at home she suddenly fell into a hypoglycemic coma and quickly deteriorated in her intellectual level and manifested signs of a Klüver-Bucy syndrome (especially an increased oral activity). Autopsy revealed a reduced volume of the cranium and the brain. Nevertheless the principal macroscopical abnormality was a bilateral reduction in the size of the hippocampal formation. No senile plaques were found. On the light-microscopical level the only serious changes again were found bilaterally in the Ammon's horns.

Grünthal emphasized that after the successful treatment of the infection (including a three months stay at the hospital) the patient was not dementic, but well-oriented and reasonable and it was not until her insulin coma, which occurred three days later, that she deteriorated intellectually; furthermore he mentioned that apart from the destruction of the Ammon's horn the other observable changes in the brain were age-related and could not have caused the severe intellectual deterioration.

Grünthal included altogether 11 photographs in his article, of which seven showed portions of the damaged hippocampal formation. The following is the English summary of his report (p. 15): "Dementia of high rate after acute circumscribed destruction of the cornu ammonis formation on both sides is described. Thence is to be concluded that the normal functioning of the cortex of the cornu ammonis is a necessary preliminary condition to the intellectual production of the cerebrum."

The next cases then were those of Conrad and Ule (1951), Ule (1951), Glees and Griffith (1952), and Hegglin (1953) (all with mental deterioration), and the case of Nathan and Smith (1950) with no deterioration of memory.

Glees and Griffith described the case of an older woman (58 years old) who had been hospitalized, however, for the 15 years before she died. During her stay she deteriorated progressively in cognitive behavior, with anterograde and retrograde amnesia being the most prominent symptoms. As in the case of Zingerle (1912 a), a cyst occupied the region of each of the two medial and anterior temporal lobe areas, where the respective neuronal tissue was completely missing. The rest of the temporal lobe was preserved and showed "a normal cortical arrangement in layers". The fornix was densely gliosed (75% of its fibers were degenerated), while the amygdala appeared normal in structure, as did the thalamus, hypothalamus, the basal ganglia and the rest of the cerebral cortex. The authors considered the damage to be of vascular origin, but emphasized the normal appearance of the mammillary bodies, which again corresponded to Grünthal's case (and furthermore to another case with hippocampal damage and an absent fornix: Nathan & Smith, 1950).

Hegglin's (1953) case was similar to that of Zingerle (1912 a) in that hippocampal softening was again only unilateral and nevertheless apparently led to pre-senile dementia. On the basis of sclerosis of the basal artery, Hegglin assumed that vascular damage was the origin of the insult. The 63-year old patient was observed for about three months during which time he was found to have marked anterograde amnesia, extensive remote memory gaps and disorientation in space and time. In his discussion of the case, Hegglin was among the first authors to ask whether an acute destruction of the hippocampus alone might be able to cause dementia (and in his case it was only a unilateral destruction of the pyramidal cells of the Ammon's horn). While he did not have confidence enough to give a positive answer from his case with unilateral damage only, he cited Grünthal's case (and that of Conrad & Ule, 1951) as support for the likelihood that an acute, massive destruction of the Ammon's horn might result in amnesia.

The Discovery of Medial Temporal Lobe Amnesia

The case descriptions on temporal lobe tumors in the decades before and after the turn of the century most clearly demonstrate how unsure neurology was at that time with respect to the diagnosis of brain tumors in the so-called silent areas. Once given, diagnoses were frequently taken up without criticism as labels so that language disturbances were considered to be the dominant symptom for left lateral temporal cases. The hippocampal region was usually regarded as an olfactory area (e.g., Ulrich, 1910).

Contrary to diencephalic amnesia which had quite a long history (e.g., Gudden, 1896), the advent of hypothesizing about the existence of a medial temporal lobe amnesia came only around the time of the Second World War. There may be many reasons for this, among others the hidden and complicated anatomy of the hippocampal formation (cf., e.g., the figures in the recent overviews of Rolls, 1990, and Witter, Groenewegen, Lopes da Silva, & Lohman, 1989), the blood supply, the proximity of the overlying and surrounding cortex, the malignity of the temporal lobe tumors, and the richness of the possible concomitant symptomatology (e.g., epilepsy).

The zig-zag course in anatomical localization of the amnesia-relevant medial temporal lobe location is still apparent: Over the last few decades there has been a continous shift and backshift in the extent to which amnesic disturbances have been related to the damage of particular brain structures, with gray matter regions dominating. To take the medial temporal lobe area as an example: Scoville and Milner (1957) stressed the hippocampus and hippocampal gyrus, but de-emphasized the amygdala; Mishkin (1978) highlighted the combined role of amygdala and hippocampus, and more recently Zola-Morgan and co-workers again de-emphasized the memory-related role of the amygdala (Zola-Morgan, Squire, & Amaral, 1989) and of the temporal stem (Zola-Morgan, Squire, & Mishkin, 1982), and stressed that of field CA1 of the hippocampus proper (Zola-Morgan, Squire, & Amaral, 1986). The temporal stem had been a favorite candidate for Horel (1978). Finally, in this tour through the temporal lobe, the perirhinal and parahippocampal cortices have also been considered as centrally important for memory processing (Zola-Morgan, Squire, Amaral, & Suzuki, 1989). Recent commentaries on memory related circuits in the brain have been provided by Cramon, Hebel, and Ebeling (1990), Cramon and Markowitsch (1992), and Markowitsch (1991 a).

We still have to solve a number of riddles and to complete a number of puzzles when trying to analyze how different portions of the brain participate in information processing.

Chapter 10: Final Remarks

I had started writing this book with the naive aim of presenting research published on the relations of intellectual, in particular mnestic functions, to the mammalian brain. During the work, there were continuous shifts: I learned that in comparison to today's position, the emphasis was very different three generations ago. The ability to localize brain damage (especially in tumor cases) was low, as was the survival rate for infarct and tumor cases. Philosophy influenced psychology, psychiatry, and neurology (e. g., Ziehen, 1901 c, 1902, 1907, 1913, 1921, 1934, 1939); the soul and consciousness were central themes (e. g., Bain, 1881; Flügel, 1902; James, 1892, 1909; Lazarus, 1876, 1878, 1882; Raue, 1850; Rehmke, 1891; Semon, 1920; R. Sommer, 1891). Affective and emotional disturbances and altered states of consciousness and thought were regarded as central (Hofmann, 1921; Jahrreis, 1928 a, 1928 b; Kretschmer, 1928; Semon, 1920), more than memory itself.

The neurosciences were much more interwoven than was the case for the generation of scientists after the Second World War. This is reflected in the existence of journals such as the *Journal of Comparative Neurology and Psychology*, and the *Journal für Psychologie und Neurologie*. Several of the first researchers who held professorships in psychology were neurologists by training (cf. Markowitsch, 1986), or worked in several fields of the neurosciences simultaneously or successively. A good example is Freud, who wrote a number of influential contributions in the fields of neurology and neuroanatomy (e. g., Freud, 1891; cf. Amacher, 1965; Freud, 1884; Triarhou & del Cerro, 1985). Other examples are Paul Broca (Broca, 1861 a, 1861 b, 1878), Korbinian Brodmann, Ramón y Cajal (Cajal, 1895, 1896, 1909-11, 1935), Ludwig Edinger, Paul Flechsig (cf. Busse, 1989; Schröder, 1930), Karl S. Lashley (cf. Lashley, 1929, 1937; Lashley & Clark, 1946), Konstantin von Monakow (cf. Goldstein, 1931), and Ziehen (e. g., Ziehen, 1891, 1901 a, 1901 c, 1902, 1903, 1907).

I was also learning that certain labels were given with high preference, though the exact nature of the respective process and its underlying neuroanatomical damage were not very clear (e. g., Korsakoff's psychosis; aphasic-amnesic syndrome; progressive paralysis), and that there were some early, very important results which, however, were forgotten, not accepted, or not realized. Among them were Gudden's (1896) and Gamper's (1928 a, 1928 b, 1929) cases on diencephalic amnesia and the possible role of the mammillary bodies in amnesia, or, for medial temporal lobe amnesia, Bechterew's (1900 a) abstract of a severely amnesic case with bilateral hippocampal destruction. Even when Scoville in 1953 performed his medial temporal lobe resections in amnesics (cf. Corkin, 1984; Markowitsch, 1985; Milner, 1959, 1966, 1970; Scoville, Dinsmoore, Liberson, Henry, & Pepe, 1953; Scoville, 1954 a, 1968; Scoville & Milner, 1957) he was probably unaware of the severe consequences which had been reported earlier to follow damage of this brain region (aside from Bechterew's findings there were those of Grünthal, 1947, Conrad & Ule, 1951, Ule, 1951, Glees & Griffith, 1952, and Hegglin, 1953). For instance, in his 1954 a report on "The limbic lobe in man", Scoville did not mention any of the just mentioned reports (but he did mention two of the above in 1957). As being really surprised from the outcome of a "bilateral resection of the uncus and amygdalum alone, or in conjunction with the entire pyriform amygdaloid hippocampal complex" (p. 64), he wrote that this surgery "has resulted in no marked physiologic or behavioral changes with the one exception of *a very grave, recent memory loss*, so severe as to prevent the patient from remembering the locations of the rooms in which he lives, the names of his close associates, or even the way to toilet and urinal" (Scoville, 1954 a, p. 64 f; his emphasis). It is unfortunate that Bechterew (1900 a) did not take up his findings to include them in a full report (at least not in a non-Russian language).

A number of rather early (and partly even well documented) findings disappeared from common scientific knowledge and were only re-studied recently (cf. also Patten, 1972, 1990). This holds true for possible relations between changes in brain anatomy and psychotic disturbances, for the investigation of different kinds of memories (declarative, non-declarative), and for the functions of the frontal lobes. It is the hope that this book will alert present-day scientists to the existence of such old results.

References

Aall, A. (1913). Ein neues Gedächtnisgesetz? Experimentelle Untersuchung über die Bedeutung der Reproduktionsperspektive [A new law of memory? Experimental investigation on the significance of the perspective of reproduction]. *Zeitschrift für Psychologie und Physiologie der Sinnesorgane, 66*, 1–50.

Abeles, M., & Schilder, P. (1935). Psychogenic loss of personal identity: amnesia. *A.M.A. Archives of Neurology and Psychiatry, 34*, 587–604.

Ach, N. (1901). Ueber die Beeinflussung der Auffassungsfähigkeit durch einige Arzneimittel [On the influence of some drugs on comprehension ability*]. In E. Kraepelin (Ed.), *Psychologische Arbeiten (Vol. 3)* (pp. 203–288). Leipzig: Barth.

Ackerknecht, E.H. (1985). *Kurze Geschichte der Psychiatrie* [Short history of psychiatry]. (3rd ed.). Stuttgart: Enke.

Ackerly, S. (1935). Instinctive, emotional and mental changes following prefrontal lobe extirpation. *American Journal of Psychiatry, 92*, 717–729.

Adler, (n.n.g.)** (1875). Ueber einige pathologische Veränderungen im Gehirne Geisteskranker.[On some pathologic changes in the brains of mental patients]. *Archiv für Psychiatrie und Nervenkrankheiten, 5*, 346–378 (and 1 Table).

Adler, (n.n.g.) (1901). Ueber die Beziehungen des Kleinhirns zur multiplen Sklerose [On the relations of the cerebellum to multiple sclerosis]. *Deutsche medizinische Wochenschrift, 8*, 121.

Adler, M., & Saupe, R. (1979). *Psychochirurgie* [Psychosurgery]. Stuttgart: Enke.

Aichner, F. (1984). Die Phänomenologie des nach Klüver und Bucy benannten Syndroms beim Menschen [The phenomenology of the syndrome, named after Klüver and Bucy, in humans]. *Fortschritte der Neurologie und Psychiatrie, 52*, 375–397.

Allers, R. (1916). *Ueber Schädelschüsse. Probleme der Klinik und der Fürsorge* [On cranial shots. Problems for the clinic and medical care]. Berlin: Springer.

Allison, H.W., & Allison, S.G. (1954). Personality changes following transorbital lobotomy. *Journal of Social Psychology, 49*, 219–223.

Altschul, R. (1935). Der Uncus als Index der Entwicklungshöhe des Gehirnes [The uncus as an index of the developmental stage of the brain]. *Zeitschrift für die gesamte Neurologie und Psychiatrie, 152*, 451–479.

Altshuler, L.L., Casanova, M.F., Goldberg, T.E., & Kleinman, J.E. (1990). The hippocampus and parahippocampus in schizophrenic, suicide, and control brains. *Archives of General Psychiatry, 47*, 1029–1034.

Alzheimer, A. (1897). Ueber rückschreitende Amnesie bei der Epilepsie [On retrogressive amnesia in epilepsy]. *Allgemeine Zeitschrift für Psychiatrie, 53*, 483–499.

Alzheimer, A. (1904 a). Einiges über die anatomischen Grundlagen der Idiotie [Some remarks on the anatomical bases of idiocy]. *Centralblatt für Nervenheilkunde und Psychiatrie, 27 (N.F. 15)*, 497–505.

Alzheimer, A. (1904 b). Histologische Studien zur Differentialdiagnose der progressiven Paralyse [Histological studies on the differential diagnosis of progressive paralysis]. In F. Nissl (Ed.) *Histologische und histopathologische Arbeiten über die Grosshirnrinde mit besonderer Berücksichtigung der Pathologischen Anatomie der Geisteskranken. Band 1.* (pp. 18–314). Jena: Gustav Fischer.

Alzheimer, A. (1907). Ueber eine eigenartige Erkrankung der Hirnrinde [On a peculiar disease of the cortex]. *Allgemeine Zeitschrift für Psychiatrie, 64*, 146–148.

Alzheimer, A. (1911). Ueber eigenartige Krankheitsfälle des späteren Alters [On peculiar cases of disease of late aging]. *Zeitschrift für die gesamte Neurologie und Psychiatrie, 4*, 356–385.

---

* In a few cases the English title translations of the respective authors were taken, even when I think they did not strictly conform to the German-language title.

** (n.n.g.) is used whenever no first name(s) was or were given in the respective publication and could not be inferred with certainty from other sources.

Amacher, P. (1965). *Freud's neurological evaluation and its influence on psychoanalytic theory*. New York: International Universities Press.

Anderson, A.L. (1949). Personality changes following prefrontal lobotomy in a case of severe psychoneurosis. *Journal of Consulting Psychology, 13*, 105–107.

Anderson, E.W., & Mallinson, W.P. (1941). Psychogenic episodes in the course of major psychoses. *Journal of Mental Science, 87*, 383–396.

Andreasen, N.C., Ehrhardt, J.C., Swayze II, V., Alliger, R.J., Yuh, W.T.C., Cohen, G., & Ziebell, S. (1990). Magnetic resonance imaging of the brain in schizophrenia. *Archives of General Psychiatry, 4*, 35–44.

Angell, E.B. (1906). A case of double consciousness-amnesic type, with fabrication of memory. *Journal of Abnormal Psychology, 1*, 155–169.

Annan, S. (1840). Idiocy from alcoholism. *Maryland Medical and Surgical Journal, 1*, 333–334.

Anton, D.G. (1899). Beiderseitige Erkrankung der Scheitelgegend des Grosshirnes [Bilateral disease of the parietal areas of the cerebrum]. *Wiener klinische Wochenschrift, 12*, 1193–1199.

Anton, G. (1898). Ueber Herderkrankungen des Gehirnes [On focal diseases of the brain]. *Wiener medizinische Wochenschrift, 48*, 1282–1283.

Anton, G. (1899). Ueber die Selbstwahrnehmung der Herderkrankungen durch den Kranken bei Rindenblindheit und Rindentaubheit [On self-observation of focal brain diseases in cases with optic and acoustic agnosia]. *Archiv für Psychiatrie und Nervenkrankheiten, 32*, 86–127 (and 2 tables).

Anton, G. (1906). Symptome der Stirnhirnerkrankung [Symptoms of frontal lobe disease]. *Münchener medizinische Wochenschrift, 53*, 1289–1291.

Anton, G. (1914). Nachruf auf E. Hitzig [Obituitary for E. Hitzig]. *Archiv für Psychiatrie und Nervenkrankheiten, 54*, 1–7.

Anton, G., & Zingerle, H. (1902). *Bau, Leistung und Erkrankung des menschlichen Stirnhirnes* [Construction, performance, and diseases of the frontal lobe]. Graz, Austria: Leuschner and Lubensky.

Arndt, M., & Sklarek, F. (1903). Ueber Balkenmangel im menschlichen Gehirn [On callosal lack in the human brain]. *Archiv für Psychiatrie und Nervenkrankheiten, 37*, 756–799 (and 2 tables).

Arnett, L.D. (1904). The soul – a study of past and present beliefs. *American Journal of Psychology, 15*, 347–382.

Arnold, F. (1838). *Bemerkungen über den Bau des Hirns und Rückenmarks nebst Beiträgen zur Physiologie des zehnten und eilften Hirnnerven, mehrern kritischen Mittheilungen so wie verschiedenen pathologischen und anatomischen Beobachtungen.* [Remarks on the construction of the brain and spinal cord, together with contributions on the physiology of the tenth and eleventh brain nerve, several critical comments and several pathological and anatomical observations]. Zürich: S. Höhr.

Arnold, S.E., Hyman, B.T., & Van Hoesen, G.W. (1989). Cytoarchitectonic abnormalities of the entorhinal cortex in schizophrenia. *Society for Neuroscience Abstracts, 15*, 1223 (Abstr. No. 449.7).

Artom, G. (1923). Die Tumoren des Schläfenlappens [Tumors of the parietal lobe]. *Archiv für Psychiatrie und Nervenkrankheiten, 69*, 47–242.

Ascenzi, O. (1908). Una cisti emorragica del corpo calloso [A hemorrhagic cyst of the corpus callosum]. *Rivista di Patologia nervosa e mentale, 13*, 1–15.

Aschaffenburg, G. (1895). Experimentelle Studien über Associationen [Experimental studies on associations]. *Psychologische Arbeiten, 1*, 209–299.

Aschaffenburg, G. (1899). Experimentelle Studien über Associationen [Experimental studies on associations]. *Psychologische Arbeiten, 2*, 1–83.

Aschner, B. (1914). Ueber die posteklamptische Amnesie [On posteclamsic amnesia]. *Zeitschrift für Geburtshilfe und Gynäkologie, 75*, 405–410.

Auerbach, S. (1902). Beitrag zur Diagnostik der Geschwülste des Stirnhirns [Contribution to the diagnosis of the tumors of the frontal lobe]. *Deutsche Zeitschrift für Nervenheilkunde*, 312–332.

Auerbach, S. (1904). Bemerkungen zu dem Aufsatz: „Zur Aetiologie und pathologischen Anatomie der Geschwülste des Stirnhirns" von Dr. Ed. Müller [Remarks on the essay: "On the etiology and pathological anatomy of the tumors of the frontal lobe" of Dr. Ed. Müller]. *Deutsche Zeitschrift für Nervenheilkunde, 24*, 320–3222.

Auerbach, S. (1906). Beitrag zur Lokalisation des musikalischen Talentes im Gehirn und am Schädel [Contribution to the localization of musical talent in the brain and skull]. *Archiv für Anatomie und Physiologie, Anatomische Abteilung*, 197–230.

Austregesilo, A. (1927). Des troubles nerveux dans quelques maladies tropicales [Neuronal damage after certain tropical diseases]. *Revue neurologique, 34*, 1–21.

Axhausen, G., & Kramer, F. (1920). Die Kriegsschussverletzungen des Hirnschädels [The war-caused shot injuries of the cranium]. In A. Borchard & V. Schmieden (Eds.), *Die deutsche Chirurgie im Weltkrieg 1914 bis 1918* (pp. 345–427). Leipzig: Barth.

Azam, M. (1876). Periodical amnesia; or, double consciousness. *Journal of Nervous and Mental Disease, 3*, 584–612.

Babcock, H. (1947). A case of anxiety neurosis before and after lobotomy. *Journal of Abnormal and Social Psychology, 42*, 466–472.

Bach, C. (1907). Nekrolog Dr. G. Burckhardt [Necrology on Dr. G. Burckhardt]. *Allgemeine Zeitschrift für Psychiatrie, 64*, 529–534.

Baeyer, W. von (1947). Vergleichende Psychopathologie der Shocktherapien und der präfrontalen Lobotomie [Comparative psychopathology of shock therapies and of prefrontal lobotomy]. *Fortschritte der Neurologie . Psychiatrie und ihrer Grenzgebiete, 17*, 95–115.

Bailey, P. (1933). *Intracranial tumors*. Springfield, IL: C.C. Thomas.

Bailey, P., & Auvrey, H.A. (1928). A case of pinealoma with symptoms suggestive of compulsion neurosis. *A.M.A. Archives of Neurology and Psychiatry, 19*, 932–945.

Bain, A. (1881). *Geist und Körper. Die Theorien über ihre gegenseitigen Beziehungen* [Mind and body. The theories of their mutual relations]. (2nd ed.). Leipzig: Brockhaus.

Baldwin, J.M. (1898). *Die Entwickelung des Geistes beim Kinde und bei der Rasse (Methoden und Verfahren)* [The development of the mind in the child and in different races (Methods and techniques)]. Berlin: Reuther & Reinhard.

Bálint, R. (1909). Seelenlähmung des „Schauens", optische Ataxie, räumliche Störung der Aufmerksamkeit [Mind-paralysis of "perception", optic ataxia, spatial disturbance of attention]. *Monatsschrift für Psychiatrie und Neurologie, 25*, 51–81.

Banaye, R.S., & Davidoff, L. (1942). Apparent recovery of a sex psychopath after lobotomy. *Journal of Criminal Psychopathology, 4*, 59–66.

Barahona-Fernandes, H.J. (1950). Über die präfrontale Leukotomie [On prefrontal leucotomy]. *Fortschritte der Neurologie und Psychiatrie, 18*, 53–69.

Barahona-Fernandes, H.J. (1952). Hirnanatomie und -physiologie. Psychische Funktionsänderungen nach der präfrontalen Leukotomie [Brain anatomy and physiology. Changes in psychic functions after prefrontal leucotomy]. *Nervenarzt, 23*, 101–105.

Barahona-Fernandes, H.J. (1953). Voraussetzungen und Ergebnisse der Leukotomie [Prerequisites and results of leucotomy]. *Langenbecks Archiv für klinische Chirurgie und Deutsche Zeitschrift für Chirurgie, 276*, 109–117.

Barker, L.F. (1897). The phrenology of Gall and Flechsig's doctrine of association centers in the cerebrum. *Johns Hopkins Hospital Bulletin 8*, 7–14.

Bartholow, R. (1874). Experimental investigations into the functions of the human brain. *American Jounral of the Medical Sciences, 67 (No. 134)*, 305–313.

Bartlett, F.C. (1932). *Remembering*. Cambridge University Press, Cambridge, England.

Bartsch, W. (1953). Erfahrungen mit der Leukotomie bei schwersten chronischen Schmerzzuständen [Experiences with leucotomy in most severe conditions of pain]. *Nervenarzt, 24*, 107–112.

Bassoe, P. (1916). Tumors of the third and fourth ventricles. *Journal of the American Medical Association, 67*, 1423–1430.

Bast, T.H. (1928). Karl Friedrich Burdach. June 12, 1776 – July 16, 1847. *Annals of Medical History, 10*, 34–46.

Batten, F.E., & Collier, J.S. (1899). Spinal cord changes in cases of cerebral tumour. *Brain 22*, 473–533 (and 27 plates).

Bauer, J. (1917). Hysterische Erkrankungen bei Kriegsteilnehmern [Hysteric diseases in combatants]. *Archiv für Psychiatrie und Nervenkrankheiten, 57*, 139–168.

Baumgarten, P. von (1907). Ueber die durch Alkohol hervorzurufenden pathologisch-histologischen Veränderungen [On the pathological-histological changes evoked by alcohol]. *Berliner klinische Wochenschrift, 44*, 1331–1332.

Bay, E. (1961). Die Geschichte der Aphasielehre und die Grundlagen der Hirnlokalisation [The history of aphasia and the bases of brain localization]. *Deutsche Zeitschrift für Nervenheilkunde, 181*, 634–646.

Bayerthal, (n.n.g.) (1903). Zur Diagnose der Thalamus- und Stirnhirntumoren [On the diagnosis of thalamic- and frontal lobe tumors]. *Neurologisches Zentralblatt, 77*, 572–577 und 615–624.

Beal, M.F., Kleinman, G.M., Ojemann, R.G., & Hochberg, F.H. (1981). Gangliocytoma of third ventricle: Hyperphagia, somnolence, and dementia. *Neurology, 31*, 1224–1228.

Bechterew, W. von (1894). Unaufhaltsames Lachen und Weinen bei Hirnaffectionen [Uncontrollable laughing and crying with affections of the brain]. *Archiv für Psychiatrie und Nervenkrankheiten, 26*, 791–817.

Bechterew, W. von (1898). Ueber das Hören der eigenen Gedanken [On hearing one's own thoughts]. *Archiv für Psychiatrie und Nervenkrankheiten, 30*, 284–294.

Bechterew, W. von (1900a). Demonstration eines Gehirns mit Zerstörung der vorderen und inneren Theile der Hirnrinde beider Schläfenlappen [Demonstration of a brain with destruction of the anterior and inner portions of the cerebral cortex of both temporal lobes]. *Neurologisches Centralblatt, 19*, 990–991.

Bechterew, W. von (1900b). Ueber periodische Anfälle retroactiver Amnesie [On periodic attacks of retroactive amnesia]. *Monatsschrift für Psychiatrie und Neurologie, 8*, 353–358.

Bechterew, W. von (1901). Ueber das corticale Sehen des Hundes [On cortical vision in the dog]. *Monatsschrift für Psychiatrie und Neurologie, 10*, 432–437.

Bechterew, W. von (1907). Über persönliches und Gemeinbewusstsein [On personal and common consciousness]. *Journal für Psychologie und Neurologie, 9*, 54–80.

Bechterew, W. von, & Weinberg, R. (1909). Das Gehirn des Chemikers D.J. Mendelew [The brain of the chemist D.J. Mendelew]. In W. Roux (Ed.), *Anatomische und Entwicklungsgeschichtliche Monographien* (Heft 1, pp. 1–22 and 8 tables). Leipzig: W. Engelmann.

Beck, E., McLardy, T., & Meyer, A. (1950). Anatomical comments on psychosurgical procedures. *Journal of Mental Science, 96*, 157–167.

Becker, A.M., & Sternbach, I. (1953). Über Zeitsinnstörung bei Thalamusherden [On disturbances of the sense of time in thalamic foci]. *Wiener Zeitschrift für Nervenheilkunde, 7*, 62–67.

Becker, J.T., Furman, J.M., Panisset, M., & Smith, C. (1990). Characteristics of memory loss of a patient with Wernicke-Korsakoff's syndrome without alcoholism. *Neuropsychologia, 28*, 171–179.

Beevor, C.E. (1898). The accurate localisation of intracranial tumours, excluding tumours of the motor cortex, motor tract, pons and medulla. *Brain, 21*, 291–305.

Bench, C.J., Dolan, R.J., Friston, K.J., & Frackowiak, R.S.J. (1990). Positron emission tomography in the study of brain metabolism in psychiatric and neuropsychiatric disorders. *British Journal of Psychiatry, 157 (Suppl. 9)*, 82–95.

Bender, L., Curran, F.J., & Schilder, P. (1938). Organization of memory traces in the Korsakoff syndrome. *A.M.A. Archives of Neurology and Psychiatry, 39*, 482–487.

Benedek, L., & Juba, A. (1940). Korsakowsyndrom, Störungen der zentral-vegetativen Regulation und Hypothalamus [Korsakoff's syndrome, disturbances of the central-vegetative regulation and hypothalamus]. *Archiv für Psychiatrie, 111*, 341–372.

Benedek, L., & Juba, A. (1941). Korsakow-Syndrom bei den Geschwülsten des Zwischenhirns [Korsakoff's syndrome with tumors of the diencephalon]. *Archiv für Psychiatrie, 164*, 366–376.

Benedek, L., & Porsche, F. (1921). Amnestischer Symptomenkomplex nach Meningismus [Amnesic symptom complex after meningitis]. *Deutsche Zeitschrift für Nervenheilkunde, 70*, 320–329.

Benedikt, M. (1876). Der Raubthiertypus am menschlichen Gehirne [The carnivorous type of the human brain]. *Centralblatt für die medicinischen Wissenschaften, 42*, 930–933.

Benedikt, M. (1879). *Anatomische Studien an Verbrecher-Gehirnen* [Anatomical studies on the brains of criminals]. Wien: Wilhelm Braumüller.

Benedikt, M. (1880). Zur Frage des Vierwindungstypus [On the question of the four-gyri-type]. *Centralblatt für die medicinischen Wissenschaften, 46*, 849–852.

Benes, F.M., McSparren, J., Sangiovanni, J.P., & Vincent, S.L. (1989). Deficits in small interneurons in schizophrenic cortex. *Society for Neuroscience Abstracts, 15*, 1122 (Abstr. No. 449.6).

Bennett, A.E., Keegan, J.J., & Wilbur, C.B. (1943). Prefrontal lobotomy in chronic schizophrenia. *Journal of the American Medical Association, 123*, 809–813.

Bennett, A.H. (1878). Case of cerebral tumour-symptoms simulating hysteria. *Brain, 1*, 114–120.

Bental, D. (1957). Vergleich über den Verlauf von Psychosen bei lobotomierten und nicht lobotomierten Geschwistern [Comparison on the progress of psychoses in lobotomized and non-lobotomized brothers and sisters]. *Schweizer Archiv für Neurologie und Psychiatrie, 79*, 1–26.

Berger, H. (1900). Experimentell-anatomische Studien über die durch den Mangel optischer Reize veranlassten Entwicklungshemmungen im Occipitallappen des Hundes und der Katze [Experimental-anatomical studies on developmental retardation in the occipital lobe of dog and cat caused by a lack of optic stimuli]. *Archiv für Psychiatrie und Nervenkrankheiten, 33*, 521–567 (and 2 tables).

Berger, H. (1920). Vorstellungen eines Falles von Stirnhirntumor(?) [Demonstrations of a case with a frontal lobe tumor(?)]. *Münchener medizinische Wochenschrift*, 201.

Berger, H. (1923). Klinische Beiträge zur Pathologie des Grosshirns. I. Mitteilung: Herderkrankungen der Präfrontalregion [Clinical contributions on the pathology of the cerebrum. I. Communication: Focal diseases of the prefrontal region]. *Archiv für Psychiatrie und Nervenkrankheiten, 69*, 1–46.

Berger, H. (1926). Über Rechenstörungen bei Herderkrankungen des Grosshirns [On calculation disturbances in focal diseases of the cerebrum]. *Archiv für Psychiatrie und Nervenkrankheiten, 78*, 238–263.

Berger, H. (1929). Über das Elektroencephalogramm des Menschen. 1. Mitteilung [On the human electroencephalogram. 1. Communication].

Archiv für Psychiatrie und Nervenkrankheiten, 87, 527–570.

Berger, H. (1938). Das Elektrenkephalogramm des Menschen [The human electrencephalogram]. *Nova Leopoldina, 6*, 173–309.

Bergson, H. (1911). *Matter and memory*. New York: Macmillan.

Beringer, K. (1927). *Der Meskalinrausch* [Mescaline intoxication]. *(Monographien aus dem Gesamtgebiete der Neurologie und Psychiatrie, No. 49)*. Berlin: Springer.

Berkhan, O. (1892). Ein Fall von subcorticaler Alexie (Wernicke) [A case of subcortical alexia (Wernicke)]. *Archiv für Psychiatrie und Nervenkrankheiten, 23*, 558–564.

Berliner, B., Beveridge, R.L., Mayer-Gross, W., & Moore, J.P.N. (1945). Prefrontal leucotomy: Report on 100 cases. *Lancet, i*, 325–328.

Bernhardt, M. (1874). Zur Frage von den Funktionen einzelner Theile der Hirnrinde des Menschen [On the question of the functions of individual parts of the human cerebral cortex]. *Archiv für Psychiatrie und Nervenkrankheiten, 4*, 480–481.

Bernhardt, M. (1885). Ueber die spastische Cerebralparalyse im Kindesalter (Hemiplegia spastica infantilis), nebst einem Excurse über „Aphasie bei Kindern“ [On spastic cerebral paralysis in childhood (hemiplegia spastica infantilis), together with a disgression on "aphasia in childhood"]. *Archiv für pathologische Anatomie und Physiologie und für klinische Medicin, 10/2*, 26–80.

Bernhardt, M., & Borchardt, M. (1909). Zur Klinik der Stirnhirntumoren nebst Bemerkungen über Hirnpunktion [Clinical observations of frontal lobe tumors, together with remarks on brain puncture]. *Berliner klinische Wochenschrift, 46*, 1341–1347.

Bernstein, A. (1903). Über eine einfache Methode zur Untersuchung der Merkfähigkeiten resp. des Gedächtnisses bei Geisteskranken [On a simple method for investigating memory ability, especially memory in the mentally diseased]. *Zeitschrift für Psychologie und Physiologie der Sinnesorgane, 32*, 259–263.

Bethe, A. (1898). Dürfen wir den Ameisen und Bienen psychische Qualitäten zuschreiben? [May we attribute psychic qualities to ants and bees?] *Pflüger's Archiv für die gesammte Physiologie des Menschen und der Tiere, 70*, 15–100 (and 2 tables).

Bethe, A. (1900). Noch einmal über die psychischen Qualitäten der Ameisen [Continuing on the psychic qualities of the ants]. *Pflüger's Archiv für die gesammte Physiologie des Menschen und der Tiere, 79*, 39–52.

Betlheim, S., & Hartmann, H. (1924). Über Fehlreaktionen bei der Korsakoffschen Psychose [On parapraxes in Korsakoff psychosis]. *Archiv für Psychiatrie und Nervenkrankheiten, 72*, 275–286. (translated: see Betlheim & Hartmann, 1951)

Betlheim, S., & Hartmann, H. (1951). On parapraxes in the Korsakow psychosis]. In D. Rapaport (Ed. and Transl.), *Organization and pathology of thought* (pp. 288–307). New York: Columbia University Press. (translation of Betlheim & Hartmann, 1924)

Beyerman, T. (1912). Zur Casuistik der Thalamusherde [On the casuistry of thalamic foci]. *Folia neuro-biologica, 6*, 209–218.

Bianchi, L. (1894). Ueber die Function der Stirnlappen [On the function of the frontal lobes]. *Berliner klinische Wochenschrift, 31*, 309–310.

Bianchi, L. (1895). The functions of the frontal lobes. *Brain, 18*, 497–530.

Bianchi, L. (1922). *The mechanism of the brain and the function of the frontal lobes*. Edinburgh: E. and S. Livingstone.

Bickel, A. (1903). Beitrag zur Symptomatologie der Neubildungen des Gehirns, nach Beobachtungen an der Göttinger Medizinischen Klinik [Contribution to the symptomatology of brain tumors observated in the Göttingen Medical Clinic]. *Pathologisch-Anatomische Arbeiten. Herrn Geh. Medicinalrath Orth. Orths Festschrift*, 652–668.

Bielschowsky, M. (1915). Ueber Mikrogyrie [On micro-gyri]. *Journal für Psychologie und Neurologie, 22*, 1–47 (and 5 tables).

Bielschowsky, M., & Brodmann, K. (1905). Zur feineren Histologie und Histopathologie der Grosshirnrinde [On the more detailed histology and histo-pathology of the cerebral cortex]. *Journal für Psychologie und Neurologie, 5*, 173–199.

Bigelow, H.J. (1850). Dr. Harlow's case of recovery from the passage of an iron bar through the head. *American Journal of the Medical Sciences, 39*, 13–22 (and 1 Plate).

Binswanger, O. (1882). Ueber eine Missbildung des Gehirns [On a malformation of the brain]. *Archiv für pathologische Anatomie und Physiologie und für klinische Medicin, 87*, 427–476 (and 2 tables).

Binswanger, O. (1885). Ueber einen Fall von Porencephalie [On a case with porencephaly]. *Archiv für pathologische Anatomie und Physiologie und für klinische Medicin, 102*, 13–25 (and 1 Table).

Binswanger, O., & Berger, H. (1901). Zur Klinik und pathologischen Anatomie der postinfectiösen und Intoxicationspsychosen [Clinical observations and pathological anatomy of the post-infectious and intoxication psychoses]. *Archiv für Psychiatrie und Nervenkrankheiten, 34*, 107–139 (and 2 tables).

Birley, J.L.T. (1964). Modified frontal leucotomy: a review of 106 cases. *British Journal of Psychiatry, 110*, 211–221.

Biro, M. (1910). Die Hirntumoren: Herddiagnostik, Differentialdiagnostik mit besonderer Berücksichtigung der Meningitis serosa, Behandlung [Brain tumors: Focal diagnosis, differential diagnosis with special emphasis on the meningitis serosa, treatment]. *Deutsche Zeitschrift für Nervenheilkunde, 39*, 377–402.

Bischoff, E. (1912). Untersuchungen über das unmittelbare und mittelbare Zahlengedächtnis [Investigations of immediate and indirect memory for figures]. *Zeitschrift für die gesamte Neurologie und Psychiatrie, 11*, 63–68.

Blakemore, C., & Greenfield, S. (1987). *Mindwaves. Thoughts on intelligence, identity and consciousness*. Oxford: Basil Blackwell.

Bleuler, E. (1893). Ein Fall von aphasischen Symptomen, Hemianopsie, amnestischer Farbenblindheit und Seelenlähmung [A case with aphasic symptoms, hemianopia, amnesic color blindness, and optic agnosia]. *Archiv für Psychiatrie und Nervenkrankheiten, 25*, 32–73.

Bleuler, E. (1905). Diagnostische Assoziationsstudien V. Bewusstsein und Assoziation [Diagnostic association studies V. Consciousness and association]. *Journal für Psychologie und Neurologie, 6*, 126–154.

Bleuler, E. (1921). Über unbewusstes psychisches Geschehen [On unconscious psychic activity]. *Zeitschrift für die gesamte Neurologie und Psychiatrie, 64*, 122–135.

Blumer, D., & Benson, D.F. (1975). Personality with frontal and temporal lobe lesions. In D.F. Benson & D. Blumer (Eds.), *Psychiatric aspects of neurological disease* (pp. 151–170). New York: Gruner & Stratton.

Bochnik, H.J. (1952). „Tagesrhythmen" nach halbseitiger präfrontaler Leukotomie (Zur Analyse gestörter Funktionsstrukturen nach Beobachtung spontaner 24-Stunden-Schwankungen animaler und psychischer Vorgänge.) ["Daily rhythms" after unilateral prefrontal leucotomy (On the analysis of disturbed functional structures after observation of spontaneous 24-hour-deviations of animalian and psychic processes.)]. *Deutsche Zeitschrift für Nervenheilkunde, 168*, 95–111.

Boedeker, J. (1905). Ueber einen acuten („Polioencephalitis superior haemorrhagica") und einen chronischen Fall von Korsakow'scher Psychose [On an acute ("Polioencephalitis superior haemorrhagica") and a chronic case of Korsakoff's psychosis]. *Archiv für Psychiatrie und Nervenkrankheiten, 40*, 304–328.

Boediker, (n.n.g.) (1896). Ueber einen Fall von retro- und anterograder Amnesie nach Erhängungsversuch [On a case with retrograde and anterograde amnesia after an attempt of hanging]. *Archiv für Psychiatrie und Nervenkrankheiten, 29*, 647–650.

Boehlke, W. (1952). Ein neues Leukotomieverfahren [A new technique for leucotomy]. *Archiv für Psychiatrie und Zeitschrift Neurologie, 187*, 459–468.

Bogaert, L. van, & Helsmoortel, J., jun. (1928). Toxineurite alcoolique vestibulaire avec syndrome de Korsakow [Alcohol-based toxic neuritis of the vestibular system with Korsakoff's syndrome]. *Journal de neurologie et de psychiatrie, 28*, 213–215.

Bogerts, B. (1984). Zur Neuropathologie der Schizophrenien [On the neuropathology of schizophrenia]. *Fortschritte der Neurologie und Psychiatrie, 52*, 428–437.

Boldt, K. (1905). Studien über Merkdefekte [Studies on defects of memorizing]. *Monatsschrift für Psychiatrie und Neurologie, 17*, 97–115.

Bollinger, G. (1891). Ueber traumatische Spät-Apoplexie. Ein Beitrag zur Lehre von der Hirnerschütterung [On late traumatic apoplexia. Contribution to the study of cerebral concussion]. *Festschrift Rudolf Virchow zu seinem 71. Geburtstag gewidmet* (pp. 457–470). Berlin: Reinert.

Bolton, J.S. (1903 a). The functions of the frontal lobes. *Brain, 26*, 215–241.

Bolton, J.S. (1903 b). The histological basis of amentia and dementia. *Archives of Neurology (London), 2*, 424–620.

Bonhoeffer, K. (1901). *Die akuten Geisteskrankheiten der Gewohnheitstrinker* [Acute mental illnesses of chronic drinkers]. Fischer: Jena.

Bonhoeffer, K. (1904). Der Korsakowsche Symptomenkomplex in seinen Beziehungen zu den verschiedenen Krankheitsformen [The Korsakoff symptom complex in its relation to different forms of illnesses]. *Allgemeine Zeitschrift für Psychiatrie und psychisch-gerichtliche Medicin, 61*, 744–752.

Bonner, F., Cobb, S., Sweet, W.H., & White, J.C. (1952). Frontal lobe surgery in the treatment of pain. *Psychosomatic Medicine, 14*, 382–405.

Borrini, G., Dall'Ora, P., Della Sala, S., Marinelli, L., & Spinnler, H. (1989). Autobiographical memory. Sensitivity to age and education of a standardized enquiry. *Psychological Medicine, 19*, 215–224.

Bostroem, A. (1921). Zur Diagnose von Stirnhirntumoren [On the diagnosis of frontal lobe tumors]. *Deutsche Zeitschrift für Nervenheilkunde, 70*, 80–91.

Bouman, L., & Gruenbaum, A.A. (1929). Eine Störung der Chronognosie und ihre Bedeutung im betreffenden Symptomenbild [A disturbance of chronosognosia and its meaning in the corresponding picture of the symptom]. *Monatsschrift für Psychiatrie und Neurologie, 73*, 1–39.

Bowen, M. (1989). Frontal lobe function. *Brain Injury, 3*, 109–128.

Bowman, K.M., Goodhart, R., & Jolliffe, N. (1939). Observations of the role of vitamin B1 in the etiology and treatment of Korsakoff psychosis. *Journal of Nervous and Mental Disease, 90*, 569–575.

Bramwell, B. (1899). On the localisation of intracranial tumours. *Brain, 22*, 1–70.

Bramwell, B., & Edin, F.R. (1898). A remarkable case of aphasia. Acute und complete destruction by embolic softening of the left motor-vocal speech centre (Broca's convolution), in a right-handed man: transient motor aphasia, marked inability to name objects and especially persons, considerable agraphia and slight word-blindness. *Brain, 21*, 369–373.

Bratz, (n.n.g.) (1898). Ammonshornbefunde bei Epileptischen [Ammon's horn findings in epileptics]. *Archiv für Psychiatrie und Nervenkrankheiten, 31*, 820–836.

Braunmühl, A. von (1930). PICKsche Krankheit [PICK's disease]. In O. Bumke (Ed.), *Handbuch der Geisteskrankheiten, Vol. 7. Die Anatomie der Psychosen* (pp.673–715). Berlin: Springer.

Bräutigam,|W., & Czernigewycz, M. (1950). Hirnatrophischer Prozess und Leukotomie in ihrer Wirkung auf die Zwangsneurose [Brain atrophic process and leucotomy in their effect on a compulsive neurosis]. *Archiv für Psychiatrie und Zeitschrift Neurologie, 184*, 80–94.

Brazier, M.A.B. (1984). *History of neurophysiology in the 17th and 18th centuries*. New York: Raven Press.

Bregman, L.E. (1899). Ueber den „Automatisme ambulatoire" („Fugues", „Dromomania") [On the "automatisme ambulatoire" ("fugues", "dromomania")]. *Neurologisches Centralblatt, 18*, 776–781.

Breuer, J., & Freud, S. (1895). *Studien über Hysterie* [Studies on hysteria]. Wien: Deuticke.

Breukink, H. (1907). Über Patienten mit Perseveration und symbolischen und aphasischen Erscheinungen [On patients with perseveration and symbolic and aphasic symptoms]. *Journal für Psychologie und Neurologie, 9*, 113–133 and 165–185.

Brickner, R.M. (1936). *Intellectual functions of the frontal lobes: A study based upon observation of a man after partial bilateral frontal lobectomy*. New York: Macmillan Company.

Brickner, R.M. (1939). Bilateral frontal lobectomy. Follow-up report of a case. *A.M.A. Archives of Neurology and Psychiatry, 41*, 580–585.

Brickner, R.M. (1952). Brain of patient A. after bilateral frontal lobectomy; status of frontal-lobe problem. *A.M.A. Archives of Neurology and Psychiatry, 68*, 293–313.

Bridges, P.K. (1972). Psychosurgery today: Psychiatric aspects. *Proceedings of the Royal Society of Medicine, 65*, 1104–1108.

Bridges, P.K., & Goktepe, E.O. (1973). A review of patients with obsessional symptoms treated by psychosurgery. In L.V. Laitinen & K.E. Livingston (Eds.), *Surgical approaches in psychiatry* (pp. 96–100). Lancaster, UK: Medical and Technical Publ. Comp.

Bridges, P.K., Goktepe, E.O., Maratos, J., Browne, & Young, L. (1973). A comparative review of patients with obsessional neurosis and with depression treated by psychosurgery. *British Journal of Psychiatry, 123*, 663–674.

Brie, (n.n.g.). (1892). Ein Fall von Geistesstörung bei multipler Neuritis [A case of mental disturbance in multiple neuritis]. *Allgemeine Zeitschrift für Psychiatrie und ihre Grenzgebiete, 48*, 175–179.

Broca, P. (1861 a). Perte de la parole. Ramollissement chronique et destruction partielle du lobe antérieur gauche du cerveau [Loss of words. Chronic softening and partial destruction of the anterior left cerebral lobe]. *Bulletin de la Societé d'Anthropologie, 2*, 235–238.

Broca, P. (1861 b). Remarques sur le siège de la faculté du langage articulé: Suivies d'une observation d'aphémie (perte de la parole) [Remarks on the seat of the faculty of articulate language, followed by an observation on aphemia]. *Bulletin de la Société Anatomique de Paris, 36*, 330–357.

Broca, P. (1878). Anatomie comparée des circonvolutions cérébrales. Le grand lobe limbique et la scissure limbique dans la série des mammiféres [Comparative anatomy of the cerebral lobes. The grand limbic lobe and the limbic fissure throughout mammalian phylogeny]. *Revue Anthropologie, 2*, 385–498.

Brodmann, K. (1897). Zur Methodik der hypnotischen Behandlung [On the methodology of hypnotic treatment]. *Zeitschrift für Hypnotismus, Psychotherapie sowie andere psychophysiologische und psychopathologische Forschungen, 6*, 1–10, 193–214.

Brodmann, K. (1902). Experimenteller und klinischer Beitrag zur Psychopathologie der polyneuritischen Psychose [Experimental and clinical contribution to the psychopathology of the polyneuritic psychoses]. *Journal für Psychologie und Neurologie, 1*, 225–246.

Brodmann, K. (1904). Experimenteller und klinischer Beitrag zur Psychopathologie der polyneuritischen Psychose. B. Experimenteller Teil. [Experimental and clinical contribution to the psychopathology of the polyneuritic psychoses. B. Experimental part.]. *Journal für Psychologie und Neurologie, 3*, 1–48.

Brodmann, K. (1904/05). Die Rindenfelder der niederen Affen [The cortical fields of lower monkeys]. *Journal für Psychologie und Neurologie, 4*, 177–226.

Brodmann, K. (1908a). Beiträge zur histologischen Lokalisation der Grosshirnrinde. VII. Mitteilung: die cytoarchitektonische Cortexgliederung der Halbaffen (Lemuriden) [Contribution to histological localization in the cerebral cortex. VII. Communication: The cytoarchitectonic division of the cortex of the prosimians (lemurids)]. *Journal für Psychologie und Neurologie, 10*, 287–334.

Brodmann, K. (1908b). Ueber Rindenmessungen [On measurements of the cortex]. *Zentralblatt für Nervenheilkunde und Psychiatrie (N.F.), 19*, 781–798.

Brodmann, K. (1909a). Antwort an Herrn Dr. Th. Kaes [Response to Dr. Th. Kaes]. *Neurologisches Centralblatt, 28*, 635–639.

Brodmann, K. (1909b). *Vergleichende Lokalisationslehre der Grosshirnrinde in ihren Prinzipien dargestellt auf Grund des Zellenbaues* [Comparative study of the localization in the cerebral cortex, demonstrated in its principles on the basis of cytoarchitecture]. Leipzig: Barth.

Brodmann, K. (1912). Ergebnisse über die vergleichende histologische Lokalisation der Grosshirnrinde mit besonderer Berücksichtigung des Stirnhirns [Results on the comparative histological study of the cerebral cortex with special emphasis on the frontal lobe]. *Anatomischer Anzeiger (Suppl.), 41*, 157–216.

Brodmann, K. (1915). Zur Neurologie der Stirnhirnschüsse [On the neurology of frontal-lobe shots]. *Psychiatrisch-neurologische Wochenschrift, 17*, 193–194.

Brooks, C. McC., & Cranefield, P.F. (Eds.). (1959). *Historical development of physiological thought.* New York: Hafner.

Brouwer, B. (1912). Das Gehirn einer congenital tauben Katze [The brain of a congenitally deaf cat]. *Folia Neurobiologica, 6*, 197–208.

Brown, J.W. (1990). Psychology of time awareness. *Brain and Cognition, 14*, 144–164.

Brown, S., & Schäfer, E.A. (1888). An investigation into the functions of the occipital and temporal lobes of the monkey's brain. *Philosophical Transactions of the Royal Society of London, 179*, 303–327.

Browne, (n.n.g.) (1872). Cranial injuries and mental disease. *West Riding Lunatic Asylum Report London, 2*, 97–136.

Browne, C.E. (1906). The psychology of the simple arithmetical processes: a study of certain habits of attention and association. *American Journal of Psychology, 17*, 1–37.

Bruck, C. (1867). Die biologische Differenzierung von Affenarten und menschlichen Rassen durch spezifische Blutreaktion [The biological differentiation of monkey species and human races by specific blood reactions]. *Berliner klinische Wochenschrift, 44*, 793–797.

Brücke, E.T. von (1913). *Ueber die Grundlagen und Methoden der Grosshirnphysiologie und ihre Beziehungen zur Psychologie* [On the basics and methods of cerebral physiology and their relations to psychology]. Jena: G. Fischer.

Bruns, L. (1892). Ueber Störungen des Gleichgewichtes bei Stirnhirntumoren [On disturbances in balance due to frontal lobe tumors]. *Deutsche medicinische Wochenschrift, No. 7*, 138–140.

Bruns, L. (1897). *Die Geschwülste des Nervensystems* [The tumors of the nervous system]. Berlin: Karger.

Bruns, L. (1898). Zwei Fälle von Hirntumor mit genauer Localdiagnose [Two cases of brain tumor with exact locus diagnosis]. *Neurologisches Zentralblatt, 17*, 770–788 and 848–858.

Brunswik, E. (1932). *Untersuchungen zur Entwicklung des Gedächtnisses* [Studies on the development of memory]. Leipzig: J.A. Barth.

Bruton, C.J., Crow, T.J., Frith, C.D., Johnstone, E.C., Owens, D.G.C., & Roberts, G.W. (1990). Schizophrenia and the brain: a prospective clinico-neuropathological study. *Psychological Medicine, 20*, 285–304.

Buchsbaum, M.S., Nuechterlein, K.H., Haier, R.J., Wu, J., Sicotte, N., Hazlett, E., Asarnow, R., Potkin, S., & Guich, S. (1990). Glucose metabolic rate in normals and schizophrenics during the continuous performance test assessed by positron emission tomography. *British Journal of Psychiatry, 156*, 216–227.

Büchner, L. (1872). *Kraft und Stoff. Empirisch-naturphilosophishe Studien in allgemein-verständlicher Darstellung* [Energy and matter. Studies in empirical natural philosophy in general terms]. Leipzig: T. Thomas.

Bucy, P.C., & Klüver, H. (1940). Anatomic changes secondary to temporal lobectomy. *A.M.A. Archives of Neurology and Psychiatry, 44*, 1142–1146.

Bumke, O. (1920). Über unbewusstes psychisches Geschehen [On unconscious psychic activity].

Zeitschrift für die gesamte Neurologie und Psychiatrie, 56, 142–149.

Bumke, O. (1922). *Das Unterbewusstsein* [The unconscious]. Berlin: Springer.

Bumke, O. (1942). *Gedanken über die Seele* [Thoughts on the soul]. (3rd ed.). Berlin: Springer.

Burckhardt, G. (1875). *Die physiologische Diagnostik der Nervenkrankheiten* [The physiological diagnosis of nervous diseases]. Leipzig: W. Engelmann.

Burckhardt, G. (1891). Ueber Rindenexcisionen, als Beitrag zur operativen Therapie der Psychosen [On cortical excisions as a contribution to the surgical therapy of psychoses]. *Allgemeine Zeitschrift für Psychiatrie und psychiatrisch-gerichtliche Medicin, 47*, 463–548.

Burdach, K.F. (1819). *Vom Baue und Leben des Gehirns* [On the construction and life of the brain]. (Vol. 1). Leipzig: Dyk'sche Verlagsbuchhandlung.

Burdach, K.F. (1822). *Vom Baue und Leben des Gehirns* [On the construction and life of the brain]. (Vol. 2). Leipzig: Dyk'sche Verlagsbuchhandlung.

Burdach, K.F. (1826). *Vom Baue und Leben des Gehirns* [On the construction and life of the brain]. (Vol. 3). Leipzig: Dyk'sche Verlagsbuchhandlung.

Bürger, H. (1927). Zur Psychologie des amnestischen Symptomenkomplexes [On the psychology of the amnesic symptom complex]. *Archiv für Psychiatrie und Nervenkrankheiten, 81*, 348–352.

Bürger-Prinz, H., & Kaila, M. (1930). Über die Struktur des amnestischen Symptomenkomplexes [On the structure of the amnesic symptom complex]. *Zeitschrift für die gesamte Neurologie und Psychiatrie, 124*, 553–595.

Burgl, G. (1900). Eine Reise in die Schweiz im epileptischen Dämmerzustande und die transitorischen Bewusstseinsstörungen der Epileptiker vor dem Strafrichter [A journey to Switzerland done in epileptic somnolence and the transitory disturbances of consciousnes before the criminal judge]. *Münchener medizinische Wochenschrift, No. 37*, 1270–1273.

Burkle, F.M., & Lipowski, Z.J. (1978). Colloid cyst of the third ventricle presenting as a psychiatric disorder. *American Journal of Psychiatry, 135*, 373–595.

Burnett, C.T. (1925). Splitting the mind. *Psychological Monographs,34 (No. 2)*, 1–132.

Burnham, W.H. (1889 a). Memory, historically and experimentally considered. I. An historical sketch of the older conceptions of memory. *American Journal of Psychology, 2*, 39–90.

Burnham, W.H. (1889 b). Memory, historically and experimentally considered. II. Modern conceptions of memory. *American Journal of Psychology, 2*, 225–270.

Burnham, W.H. (1889 c). Memory, historically and experimentally considered. III. Paramnesia. *American Journal of Psychology, 2*, 431–464.

Burnham, W.H. (1889d). Memory, historically and experimentally considered. IV. Recent theories, experimental studies, conclusion. *American Journal of Psychology, 2*, 568–622.

Burnham, W.H. (1903). Retroactive amnesia: Illustrative cases and a tentative explanation. *American Journal of Psychology, 14*, 118–132.

Burr, C.W. (1907). Tactile amnesia. *The American Journal of the Medical Sciences, 134*, 106–112.

Busch, E. (1957). Psychosurgery. In H. Olivecrona & W. Tönnis (Eds.), *Handbuch der Neurochirurgie, Vol. 6. Chirurgie der Hirnnerven und Hirnbahnen* (pp. 137–177). Berlin: Springer.

Bushnell, M.C., & Duncan, G.H. (1989). Sensory and affective aspects of pain perception: is medial thalamus restricted to emotional issues? *Experimental Brain Research, 78*, 415–418.

Busse, G. (1989). Schreber und Flechsig: der Hirnanatom als Psychiater [Schreber and Flechsig: the brain anatomist as psychiatrist]. *Medizinhistorisches Journal, 24*, 260–305.

Cairns, H., & Mosberg, W.H. (1951). Colloid cyst of the third ventricle. *Surgery, Gynecology and Obstetrics, 92*, 546–570.

Cajal, S.R. y. (1895). Einige Hypothesen über den anatomischen Mechanismus der Ideenbildung, der Association und der Aufmerksamkeit [Some hypotheses on the anatomical mechanism of creating ideas, associations, and attention]. *Archiv für Anatomie und Physiologie. Anatomische Abteilung*, 367–378.

Cajal, S.R. y (1896). Beitrag zum Studium der Medulla oblongata, des Kleinhirnes und des Ursprunges der Gehirnnerven [Contribution to the study of the medulla oblongata, the cerebellum, and the origin of the brain nerves]. Leipzig: Barth.

Cajal, S.R. y. (1909–1911). *Histologie du systeme nerveux de l'homme et de vertébrès* [Histology of the nervous system in man and vertebrates]. Paris: Maloine.

Cajal, S.R. y. (1935). Die Neuronenlehre [The neuron doctrine]. In O. Bumke & O. Foerster (Eds.), *Handbuch der Neurologie. (Vol. 1/1)* (pp. 887–994). Berlin: Springer.

Calderwood, H. (1879). *The relations of mind and brain.* London: Macmillan.

Cambier, J. (1954). L'encephalopathie de Gayet-Wernicke et les encephalopathies carentielles des alcooliques [The encephalopathy of Gayet-Wernicke and the deficiency-caused encephalopathies of alcoholics]. *Presse Medicale, 62*, 859–861.

Campbell, D. (1909). Störungen der Merkfähigkeit und fehlendes Krankheitsgefühl bei einem Fall von Stirnhirntumor [Disturbances in memory and lack of insight into the disease in a case of frontal lobe tumor]. *Monatsschrift für Psychiatrie und Neurologie, 26 (Suppl.)*, 33–41.

Campbell, A.C.P., & Biggart, J.H. (1939). Wernicke's encephalopathy (Polioencephalitis haemorrhagica superior): its alcoholic and non-alcoholic incidence. *Journal of Pathology and Bacteriology, 48*, 245–262.

Campbell, A.W. (1905). *Histological studies on the localization of cerebral function*. Cambridge: Cambridge University Press.

Camper, P., & Pringle, J. (1779). XIV. Account of the organs of speech of the Orang Outang. *Philosophical Transactions of the Royal Society of London, 69*, 139–159.

Canton, (n.n.g.) (1860). Chronic alcoholism with impending delirium tremens treated by suspension of the stimulus. *Lancet, ii*, 237–238.

Carmel, P.W. (1985). Tumours of the third ventricle. *Acta Neurochirurgica, 75*, 136–146.

Carmichael, E.A., & Stern, R.O. (1931). Korsakoff's syndrome: its histopathology. *Brain, 54*, 189–213.

Carney, M.W.P., Charty, T.K.N., Robotis, P., & Childs, A. (1987). Ganser syndromes and its management. *British Journal of Psychiatry, 151*, 697–700.

Carscallen, H.B., Buck, C.W., & Hobbs, G.E. (1951). Clinical and psychological investigation of prefrontal lobotomy in chronic schizophrenia. *A.M.A. Archives of Neurology and Psychiatry, 65*, 206–220.

Caton, R. (1875). The electric currents of the brain. *British Medical Journal, 2*, 278.

Centres, J.L. (1914). Ueber den Schädelinhalt Geisteskranker [On the cranial volume of mental patients]. *Archiv für Psychiatrie und Nervenkrankheiten, 54*, 1015–1030.

Chapman, W.P., Livingston, R.B., & Livingston, K.E. (1949). Frontal lobotomy and electrical stimulation of orbital surface and frontal lobes. *A.M.A. Archives of Neurology and Psychiatry, 62*, 701–716.

Chapman, W.P., Rose, A.S., & Solomon, H.S. (1948). Measurements of heat stimulus producing motor withdrawal reaction in patients following frontal lobotomy. In J.F. Fulton, W.C. Aring, & S.B. Wortis (Eds.), *The frontal lobes. (Research publications of the association for research in nervous and mental disease, Vol. 27)* (pp. 754–768). Baltimore: Williams & Wilkins.

Charcot, J.M. (1878). *Ueber die Localisationen der Gehirn-Krankheiten* [On the localization of brain diseases]. Stuttgart: Bonz & co.

Charcot, J.M. (1892). Sur un cas d'amnesie retro-anterograde [On a case with retro- and anterograde amnesia]. *Revue de medicine, 12*, 81–96.

Chaussier, F.B. (1807). *Exposition sommaire de la structure et des différentes parties de l'encéphale du cerveau* [Overview of the structure and the different parts of the cerbral cortex]. Paris: Barrois.

Cheek, W.R., & Taveras, J.M. (1966). Thalamic tumors. *Journal of Neurosurgery, 24*, 505–513.

Chiarello, C. (1980). A house divided? Cognitive functioning with callosal agenesis. *Brain and Language, 11*, 128–158.

Choroschko, W.K. (1923). Die Stirnlappen des Gehirns in funktioneller Beziehung [The frontal lobes of the brain in functional relation]. *Zeitschrift für die gesamte Neurologie und Psychiatrie, 83*, 291–302.

Chotzen, F. (1902). Zur Kenntnis der polyneuritischen Psychose [On our understanding of the polyneuritic psychosis]. *Allgemeine Zeitschrift für Psychiatrie und ihre Grenzgebiete, 59*, 498–534.

Christoffel, H., & Grossmann, E. (1923). Über die expressionistische Komponente in Bildnereien geistig minderwertiger Knaben. (Vorläufige Mitteilung nach einem Demonstrationsversuch in der Frühjahrsversammlung 1923 des Schweizer Vereins für Psychiatrie) [On the expressionistic component in the pictures of mentally inferior boys. (Preliminary communication after a demonstration on the spring meeting 1923 of the Swiss Society of Psychiatry)]. *Zeitschrift für die gesamte Neurologie und Psychiatrie, 87*, 372–376.

Churchland, P.S. (1986). *Neurophilosophy. Toward a unified science of the mind/brain*. Cambridge, MA: MIT Press.

Ciarla, E. (1915). Ein Beitrag zum histologischen Bild der senilen Hirnrinde [A contribution to the histological picture of the senile cerebral cortex]. *Archiv für Psychiatrie und Nervenkrankheiten, 55*, 223–240.

Claparede, E. (1911). Recognition et moiite [Recognition and me-ness]. *Archives de Psychologie, 11*, 79–90.

Clapham, C. (1879). On skull mapping. *Brain 1*, 97–100.

Clark, C.R., & Geffen, G.M. (1989). Corpus callosum surgery and recent memory. *Brain, 112*, 165–175.

Clarke, E., & Dewhurst, K. (1972). *An illustrated history of brain function*. New York: Sanford.

Clarke, E., & Jacyna, L.S. (1987). *Nineteenth-century origins and neuroscientific concepts*. Berkeley, CA: University of California Press.

Clarke, J.M. (1898). The accurate localisation of intracranial tumours, excluding tumours of the motor cortex, motor tract, pons and medulla. *Brain, 21*, 305–319.

Cochrane, W.A., Collins-Williams, C., & Donohue, W.L. (1961). Superior hemorrhagic polioencephalitis (Wernicke's disease) occurring in an infant – probably due to thiamine deficiency from use of a soya bean product. *Pediatrics, 28*, 771–777.

Cocores, J.A., Santa, W.G., & Patel, M.D. (1984). The Ganser syndrome: Evidence suggesting its classification as a dissociative disorder. *International Journal of Psychiatry in Medicine, 14*, 47–56.

Cohen, L.H., Novick, R.G., & Ettleson, A. (1942). Frontal lobotomy in the treatment of chronic psychotic overactivity: Report of six cases. *Psychosomatic Medicine, 4*, 96–103.

Cohn, J. (1897). Experimentelle Untersuchungen über das Zusammenwirken des akustisch-motorischen und des visuellen Gedächtnisses [Experimental investigations on cooperation between acoustic-motoric and visual memory]. *Zeitschrift für Psychologie und Physiologie der Sinnesorgane, 15*, 161–183.

Cole, S.J. (1902). On changes in the central nervous system in the neuritic disorders of chronic alcoholism. *Brain, 25*, 326–363.

Cole, S.J. (1911). The comparative anatomy of the frontal lobe and its bearing upon the pathology of insanity. *Journal of Mental Science, 57*, 52–55.

Colmant, H.J. (1965). *Enzephalopathien bei chronischem Alkoholismus, insbesondere Thalamusbefunde bei Wernickescher Enzephalopathie* [Encephalopathies in chronic alcoholism, especially thalamic findings in Wernicke's encephalopathy]. *(Forum der Psychiatrie, 12*, 1–86.) Stuttgart: Enke.

Compston, A. (1988). The 150th anniversary of the first depiction of the lesions of multiple sclerosis. *Journal of Neurology, Neurosurgery, and Psychiatry, 51*, 1249–1252.

Conkey, R.C. (1938). Psychological changes associated with head injuries. *Archives of Psychology (New York),No. 232*, 1–62.

Conrad, K. & Ule, G. (1951). Ein Fall von Korsakow-Psychose mit anatomischem Befund und klinischen Betrachtungen [A case with Korsakoff's psychosis and clinical considerations]. *Deutsche Zeitschrift für Nervenheilkunde, 165*, 430–445.

Constantinides, C.D., & Stroussopoulos, B. (1954). Prefrontal leucotomy. Remarks on the pathophysiology of the brain. *American Journal of Psychiatry, 111*, 196–197.

Corkin, S. (1984). Lasting consequences of bilateral medial temporal lobectomy: Clinical course and experimental findings in H.M. *Seminars in Neurology, 4*, 249–259.

Corsellis, J.A.N., & Jack, A.B. (1973). Neuropathological observations on Yttrium implants and on undercutting in the orbito-frontal areas of the brain. In L.V. Laitinen & K.E. Livingston (Eds.), *Surgical approaches in psychiatry* (pp. 90–95). Lancaster, UK: Medical and Technical Publ. Comp.

Cortesi, T. (1908). Tumore cerebrale del lobo prefrontale sinistro. Osservazione-clinica ed anatomica [Cerebral tumor of the left prefrontal lobe. Clinical and anatomical observations]. *Il Morgagni, 50*, 65–81.

Cowen, T.P. (1902). A case of tumour of the frontal lobes of the cerebrum in which sleep was a marked symptom. *Journal of the Mental Sciences, 48*, 327–328.

Cowles, E. (1900). Epilepsy with retrograde amnesia. *American Journal of Insanity, 56*, 593–614.

Cramer, A. (1899). Neuere Arbeiten über die Localisation geistiger Vorgänge [Recent work on the localization of mental acts]. *Zentralblatt für allgemeine Pathologie und pathologische Anatomie, 10*, 441–448.

Cramon, D.Y. von, Hebel, N., & Ebeling, U. (1990). Anatomical considerations on memory and learning deficits due to focal cerebral lesions in man. In L.R. Squire & E. Lindenlaub (Eds.), *The biology of memory* (pp. 527–540). Stuttgart: F.K. Schattauer.

Cramon, D.Y. von, & Markowitsch, H.J. (1992). The problem of "localizing" memory in focal cerebrovascular lesions. In L.R. Squire & N. Butters (Eds.), *Neuropsychology of memory* (2nd ed.). (in press). New York: Guilford Press.

Crawford, M.P., Fulton, J.F., Jacobsen, C.F., & Wolf, J.B. (1948). Frontal lobe ablation in chimpanzee: A resumé of "Becky" and "Lucy". In J.F. Fulton, W.C. Aring & S.B. Wortis (Eds.), *The frontal lobes. (Research publications for the association for research in nervous and mental disease, Vol. 27)* (pp. 3–58). Baltimore: Williams & Wilkins.

Creutzfeldt, H.G. (1928). Hirnveränderungen bei Gewohnheitstrinkern [Brain changes in chronic alcoholics]. *Zentralblatt für Neurologie, 50*, 321.

Crichton-Browne, J. (1879). On the weight of the brain and its component in the insane. *Brain, 1*, 504–518.

Crovitz, H.F., & Schiffman, H. (1974). Frequency of episodic memories as a function of their age. *Bulletin of the Psychonomic Society, 4*, 517–518.

Crown, S. (1951). Psychological changes following prefrontal leucotomy: a review. *Journal of Mental Science, 97*, 49–83.

Crown, S. (1952). An experimental study of psychological changes following prefrontal lobotomy. *Journal of General Psychology, 47*, 3–41.

Cruickshank, E.K. (1950). Wernicke's encephalopathy. *Quarterly Journal of Medicine, 19*, 327–338.

Curran, F.J., & Schilder, P. (1937). Experiments in repetition and recall. *Pedagogical Seminary and Journal of Genetic Psychology, 51*, 163–187.

Cushing, H. (1922). Distortions of the visual fields in cases of brain tumour: The field defects produced by temporal lobe lesions. *Brain, 44*, 341–396.

Cutting, J. (1978). The relationship between Korsakov's syndrome and 'alcoholic dementia'. *British Journal of Psychiatry, 132*, 240–251.

Da Fano, C. (1909). Studien über die Veränderungen im Thalamus opticus bei Defektpsychosen [Studies on changes in the optic thalamus in defect psychoses]. *Monatsschrift für Psychiatrie und Neurologie, 26*, 4–36.

Dahl, F. (1922). *Vergleichende Psychologie oder Die Lehre von dem Seelenleben des Menschen und der Tiere* [Comparative psychology or the doctrine of the life of the soul in man and animals]. Jena: G. Fischer.

Dahlmann, W., & Schaefer, K.-P. (1979). Klüver-Bucy Syndrom und Greifreflexe (oral, cheiral, podal) nach schwerer Hirnkontusion [Klüver-Bucy syndrome and primitive motor reflexes after severe brain trauma]. *Archiv für Psychiatrie und Nervenkrankheiten, 226*, 229–239.

Dal Bianco, P. (1950). Transorbitale Leukotomie, zur Technik und Problematik der ihrer Indikationsstellung zugrunde liegenden Modellvorstellung [Transorbital leucotomy, techniques and problems in the rationale, on which its indication is based]. *Archiv für Psychiatrie und Nervenkrankheiten, 184*, 278–282.

Dall'Ora, P., Della Sala, S., & Spinnler, H. (1989). Autobiographical memory. Its impairment in amnesic syndromes. *Cortex, 25*, 197–217.

Damasio, A.R. (1989). Neural substrates of memory at systems level. Paper presented at the First Annual Meeting of the Memory Disorders Research Society, Boston, MA, October 26–27.

Damasio, A.R., & Tranel, D. (1989). Knowing that "Colorado" goes with "Denver" does not imply knowledge that "Denver" *is* in "Colorado". *Society for Neuroscience Abstracts, 15*, 303 (No. 121.9).

Dana, C.L. (1874). The study of a case of amnesia or 'double consciousness'. *Psychological Review, 1*, 570–580.

Dandy, W.E. (1922). Treatment of non-encapsulated brain tumors by extensive resection of contiguous brain tissue. *Johns Hopkins Hospital Bulletin, 375*, 188–190.

Dandy, W.E. (1925). Contributions to brain surgery. *Annals of Surgery, 4*, 89–93.

Dandy, W.E. (1933). *Tumours of the third ventricle.* London: Baillière, Tindal, and Cox.

Darwin, C. (1877/1971). A biographical sketch of an infant. *Developmental Medicine and Child Neurology, Suppl. 24*, 3–8.

Dax, E.C., Cunningham, E., & Ridley-Smith, E.J. (1945/46). Discussion: Prefrontal leucotomy with reference to indications and results. *Proceedings of the Royal Society of Medicine 39*, 448–449.

Dax, E.C., & Ridley-Smith, E.J. (1943). The early effects of prefrontal leucotomy on disturbed patients with mental illness of long duration. *Journal of mental Science, 89*, 182–185.

de Crinis, M. (1934). *Aufbau und Abbau der Grosshirnleistungen und ihre anatomischen Grundlagen* [Construction and destruction of cerebral cortical functions and their anatomical base]. Berlin: S. Karger.

de Groot, A.D. (1946). *Het denken van den schaker* [Thinking in chess players]. Amsterdam: North-Holland.

de Groot, A.D. (1965). *Thought and choice in chess.* The Hague: Mouton.

Dehnen, W. (1961). Psychopathologische Erfahrungen bei ein- und beidseitigen psychochirurgischen Eingriffen [Psychopathological experiences after uni- and bilateral psychosurgical interventions]. *Fortschritte der Neurologie, Psychiatrie und ihrer Grenzgebiete, 7*, 353–422.

Deisinger, K., & Markowitsch, H.J. (1991). Die Wirksamkeit von Gedächtnistrainings in der Behandlung von Gedächtnisstörungen [The effectivity of memory training in the treatment of memory disturbances]. *Psychologische Rundschau, 42*, 55–65.

Dejerine, J., & Roussy, G. (1906). Le syndrome thalamique [The thalamic syndrome]. *Revue Neurologique, 14*, 521–532.

Delacour, J., & Levy, J.C.S. (Eds.). (1988). *Systems with learning and memory abilities.* Amsterdam: Elsevier.

Delay, J., & Brion, S. (1969). *Le syndrome de Korsakoff* [Korsakoff's syndrome]. Paris: Masson.

Delgado, J.M.R., & Livingston, R.B. (1948). Some respiratory, vascular and thermal responses to stimulation of orbital surface of frontal lobe. *Journal of Neurophysiology, 11*, 39–55.

Dercum, F.X. (1907). A case of aphasia, both "motor" and "sensory", with integrity of the left third frontal convolution: lesion in the lenticular zone and inferior longitudinal fasciculus. *Journal of Nervous and Mental Disease, 35*, 681–690.

Dercum, F.X. (1910). A report of three pre-frontal tumors. *Journal of Nervous and Mental Disease, 37*, 465–480.

Dercum, F.X. (1925). The thalamus in the physiology and pathology of the mind. *A.M.A. Archives of Neurology and Psychiatry, 14*, 289–302.

DeWardener, H.E., & Lennox, B. (1947). Cerebral beriberi (Wernicke's encephalopathy). *Lancet,i*, 11–17.

Diamond, M.C., Scheibel, A.B., Murphy, G.M., & Harvey, T. (1985). On the brain of a scientist: Albert Einstein. *Experimental Neurology, 88*, 198–204.

Diehl, A. (1902). *Zum Studium der Merkfähigkeit* [On studying the ability to remember]. Berlin: Karger.

Diepgen, P. (1965). *Geschichte der Medizin. Die historische Entwicklung der Heilkunde und des ärztlichen Lebens (Vol. 2)* [History of medicine. The historical development of medical science and the life of physicians (Vol. 2)]. Berlin: Walter de Gruyter.

Divac, I. (1988). A note on the history of the term 'prefrontal'. *IBRO News, 16 (2)*, 2.

Dodds, W.J. (1878). On the localisation of the functions of the brain: Being an historical and critical analysis of the question. *Journal of Anatomy, 12*, 340–363.

Donaldson, H.H. (1890). Anatomical observations on the brain and several sense-organs of the blind and deaf-mute, Laura Dewey Bridgman. *American Journal of Psychology, 3*, 293–242 (and 2 plates).

Donaldson, H.H. (1891). Report of six lectures on cerebral localization. *American journal of Psychology, 4*, 113–130.

Donath, J. (1899). Der epileptische Wandertrieb (Poriomanie) [The epileptic drive to wander (poriomania)]. *Archiv für Psychiatrie und Nervenkrankheiten, 32*, 335–355.

Donath, J. (1907). Weitere Beiträge zur Poriomanie [Further contributions on poriomania]. *Archiv für Psychiatrie und Nervenkrankheiten, 42*, 752–760.

Donath, J. (1908). Ueber hysterische Amnesie [On hysterical amnesia]. *Archiv für Psychiatrie und Nervenkrankheiten, 44*, 559–575.

Donath, J. (1912). Gliom des linken Stirnlappens. Operation; Besserung. Gleichzeitig ein Beitrag zur Bedeutung des Stirnhirns [Glioma of the left frontal lobe. Surgery; improvement. At the same time a contribution on the importance of the frontal lobe]. *Zeitschrift für die gesamte Neurologie und Psychiatrie, 13*, 205–216.

Donath, J. (1923). Die Bedeutung des Stirnhirns für die höheren seelischen Leistungen [The importance of the frontal lobe for higher psychic processess]. *Deutsche Zeitschrift für Nervenheilkunde, 23*, 282–306.

Dorman, C. (1991). Exceptional calculation ability after early left hemispherectomy. *Brain and Cognition, 15*, 26–36.

Down, J.L. (1886). Observations on an ethnic classification of idiots. *London Hospital Clinical Lectures and Reports, 3*, 259–262 [reprinted in *Archives of Neurology, 25*, 89–90].

Down, J.L. (1887). *On some of the mental affections of childhood and youth*. London: J. & A. Churchill.

Dräseke, J. (1901). Gehirnwägungen. Wägungen des Centralnervensystems des Hamsters [Weighing brains. Weights of the central nervous systems of hamsters]. *Monatsschrift für Psychiatrie und Neurologie, 10*, 76.

Dräseke, J. (1906). Gehirngewicht und Intelligenz [Brain weight and intelligence]. *Archiv für Rassen- und Gesellschaftsbiologie, 3*, 499–522.

Drennan, A.M. (1929). Impacted cyst in third ventricle of brain. *British Medical Journal, 2*, 47.

Dreschfeld, J. (1884). On alcoholic paralysis. *Brain 7*, 200–211.

Dresel, K. (1924). Die Funktionen eines Grosshirn- und striatumlosen Hundes [The functions of a dog without cerebral cortex and striatum] . *Klinische Wochenschrift, 3*, 2231–2233.

Droste-Hülshoff, A. von (1925). *Sämtliche Werke* [Collected works]. München: G. Müller.

Dupont, R.M., Jernigan, T.L., Butters, N., Delis, D., Hesselink, J.R., Heindel, W., & Gillin, J.C. (1990). Subcortical abnormalities detected in bipolar affective disorder using magnetic resonance imaging. *Archives of General Psychiatry, 47*, 55–59.

Duus, P. (1939). Über psychische Störungen bei Tumoren des Orbitalhirns [On psychic disturbances in tumors of the orbital brain]. *Archiv für Psychiatrie und Nervenkrankheiten, 109*, 596–648.

Duus, P. (1980). *Neurologisch-topische Diagnostik. Anatomie, Physiologie, Klinik* [Neurological-topical diagnosis. Anatomy, physiology, and clinical aspects]. (2nd ed.) Stuttgart: Thieme.

Dwight, T. (1878). Remarks on the brain, illustrated by the description of the brain of a distinguished man. *Proceedings of the American Academy of Arts and Sciences (N.S.), 5*, 210–215.

Dziembowski, S. von (1916). Stirnhirnverletzung mit psychischen Ausfallserscheinungen [Prefrontal damage with psychic disturbances]. *Deutsche medizinische Wochenschrift, 42*, 630–632.

Ebbinghaus, H. (1885). *Über das Gedächtnis* [On memory]. Leipzig: Duncker & Humblot.

Ebbinghaus, H. (1897). Ueber eine neue Methode zur Prüfung geistiger Fähigkeiten und ihre Anwendung bei Schulkindern [On a new method for studying mental abilities, and its application on pupils]. *Zeitschrift für Psychologie und Physiologie der Sinnesorgane, 13*, 401–459.

Ebbinghaus, H. (1902). *Grundzüge der Psychologie* [Principles of psychology]. Leipzig: Veit & Co.

Ebbinghaus, H. (1905). Ein neuer Fallapparat zur Kontrolle des Chronoskopes [A new falling apparatus for controling the chronoscope]. *Zeitschrift für Psychologie, 30*, 292–305.

Eberstaller, (n.n.g.) (1890). *Das Stirnhirn. Ein Beitrag zur Anatomie der Oberfläche des Grosshirns.* [The frontal lobe. A contribution to the anatomy and surface of the cerebral cortex]. Wien and Leipzig: Urban & Schwarzenberg.

Ebert, E., & Meumann, E. (1905). Ueber einige Grundfragen der Psychologie der Uebungsphänomene im Bereiche des Gedächtnisses [On some basic questions of the psychology of practice phenomena in the field of memory]. *Archiv für die gesamte Psychologie, 4*, 1–232.

Eccles, J.C., & Robinson, D.N. (1984). *The wonder of being human. Our brain and our mind.* New York: Free Press.

Ecker, A.D., & Woltman, H.W. (1939). Is nutritional deficiency the basis of Wernicke's disease? Report of case. *Journal of the American Medical Association, 112*, 1794–1796.

Ederle, W. (1948). Ein schizophrener vor und nach der präfrontalen Leukotomie [A schizophrenic before and after prefrontal leucotomy]. *Archiv für Psychiatrie und Nervenkrankheiten, 181*, 319–324.

Ederle, W. (1951). Erfahrung mit der präfrontalen Leukotomie bei Psychosen [Experience with prefrontal leucotomy in psychoses]. *Archiv für Psychiatrie und Zeitschrift Neurologie, 187*, 337–352.

Edinger, L. (1893). Über die Bedeutung der Hirnrinde [On the role of the cerebral cortex]. *Neurologisches Zentralblatt, 21*, 327.

Edinger, L. (1899). Studien über das Gedächtnis der niederen Vertebraten [Studies on the memory of the low vertebrates]. *Neurologisches Centralblatt, 18*, 956–957.

Edinger, L. (1902). Geschichte eines Patienten, dem operativ der ganze Schläfenlappen entfernt war, ein Beitrag zur Kenntniss der Verbindungen des Schläfenlappens mit dem übrigen Gehirne [Case of a patient with surgical removal of the complete temporal lobe, a contribution to the knowledge of the connections of the temporal lobe with the rest of the brain]. *Deutsches Archiv für klinische Medizin, 73*, 304–323.

Edinger, L. (1905). Ueber die Herkunft des Hirnmantels in der Tierreihe [On the origin of the cerebral mantle in the animal kingdom]. *Berliner Klinische Wochenschrift, 42*, 1357–1361.

Edinger, L. (1913). Zur Funktion des Kleinhirns [On the functions of the cerebellum]. *Deutsche Medizinische Wochenschrift, 39*, 633–637.

Edinger, L. (1914). Die Entstehung des Menschenhirnes [The ontogeny of the human brain]. *Wiener Medizinische Wochenschrift, 64*, 2242–2253.

Edinger, L., & Fischer, B. (1913). Ein Mensch ohne Grosshirn [A human without cerebrum]. *Pflüger's Archiv für die gesamte Physiologie des Menschen und der Tiere, 152*, 535–561.

Edinger, L., & Wallenberg, A. (1902). Untersuchungen über den Fornix und das Corpus mamillare [Investigations on the fornix and the mamillary bodies]. *Archiv für Psychiatrie und Nervenkrankheiten, 35*, 1–21.

Egan, G. (1949). Results of isolation of the orbital lobes in leucotomy. *Journal of Mental Science, 95*, 115–123.

Ehrenwald, H. (1931). Über den Zeitsinn und die gnostische Störung der Zeitauffassung beim Korsakow [On the sense of time and the gnostic disturbance of time comprehension in Korsakoff's syndrome]. *Zeitschrift für die gesamte Neurologie und Psychiatrie, 134*, 512–521.

Eichler, G. (1878). Ein Fall von Balkenmangel im menschlichen Gehirn [A case of callosal agenesis in the human brain]. *Archiv für Psychiatrie und Nervenkrankheiten, 8*, 355–366.

Ekehorn, G. (1901). Die Brüche des Meckel'schen Divertikels [Hernias in the diverticulum of Meckel]. *Archiv für klinische Chirurgie, 64*, 115–133.

Elder, W., & Miles, A. (1902). A case of tumour of the left prefrontal lobe removed by operation. *Lancet, i*, 363–366.

Elithorn, A., Piercy, M.F., & Crosskey, M.A. (1954). Autonomic changes after unilateral leucotomy. *Journal of Neurology, Neurosurgery, and Psychiatry, 17*, 139–144.

Elmiger, J. (1902). Neurogliabefunde in 30 Gehirnen von Geisteskranken [Results on neuro-glia in the brains of 30 mentally ill subjects]. *Archiv für Psychiatrie und Nervenkrankheiten, 35*, 153–158.

Ely, F.A. (1922). Memory defect of Korsakoff type, observed in multiple neuritis following toxaemia of pregnancy. *Journal of Nervous and Mental Disease, 56*, 115–125.

Elzholz, A. (1900). Ueber Beziehungen der Korsakoff'schen Psychose zur Polioencephalitis acuta haemorrhagica superior [On relations of Korsakoff's psychosis and polioencephalitis acuta haemorrhagica superior]. *Wiener klinische Wochenschrift, 13*, 337–344.

Engerth, G., & Hoff, H. (1930). Ein weiterer Beitrag zur Lehre von der Stirnhirnfunktion [Another contribution to the study of frontal lobe function]. *Zeitschrift für die gesamte Neurologie und Psychiatrie, 129*, 332–341.

Ephrussi, P. (1904). Experimentelle Beiträge zur Lehre vom Gedächtnis [Experimental contributions to the study of memory]. *Zeitschrift für Psychologie, 37*, 56–103 and 161–234.

Erb, W. (1880). Zur Abwehr und Berichtigung [Defense and correction]. *Archiv für Psychiatrie und Nervenkrankheiten, 10*, 289–291.

Ettlinger, G. (1971). Unterschiede und Übereinstimmungen zwischen der Organisation des Menschen- und Affengehirns im Licht neuropsychologischer Erkenntnisse [Differences and commonalities in the organization of the human and monkey brain viewed on the basis of neuropsychological findings]. *Klinische Wochenschrift, 49*, 786–790.

Evans, P. (1971). Failed leucotomy with misplaced cuts: A clinico-anatomical study of two cases. *British Journal of Psychiatry, 118*, 165–170.

Ewald, G. (1940). Zur Frage der Lokalisation des amnestischen Symptomenkomplexes [On the question of the localization of the amnesic symptom complex]. *Allgemeine Zeitschrift für Psychiatrie und ihre Grenzgebiete, 115*, 220–237.

Exner, S. (1881). *Untersuchungen über die Localisation der Funktionen in der Grosshirnrinde des Menschen* [Investigations on the localization of functions in the human cerebral cortex]. Wien: Braumüller.

Exner, S. (1894). *Entwurf zu einer physiologischen Erklärung der psychischen Erscheinungen* [Outline of a physiological explanation of psychic phenomena]. Leipzig und Wien: Franz Deuticke.

Exner, S., & Paneth, J. (1888). Versuche über die Folgen der Durchschneidung von Associationsfasern am Hundehirn [Experiments on the consequences of severing association fibers in the dog brain]. *Pflüger's Archiv für die gesamte Physiologie des Menschen und der Thiere, 44*, 544–555.

Falconer, M.A. (1948). Relief of intractable pain of organic origin by frontal lobotomy. In J.F. Fulton, W.C. Aring, & S.B. Wortis (Eds.), *The frontal lobes. (Research publications of the association for research in nervous and mental disease, Vol. 27)* (pp. 706–714). Baltimore: Williams & Wilkins.

Feeney, D.M., & Baron, J.C. (1986). Diaschisis. *Stroke, 17*, 817–830.

Feinstein, A., & Hattersley, A. (1988). Ganser symptoms, dissociation, and dysprosody. *Journal of Nervous and Mental Disease, 176*, 692–693.

Ferrier, D. (1874). The localisation of function in the brain. *Proceedings of the Royal Society, London, B, 22*, 229–232.

Ferrier, D. (1875). Experiments on the brain of monkeys (Second series). *Philosophical Transactions of the Royal Society (London), 165*, 433–488.

Ferrier, D. (1878 a). Munk on localization of function in the brain. *Brain, 1*, 229–231.

Ferrier, D. (1878 b). *The localisation of cerebral disease*. London: Elder & Co.

Ferrier, D. (1881). Cerebral amblyopia and hemianopia. *Brain, 3*, 456–477 (and 3 plates).

Ferrier, D. (1886). *The functions of the brain* (2nd ed.). London: Smith, Elder & Comp.

Ferrier, D. (1888). Schäfer on the temporal and occipital lobes. *Brain, 7*, 7–30.

Ferrier, D. (1889). Cerebral localisation in its practical relations. *Brain 12*, 36–58.

Ferrier, D., & Yeo, G.F. (1884). A record of experiments on the effects of lesion of different regions of the cerebral hemispheres. *Philosophical Transactions of the Royal Society, 175*, 479–565.

Ferris, G.S., & Dorsen, M.M. (1975). Agenesis of the corpus callosum 1. Neuropsychological studies. *Cortex, 11*, 95–122.

Feuchtwanger, E. (1923). *Die Funktionen des Stirnhirns. Ihre Pathologie und Psychologie* [The functions of the frontal lobes. Their pathology and psychology]. Berlin: Springer.

Fiamberti, A.M. (1937). Proposta di una tecnica operatoria modificata e semplificata per gli interventi alla Moniz sui lobi frontali in malati di mente [Demonstration of the technical modification and simplication of a surgical intervention according to Moniz for the frontal lobes in mental patients]. *Rassegna di Studi Psichiatrici, 26*, 797.

Finesinger, J.E. (1949). Prefrontal lobotomy as a therapeutic procedure. *American Journal of Psychiatry, 105*, 790–791.

Finger, S., & Stein, D.G. (Eds.). (1982). *Brain damage and recovery. Research and clinical perspectives*. New York: Academic Press.

Finzi, J. (1901). Zur Untersuchung der Auffassungsfähigkeit und Merkfähigkeit [On the investigation of the abilities of comprehension and memory]. In E. Kraepelin (Ed.), *Psychologische Arbeiten (Vol. 3)* (pp. 289–384). Leipzig: Engelmann.

Fischer, G. (1882). Ueber eine eigenthümliche Spinalerkrankung bei Trinkern [On a peculiar spinal cord disease in alcoholics]. *Archiv für Psychiatrie und Nervenkrankheiten, 13*, 1–49.

Fischer, G. (1904 a). Ueber hochgradige generelle Störung der Merkfähigkeit bei beginnender Paralyse [On severe general memory disturbances in early paralysis]. *Muenchener medizinische Wochenschrift, No. 4*, 153–155.

Fischer, G. (1904b). Ueber hochgradige generelle Störung der Merkfähigkeit bei beginnender Paralyse [On severe general memory disturbances in early paralysis]. *Muenchener medizinische Wochenschrift, No. 5*, 215–218.

Fischer, O. (1907). Miliare Nekrosen mit drusigen Wucherungen der Neurofibrillen, eine regelmässige Veränderung der Hirnrinde bei seniler Demenz [Miliar necrosis with neurofibrillary tangles, a common change in the cerebral cortex in senile dementia]. *Monatsschrift für Psychiatrie und Neurologie, 22*, 361–372.

Fischer, R. (1946). Selbstbeobachtungen im Mezkalin-Rausch [Self-observations in mescaline delirium]. *Schweizer Zeitschrift für Psychologie, 5*, 308–313.

Flatau, G. (1913). Über den Ganserschen Symptomenkomplex [On the syndrome of Ganser]. *Zeitschrift für die gesamte Neurologie und Psychiatrie, 15*, 122–137.

Flechsig, P. (1894). Ueber ein neues Eintheilungsprinzip der Grosshirn-Oberfläche [On a new principle of subdividing the cerebral cortex]. *Neurologisches Centralblatt, 13*, 674–676.

Flechsig, P. (1896a). *Die Lokalisation der geistigen Vorgänge, insbesondere der Sinnesempfindungen des Menschen* [The localization of mental acts, especially of sensorial perceptions in humans]. Leipzig: Veit & Co.

Flechsig, P. (1896b). *Gehirn und Seele* [Brain and soul]. Leipzig: Veit & Comp.

Flechsig, P. (1898). Neue Untersuchungen über die Markbildung in den menschlichen Grosshirnlappen [New investigations on myelinization of the human cerebral cortical lobes]. *Neurologisches Centralblatt, 17*, 977–996.

Flechsig, P. (1900). Uber Projections- und Associationscentren des menschlichen Gehirns [On projection and association centers of the human brain]. *Wiener medizinische Blätter, 23*, 583–584.

Flechsig, P. (1901). Developmental (myelogenetic) localisation of the cerebral cortex in the human subject. *Lancet, i*, 1027–1029.

Fleming, G.W.T.H. (1944). Prefrontal leucotomy. *Journal of Mental Science, 90*, 486–500.

Flor-Henry, P. (1975). Psychiatric surgery – 1935 – 1973. Evolution and current perspectives. *Journal of the Canadian Psychiatric Association, 20*, 157–167.

Flourens, M.J.P. (1842). *Examen de phrénologie* [Phrenological proof]. Paris: Hachette.

Flügel, O. (1902). *Die Seelenfragen mit Rücksicht auf die neueren Wandlungen gewisser naturwissenschaftlicher Begriffe* [Questions on the soul in light of recent changes of certain scientific terms]. (3rd ed.). Köthen: Schulze.

Fontaine, R., Breton, G., Dery, R., Fontaine, S., & Elie, R. (1990). Temporal lobe abnormalities in panic disorder: An MRI study. *Biological Psychiatry, 27*, 304–310.

Foerster, O., & Gagel, O. (1934). Ein Fall von Ependymcyste des III. Ventrikels. Ein Beitrag zur Frage der Beziehung psychischer Störungen zum Hirnstamm [A case of ependymal cyst in the III. ventricle. A contribution to the question on the relations of psychic disturbances to the brain stem]. *Zeitschrift für die gesamte Neurologie und Psychiatrie, 149*, 312–344.

Forel, A. (1885). *Das Gedächtnis und seine Abnormitäten* [Memory and its abnormal states]. Zürich: Orell Füssli & Co.

Forel, A. (1887). Einige hirnanatomische Betrachtungen und Ergebnisse [Some brain anatomical considerations and results]. *Archiv für Psychiatrie und Nervenkrankheiten, 18*, 162–198.

Forel, A. (1901). *Die psychologischen Fähigkeiten der Ameisen* [The psychic abilities of ants]. München: Ernst Reinhardt.

Forel, A. (1903). Nochmals Herr Dr. Bethe und die Insekten-Psychologie [Further views on Dr. Bethe and insect psychology]. *Biologisches Centralblatt, 23*, 1–3.

Forel, A. (1922). *Gehirn und Seele* [Brain and soul]. (13th ed.). Leipzig: Kröner.

Forster, E. (1919a). Agrammatismus (erschwerte Satzfindung) und Mangel an Antrieb nach Stirnhirnverletzung [Agrammatism (impeded sentence finding) and lack of drive after frontal lobe injury]. *Monatsschrift für Psychiatrie und Neurologie, 46*, 1–43.

Forster, E. (1919b). Die psychischen Störungen der Hirnverletzten [The psychic disturbances of the brain injured]. *Monatsschrift für Psychiatrie und Neurologie, 46*, 61–105.

Fraenkel, M. (1886). Ueber Degenerationserscheinungen bei Psychose [On degeneration phenomena in psychosis]. *Allgemeine Zeitschrift für Psychiatrie und psychisch-gerichtliche Medicin, 42*, 76–82.

Fraenkel, M. (1911). Beitrag zur Aetiologie des Korsakowschen Symptomenkomplexes [Contribution to the etiology of the Korsakoff symptom complex]. *Archiv für Psychiatrie und Nervenkrankheiten, 48*, 756–775.

Frank, J. (1946). Clinical survey and results of 200 cases of prefrontal leucotomy. *Journal of Mental Science, 92*, 497–508.

Frankl, L., & Mayer-Gross, W. (1947). Personality change after prefrontal leucotomy. *Lancet, ii*, 820–824.

Franz, S.I. (1902). On the functions of the cerebrum: I.- The frontal lobes in relation to the production and retention of simple sensory-motor habits. *American Journal of Physiology, 8*, 1–22.

Franz, S.I. (1906). Observations on the functions of the association areas (cerebrum) in monkeys. *Journal of the American Medical Association, 47*, 1464–1467.

Franz, S.I. (1907). On the functions of the cerebrum. The frontal lobes. *Archives of Psychology, 2*, 1–64.

Franz, S.I. (1912). New phrenology. *Science (N.S.), 35*, 321–328.

Franz, S.I. (1933). *Persons one and three. A study in multiple personalities*. New York: Whittlesey House, 1933.

Fraser, J., Mitchell, A. (1876). Kalmuc idiocy: report of a case with autopsy, with notes on sixty-two cases. *Journal of Mental Science, 22*, 161–179.

Frazier, C.H. (1936). Tumor involving the frontal lobe alone. A symptomatic survey of one hundred and five verified cases. *A.M.A. Archives of Neurology and Psychiatry, 35*, 525–571.

Freeman, W. (1941). Brain-damaging therapeutics. *Diseases of the Nervous System, 2*, 91–94.

Freeman, W. (1942). Discussion of the contribution of Strecker, Palmer, and Grant. *American Journal of Psychiatry, 98*, 531–532.

Freeman, W. (1948). Transorbital leucotomy. *Lancet, ii*, 371–373.

Freeman, W. (1949 a). Transorbital lobotomy: the deep frontal cut. *Proceedings of the Royal Society of Medicine, 42 (Suppl.)*, 8–12.

Freeman, W. (1949 b). Mass action versus mosaic function of the frontal lobe. *Journal of Nervous and Mental Disease, 10*, 360–363.

Freeman, W. (1950). Die thalamo-frontalen Verbindungen im Licht der präfrontalen Lobotomie [The thalamo-frontal connections after prefrontal lobotomy]. *Archiv für Psychiatrie und Neurologie, 185*, 624–626.

Freeman, W. (1953 a). Level of achievement after lobotomy. A study of 1000 cases. *American Journal of Psychiatry, 110*, 269–276.

Freeman, W. (1953 b). Hazards of lobotomy. Report on 2000 operations. *A.M.A. Archives of Neurology and Psychiatry, 69*, 640–643.

Freeman, W. (1954). Changes in behavior following lobotomy. The Malamud rating scale. *Journal of Neuropathology and Experimental Neurology, 8*, 90–104.

Freeman, W. (1957). Frontal lobotomy 1953–1956. A follow-up of 3000 patients from one to twenty years. *American Journal of Psychiatry. 113*, 877–886.

Freeman, W. (1971). Frontal lobotomy in early schizophrenia: long follow-up in 415 cases. *British Journal of Psychiatry, 119*, 621–624.

Freeman, W., Davis, H.W., East, I.T.C., Tait, H.S., & Rogers, W.B. (1954). The West Virginia lobotomy project. *Journal of the American Medical Association, 156*, 939–941.

Freeman, W., Tarumianz, M.A., Erickson, T.C., Lyerly, J.G., Palmer, H.D., & Grinker, R.R. (1941). Neurosurgical treatment of certain abnormal mental states. *Journal of the American Medical Association, 117*, 517–527.

Freeman, W., & Watts, J.W. (1939). Interpretation of functions of frontal lobe based upon observations in 48 cases of prefrontal lobotomy. *Yale Journal of Biology and Medicine, 11*, 527–539.

Freeman, W., & Watts, J.W. (1941). The frontal lobes and consciousness of the self. *Psychosomatic Medicine, 3*, 111–119.

Freeman, W., & Watts, J.W. (1942 a). Radical treatment of psychoses and neuroses: alterations in personality following prefrontal lobotomy. *Diseases of the Nervous System, 3*, 6–15.

Freeman, W., & Watts, J.W. (1942 b). *Psychosurgery: Intelligence, emotion and social behavior following prefrontal lobotomy for mental disorders*. Springfield, IL: C.C. Thomas.

Freeman, W., & Watts, J.W. (1943). Prefrontal lobotomy: Convalescent care and aids to rehabilitation. *American Journal of Psychiatry, 99*, 798–806.

Freeman, W., & Watts, J.W. (1944). Psychosurgery: evaluation of 200 cases over seven years. *Journal of Mental Science, 90*, 532–537.

Freeman, W., & Watts, J.W. (1945). Prefrontal lobotomy: The problem of schizophrenia. *American Journal of Psychiatry, 101*, 739–748.

Freeman, W., & Watts, J.W. (1946 a). Pain of organic disease relieved by prefrontal lobotomy. *Lancet, i*, 953–955.

Freeman, W., & Watts, J.W. (1946 b). Prefrontal lobotomy: Survey of 331 cases. *American Journal of the Medical Sciences, 211*, 1–8.

Freeman, W., & Watts, J.W. (1946 c). *Psychosurgery*. London: Baillière, Tindall and Cox.

Freeman, W., & Watts, J.W. (1947 a). Psychosurgery during 1936–46. *A.M.A. Archives of Neurology and Psychiatry, 58*, 417–425.

Freeman, W., & Watts, J.W. (1947 b). Retrograde degeneration of the thalamus following prefrontal lobotomy. *Journal of Comparative Neurology, 86*, 65–93.

Freeman, W., & Watts, J.W. (1948). Pain mechanisms and the frontal lobes: A study of prefrontal lobotomy for intractable pain. *Annals of Internal Medicine, 28*, 747–754.

Freud, S. (1884). Eine neue Methode zum Studium des Faserverlaufs im Centralnervensystem [A new method for studying the course of fibers in the central nervous system]. *Centralblatt für die medicinischen Wissenschaften 22*, 161–163.

Freud, S. (1891). *Zur Auffassung der Aphasien. Eine kritische Studie* [Towards an understanding of the aphasias. A critical study]. Leipzig and Wien: Franz Deuticke.

Freud, S. (1898). Zum psychischen Mechanismus der Vergesslichkeit [On the psychic mechanism of forgetfulness]. *Monatsschrift für Psychiatrie und Neurologie, 1*, 436–443.

Freud, S. (1899). Ueber Deckerinnerungen [On covered memories]. *Monatsschrift für Psychiatrie und Neurologie, 2*, 215–230.

Freud, S. (1900). *Die Traumdeutung* [The interpretation of dreams]. Leipzig and Wien: Franz Deuticke.

Freud, S. (1901 a). Zum psychischen Mechanismus der Vergesslichkeit [On the psychic mechanism of forgetfulness]. *Monatsschrift für Psychiatrie und Neurologie, 4/5*, 436–443.

Freud, S. (1901 b). Zur Psychopathologie des Alltagslebens (Vergessen, Versprechen, Vergreifen) nebst Bemerkungen über eine Wurzel des Aberglaubens [On the psychopathology of daily life (forgetting, slips of the tongue, mistakes) together with remarks on the root of superstititon]. *Monatsschrift für Psychiatrie und Neurologie, 10*, 1–32 and 95–143.

Freud, S. (1910). *Über Psychoanalyse. Fünf Vorlesungen gehalten zur 20jährigen Gründungsfeier der Clark University in Worcester Mass. September 1909.* [On psychoanalysis. Five lectures given on the occasion of the celebration of the 20th anniversary of the foundation of Clark University in Worcester Mass. September 1909]. Leipzig and Vienna: F. Deuticke.

Freud, S., & Breuer, J. (1970). *Studien über Hysterie* [Studies on hysteria]. (Enlarged reprint of the 1895 texts of Breuer & Freud). Frankfurt/M.: Fischer.

Freund, C.S. (1889 a). Klinische Beiträge zur Kenntnis der generellen Gedächtnisschwäche [Clinical contributions to understanding general memory weakness]. *Archiv für Psychiatrie und Nervenkrankheiten, 20*, 441–457.

Freund, C.S. (1889 b). Ueber optische Aphasie und Seelenblindheit [On optical aphasia and optic agnosia]. *Archiv für Psychiatrie und Nervenkrankheiten, 20*, 276–297.

Freund, C.S. (1889 c). Ueber optische Aphasie und Seelenblindheit [On optical aphasia and optic agnosia]. *Archiv für Psychiatrie und Nervenkrankheiten, 20*, 371–416.

Freund, C.S. (1891). Ueber das Vorkommen von Sensibilitätsstörungen bei multipler Herdsklerose [On the occurrence of disturbances in sensibility in cases with focal sclerosis]. *Archiv für Psychiatrie und Nervenkrankheiten, 22*, 317–344 and 588–614.

Freyhan, F.A. (1954). Prefrontal lobotomy and transorbital leucotomy: A comparative study of 175 patients. *American Journal of Psychiatry, 111*, 22–32.

Friedlaender, E. (1919/20). Ein Fall von absonderlicher retrograder Amnesie [A case of unusual retrograde amnesia]. *Psychiatrisch-Neurologische Wochenschrift, 13/14*, 85–88, 99–102.

Friedmann, M. (1890). Studien zur pathologischen Anatomie der acuten Encephalitis [Studies on pathological anatomy of acute encephalitis]. *Archiv für Psychiatrie und Nervenkrankheiten, 21*, 836–862.

Friedmann, M. (1906). Zur Lehre von den psychischen Störungen nach Gehirnerschütterung [On the theory of psychic disturbances after cerebral concussion]. *Neurologisches Zentralblatt, 25*, 631–632.

Friedrich, (n.n.g.) (1902). Ueber die physiologischen und pathologischen Funktionen des Stirnhirns [On the physiological and pathological functions of the frontal lobe]. *Münchener medicinische Wochenschrift, 99*, 17–25.

Fritsch, G. (1884). Herrn Prof. Goltz' Feldzug gegen die Grosshirnlocalisation [Prof. Goltz' campaign against cerebral cortical localization]. *Berliner klinische Wochenschrift, 21*, 299–301.

Fritsch, G., & Hitzig, E. (1870). Ueber die elektrische Erregbarkeit des Grosshirns [On the electrical excitability of the cerebrum]. *Archiv für Anatomie, Physiologie und Wissenschaftliche Medizin, 37*, 300–332.

Fukuda, T. (1919). Über die faseranatomischen Beziehungen zwischen den Kernen des Thalamus opticus und den frontalen Windungen (Frontalregion) des Menschen [On the fiber-anatomical relations between the nuclei of the optic thalamus and the frontal gyri (frontal region) of man]. *Schweizer Archiv für Neurologie und Psychiatrie, 5*, 325–377.

Fulton, J.F. (1947). Physiological basis of frontal lobotomy. *Acta Medica Scandinavica, 196 (Suppl.)*, 615–625.

Fulton, J.F. (1949). *Functional localization in the frontal lobes and cerebellum.* Oxford: Clarendon Press.

Fulton, J.F. (1951). *Frontal lobotomy and affective behavior. A neurophysiological analysis.* New York: Norton.

Fulton, J.F. (1966). *Selected readings in the history of physiology.* (2nd ed.). Springfield, IL: C.C. Thomas.

Fulton, J.F., Aring, C.D., & Wortis, S.B. (1948). (Eds). *The Frontal Lobes.* (*Research publications of the association for research in nervous and mental disease, Vol. XXVII*). Baltimore: Williams & Wilkins.

Fünfgeld, E. (1937). Bemerkungen zur Histopathologie der Schizophrenie [Remarks on the histopathology of schizophrenia]. *Zeitschrift für die gesamte Neurologie und Psychiatrie, 158*, 232–244.

Furtado, D., Rodrigues, M., Marques, V., Alvim, F., & De Vasconcelos, A. (1949). Personality changes after lobotomy. *Monatsschrift für Psychiatrie und Neurologie, 117*, 65–76.

Fuster, J.Q. (1989). *The prefrontal cortex. Anatomy, physiology and neuropsychology.* (2nd ed.). New York: Raven Press.

Gall, F.J. (1825). *Sur les fonctions du cerveau et sur celles de chacune de ses parties* [On the functions of the brain and on some of its parts]. (6 vols.). Paris: Baillière.

Galton, F. (1879). Psychometric experiments. *Brain, 2*, 149–162.

Galton, F. (1883). *Inquiries into human faculty and its development.* New York: Macmillan.

Gamble, E.A.McC., & Calkins, M.W. (1903). Die reproduzierte Vorstellung beim Wiedererkennen und beim Vergleichen [Reproduced imagination in recognizing and comparing]. *Zeitschrift für Psychologie und Physiologie der Sinnesorgane, 32*, 177–199.

Gamper, E. (1928 a). Zur Frage der Polioencephalitis haemorrhagica der chronischen Alkoholiker. Anatomische Befunde beim alkoholischen Korsakow und ihre Beziehungen zum klinischen Bild [On the question of polioencephalitis haemorrhagica of chronic alcoholics. Anatomical results in the chronic Korsakoff state and their relations to the clinical picture]. In: *17. Verhandlungen der Gesellschaft deutscher Nervenärzte, 1927* (pp. 122–129). Leipzig: Vogel.

Gamper, E. (1928 b). Zur Frage der Polioencephalitis haemorrhagica der chronischen Alkoholiker. Anatomische Befunde beim alkoholischen Korsakow und ihre Beziehungen zum klinischen Bild [On the question of polioencephalitis haemorrhagica of chronic alcoholics. Anatomical results in the chronic Korsakoff state and their relations to the clinical picture]. *Deutsche Zeitschrift für Nervenheilkunde, 102*, 352–359.

Gamper, E. (1929). Schlaf – Delirium tremens – Korsakowsches Syndrom [Sleep – delirium tremens – Korsakoff's syndrome]. *Zentralblatt für Neurologie, 51*, 236–239.

Gamper, E. (1931). Die Stellung des Zwischenhirns im psychozerebralen Apparat [The position of the diencephalon within the psycho-cerebral apparatus]. *Medizinische Klinik, 27*, 41–45.

Ganser, S.J. (1898). Ueber einen eigenartigen hysterischen Dämmerzustand [On a peculiar hysterical state of somnolence]. *Archiv für Psychiatrie und Nervenkrankheiten, 30*, 633–640

Ganser, S.J. (1904). Zur Lehre vom hysterischen Dämmerzustande [On the theory of the hysterical state of somnolence]. *Archiv für Psychiatrie und Nervenkrankheiten, 38*, 34–46.

Ganser, S.J. (1965). A peculiar hysterical state (transl. by C.E. Schorer). *British Journal of Criminology, Delinguency, and Deviant Social Behaviour, 5*, 120–126).

Gardner, A. (1957). Transorbital leucotomy in non-institutional cases. *American Journal of Psychiatry, 114*, 140–142.

Gascon, G.G., & Gilles, F. (1973). Limbic dementia. *Journal of Neurology, Neurosurgery, and Psychiatry, 36*, 421–430.

Gast, (n.n.g.) (1912). *Zur Lehre von den Schläfenlappentumoren* [On the theory of temporal lobe tumors]. Unpublished doctoral dissertation, Königliche Christian-Albrechts-Universität, Kiel. (cited after Artom, 1923).

Gazzaniga, M.S. (1970). *The bisected brain.* New York: Appleton-Century-Crofts.

Gazzaniga, M.S., Kutas, M., Van Petten, C., & Fendrich, R. (1989). MRI-verified neuropsychological functions. *Neurology, 39*, 942–946.

Geffen, G., Walsh, A., Simpson, D., & Jeeves, M. (1980). Comparison of the effects of transcortical and transcallosal removal of intraventricular tumours. *Brain, 103*, 773–788.

George, A.E., Raybaud, C., Salamon, G., & Kircheff, I.I. (1975). Anatomy of the thalamoperforating arteries with special emphasis on arteriography of the third ventricle: Part I. *American Journal of Roentgenology, 124*, 220–230.

Gerstmann, J. (1916). Zur Kenntnis der Störungen des Körpergleichgewichtes nach Schussverletzungen des Stirnhirns [Understanding disturbances of body balance after shot-caused wounds of the frontal lobe]. *Monatsschrift für Psychiatrie und Neurologie, 40*, 354–377.

Giacomini, C. (1881). Varietes des circonvolutions cerebrales chez l'homme [Variations in the human cerebral circumvolutions]. *Archives Italiennes de Biologie, 1*, 333–366.

Gianelli, A. (1897). Gli effetti diretti ed indiretti dei neoplasmi encefalici sulle funzioni mentali [Direct and indirect effects of cortical tumors on mental functions]. *Il Policlinico, 4*, 301–371.

Gibson, W.C. (1969). The early history of localization in the nervous system. In P.J. Vinken & G.W. Bruyn (Eds.), *Handbook oc clinical neurology. Vol. 2. Localization in clinical neurology* (pp. 4–14). Amsterdam: North-Holland Publishing Company.

Giese, G. (1911). Zur Kenntnis der psychischen Störungen nach Kohlenoxydvergiftungen [Understanding psychic disturbances after intoxication with carbon monoxide]. *Allgemeine Zeitschrift für Psychiatrie und psychisch-gerichtliche Medizin, 68*, 804–851.

Gillespie, R.D. (1937). Amnesia. *A.M.A. Archives of Neurology and Psychiatry, 37*, 748–764.

Girgis, M. (1971). The orbital surface of the frontal lobe of the brain and mental disorders. *Acta Psychiatrica Scandinavica, Suppl. 222*, 1–58.

Glass, E. (1911). Über alte Schussverletzungen des Gehirns. Ein Beitrag zur Lehre der Regenerationserscheinungen im Zentralnervensystem [On old shot wounds of the brain. A contribution to the theory of regenerative processes in the central nervous system]. *Frankfurter Zeitschrift für Pathologie, 8*, 112–134.

Glaus, A. (1953). Über Depersonalisation, nihilistische Wahnideen, Spiegelbilder, Doppelgänger und Golem im Werke Annettens von Droste-Hülshoff [On depersonalization, nihilistic delusions, mirror images, double gangers, and golems in the work of Annette von Droste-Hülshoff]. *Monatsschrift für Psychiatrie und Neurologie, 125*, 398–416.

Glees, P. (1947). The significance of the frontal lobe connections in mental diseases. *Experientia, 3*, 394–397.

Glees, P. (1948a). Anatomische und physiologische Betrachtungen zur Therapie der Geisteskrankheiten durch den frontalen Hirnschnitt. (Prefrontal leucotomy) [Anatomical and physiological considerations on the therapy of mental illnesses by prefrontal leucotomy]. *Nervenarzt, 19*, 220–223.

Glees, P. (1948b). Anatomische und physiologische Ergebnisse nach operativen Eingriffen am Frontalhirn (leucotomy frontal) [Anatomical and physiological results after surgical interventions on the frontal lobe]. *Klinische Wochenschrift, 26*, 253.

Glees, P. & Griffith, H.B. (1952). Bilateral destruction of the hippocampus (Cornu ammonis) in a case of dementia. *Monatsschrift für Psychiatrie und Neurologie, 123*, 193–204.

Gloning, I., Gloning, K., & Hoff, H. (1955). Die Störung von Zeit und Raum in der Hirnpathologie [The disturbance of time and space in brain pathology]. *Wiener Zeitschrift für Nervenheilkunde, 10*, 346–377.

Gloor, P. (1990). Experiential phenomena of temporal lobe epilepsy. Facts and hypotheses. *Brain, 113*, 1673–1694.

Goetz, C.G. (1987). Charcot at the Salpetrière: Ambulatory automatisms. *Neurology, 37*, 1084–1088.

Goldberg, E., Antin, S.P., Bilder Jr., R.M., Gerstman, L.J., Hughes, J.E.O., & Mattis, S.C. (1981). Retrograde amnesia: Possible role of mesencephalic reticular activation on long-term memory. *Science, 213*, 1392–1394.

Goldberg, E., Hughes, J.E.O., Mattis, S., & Antin, S.P. (1982). Isolated retrograde amnesia: Different etiologies, same mechanisms? *Cortex, 18*, 459–462.

Goldman-Rakic, P.S. (1987). Circuitry of primate prefrontal cortex and regulation of behavior by representational memory. In V.B. Mountcastle (Ed.), *Handbook of physiology, Section 1: The nervous system, Vol. 5. Higher functions of the brain, Part 1* (pp. 373–417). Bethesda, MD: American Physiological Society.

Goldstein, J. (1906a). Zur Frage der amnestischen Aphasie und ihrer Abgrenzung gegenüber der transcorticalen und glossopsychischen Aphasie [On the role of amnesic aphasia and its differentiation from transcortical and glossopsychic aphasia]. *Archiv für Psychiatrie und Nervenkrankheiten, 41*, 911–950.

Goldstein, K. (1906b). Merkfähigkeit, Gedächtnis und Assoziation [Memory ability, memory, and association]. *Zeitschrift für Psychologie, 41*, 38–47 und 117–144.

Goldstein, K. (1910). Einige prinzipielle Bemerkungen zur Frage der Lokalisation psychischer Vorgänge im Gehirn [Some principal remarks on the question of localization of psychic processes in the brain]. *Medizinische Klinik, No. 35*, 1363–1368.

Goldstein, K. (1911). Die amnestische und die zentrale Aphasie (Leitungsaphasie) [Amnesic and central aphasia (conduction aphasia)]. *Archiv für Psychiatrie und Nervenkrankheiten, 48*, 314–343.

Goldstein, K. (1923). Die Topik der Grosshirnrinde in ihrer klinischen Bedeutung [Topical relations of the cerebral cortex in their clinical importance]. *Deutsche Zeitschrift für Nervenheilkunde, 78*, 7–124.

Goldstein, K. (1927). Die Lokalisation in der Grosshirnrinde nach den Erfahrungen am kranken Menschen [Localization in the cerebral cortex after experiences with sick persons]. In A. Bethe, G. von Bergmann, G. Embden, & A.

Ellinger (Eds.), *Handbuch der normalen und pathologischen Physiologie, Vol. 10. Spezielle Physiologie des Zentralnervensystems der Wirbeltiere* (pp. 600–842). Berlin: Springer.

Goldstein, K. (1931). Konstantin von Monakow. *Deutsche Zeitschrift für Nervenheilkunde, 120*, 1–7.

Goldstein, K. (1944). The mental changes due to frontal lobe damage. *Journal of Psychology, 17*, 187–208.

Goldstein, K. (1949). Mental changes due to frontal lobe damage. *Journal of Psychology, 17*, 187–208.

Goldstein, K., & Reichmann, F. (1920). Ueber praktische und theoretische Ergebnisse aus den Erfahrungen an Hirnschussverletzten [Practical and theoretical results from experiences with brain injuries by shots]. *Ergebnisse der inneren Medicin und Kinderheilkunde, 18*, 405–530.

Golgi, C. (1883–84). Recherches sur l'histologie des centres nerveux [Investigations on the histology of the nervous system]. *Archives Italiennes de Biologie, 3*, 285–317, and *4*, 92–123.

Golgi, C. (1906/67). The neuron doctrine – Theory and facts. In *Nobel lectures: Physiology or medicine* (pp. 189–217). Amsterdam: Elsevier.

Golla, F.L. (1943). Range and technique of prefrontal leucotomy. *Journal of Mental Science, 89*, 189–191.

Golla, F.L. (1946). Prefrontal leucotomy with reference to indications and results. *Proceedings of the Royal Society of Medicine, 39*, 443–445.

Goltz, F. (1877). Ueber die Verrichtungen des Grosshirns. III. Abhandlung [On the functions of the cerebrum. III. Communication]. *Pflüger's Archiv für die gesammte Physiologie des Menschen und der Thiere, 20*, 1–54.

Goltz, F. (1881 a). *Ueber die Verrichtungen des Grosshirns. (Gesammelte Abhandlungen)* [On the functions of the cerebrum. (Collected communications)]. Bonn: Strauss.

Goltz, F. (1881 b). Ueber die Verrichtungen des Grosshirns. IV. Abhandlung [On the functions of the cerebrum. IV. Communication]. *Pflüger's Archiv für die gesammte Physiologie des Menschen und der Thiere, 26*, 1–49.

Goltz, F. (1884). Ueber die Verrichtungen des Grosshirns. V. Abhandlung [On the functions of the cerebrum. V. Communication]. *Pflüger's Archiv für die gesammte Physiologie des Menschen und der Tiere, 34*, 450–505.

Goltz, F. (1885). Ueber die moderne Phrenologie [On modern phrenology]. *Deutsche Rundschau, 45*, 263–283, 361–375.

Goltz, F. (1888). Ueber die Verrichtungen des Grosshirns. Sechste Abhandlung [On the functions of the cerebrum. Sixth Communication]. *Pflüger's Archiv für die gesammte Physiologie des Menschen und der Tiere, 42*, 419–467.

Goltz, F. (1892). Der Hund ohne Grosshirn. Siebente Abhandlung über die Verrichtung des Grosshirns [The dog without cerebrum. Seventh communication on the functions of the cerebrum]. *Pflüger's Archiv für die gesammte Physiologie des Menschen und der Tiere, 51*, 570–614 (and 1 Table).

Goltz, F. (1899). Beobachtungen an einem Affen mit verstümmeltem Grosshirn [Observations on a monkey with mutilated cerebrum]. *Pflüger's Archiv für die gesammte Physiologie des Menschen und der Tiere, 76*, 411–426.

Goltz, F., & Ewald, J.R. (1899). Der Hund mit verstümmeltem Rückenmark [The dog with mutilated spinal cord]. *Pflüger's Archiv für die gesammte Physiologie des Menschen und der Tiere, 63*, 362–400.

Goodhart, R., & Jolliffe, N. (1938). Effects of vitamin B (B_1) therapy on the polyneuritis of alcohol addicts. *Journal of the American Medical Association, 110*, 414–419.

Gordinier, H.C. (1899). A case of brain tumor at the base of the second left frontal convolution. *American Journal of the Medical Science, 117*, 526–535.

Gordon, A. (1906). On "double ego". *American Journal of the Medical Sciences, 131*, 480–486.

Gordon, A. (1917). Lesions of the frontal lobe simulating cerebellar involvement. Differential diagnosis. *Journal of Nervous and Mental Disease, 46*, 261–275.

Gordon, A. (1927). Tumeurs cérébrales et psychoses [Cerebral tumors and psychoses]. *Revue neurologique, 34*, 599–607.

Gordon, K. (1905). Ueber das Gedächtnis für affektiv gestimmte Eindrücke [On the memory for emotional impressions]. *Archiv für die gesamte Psychologie, 4*, 437–458.

Gott, P.S., & Saul, R.E. (1978). Agenesis of the corpus callosum: Limits of functional compensation. *Neurology, 28*, 1272–1279.

Govindaswamy, M.V., & Balakrishna, R.B.N. (1944). Bilateral prefrontal leucotomy in Indian patients. *Lancet, i*, 466–468.

Gowers, W.R. (1878 a). On some symptoms of organic brain disease. *Brain, 1*, 48–59.

Gowers, W.R. (1878 b). The brain in congenital absence of one hand. *Brain, 1*, 388–390.

Grafman, J., Weingartner, H., Newhouse, P.A., Thompson, K., Lalonde, F., Litvan, I., Molchan, S., & Sunderland, T. (1990). Implicit learning in patients with Alzheimer's disease. *Pharmacopsychiatry, 23*, 94–101.

Grage, H. (1930). Ein seltener Fall von Kopfsteckschuss im rechten Schläfenlappen mit schwerer

Stirnhirnverletzung [A rare case with a shot wound in the right temporal lobe with severe prefrontal injury]. *Journal für Psychologie und Neurologie, 40*, 356–364.

Grantham, E.g. (1951). Prefrontal lobotomy for relief of pain. With a report of a new operative technique. *Journal of Neurosurgery, 8*, 405–410.

Grassi, J.R. (1950). Impairment of abstract behavior following bilateral prefrontal lobotomy. *Psychiatric Quarterly, 24*, 74–88.

Greenblatt, M. (1950). A review of recent literature. In M. Greenblatt, R. Arnot, & H.C. Solomon (Eds.), *Psychosurgery* (pp. 7–56). New York: Grune & Stratton.

Greenblatt, M., Arnot, R., & Solomon, H.C. (1952). Survey of nine years of lobotomy investigation. *American Journal of Psychiatry, 109*, 262–265.

Greenblatt, M., Robertson, E., & Solomon, H.C. (1953). Five-year follow up of one hundred cases of bilateral prefrontal lobotomy. *Journal of the American Medical Association, 151*, 200–202.

Greenblatt, M., & Solomon, H.C. (1953). Concerning a theory of frontal lobe functioning. In M. Greenblatt, & H.C. Solomon (Eds.), *Frontal lobes and schizophrenia* (pp. 391–413). New York: Springer.

Greenblatt M., & Solomon, H.C. (1958). Studies of lobotomy. In H.C. Solomon, S. Cobb, & W. Penfield (Eds.), *The brain and human behavior. (Research publications of the association for research in nervous and mental disease, Vol. 36)* (pp. 19–34). Baltimore: Williams & Wilkins.

Greenblatt, M., Wingate, M., & Solomon, H.C. (1954). Work adjustment five to ten years after bilateral prefrontal lobotomy. (Follow-up study of 86 patients with chronic mental disease). *New England Journal of Medicine, 250*, 856–860.

Gregor, A. (1902). Beiträge zur Psychopathologie des Gedächtnisses [Contributions to the psychopathology of memory]. *Monatsschrift für Psychiatrie und Neurologie, 15*, 218–255 and 339–386.

Gregor, A. (1907). Beiträge zur Kenntnis der Gedächtnisstörung bei der Korsakoffschen Psychose [Contributions to our understanding of memory disturbance in Korsakoff's psychosis]. *Monatsschrift für Psychiatrie und Neurologie, 21*, 19–46 and 148–167.

Gregor, A. (1909). Beiträge zur Psychopathologie des Gedächtnisses [Contributions to the psychopathology of memory]. *Monatsschrift für Psychiatrie und Neurologie, 25*, 218–255 and 339–386.

Gregor, A., & Hänsel, R. (1909). Beiträge zur Kenntnis der Störung äusserer Willenshandlungen. II. Mitteilung: Schreibversuche [Contributions to our knowledge of disturbance of external acts of will. II. Communication: Attempts at writing]. *Monatsschrift für Psychiatrie und Neurologie, 26 (Suppl.)*, 87–129.

Gregor, A., & Roemer, H. (1906). Zur Kenntnis der Auffassung einfacher optischer Sinneseindrücke bei alkoholischen Geistesstörungen, insbesondere bei der Korsakoff'schen Psychose [Comprehension for simple optic sensory impressions in alcohol-based mental disturbances, especially in Korsakoff's psychosis]. *Neurologisches Zentralblatt, 25*, 339–351.

Griesinger, W. (1867/1964). *Die Pathologie und Therapie der psychischen Krankheiten für Aerzte und Studirende* [The pathology and therapy of psychic illnesses for physicians and students]. Amsterdam: Bonset (Reprint of the edition from 1867).

Grimm, E. (1868). Zur Casuistik der Tumoren in den vorderen Hirnlappen [On the casuistry of tumors in the anterior brain lobes]. *Wiener medizinische Wochenschrift, 18*, 653–655, 677–679, and 696–699.

Groenouw, A. (1892). Ueber doppelseitige Hemianopsie centralen Ursprunges [On bilateral hemianopia of central origin]. *Archiv für Psychiatrie und Nervenkrankheiten, 23*, 339–366.

Grosglik, A. (1895). Zur Physiologie der Stirnlappen [On the physiology of the frontal lobes]. *Archiv für Anatomie und Physiologie, Physiologische Abteilung*, 98–129.

Grünbaum, A.S.F., & Sherrington, C.S. (1902). Observations on the physiology of some of the higher apes. *Proceedings of the Royal Society, 69*, 206–209 (and 1 Plate).

Grünbaum, A.S.F., & Sherrington, C.S. (1903). Observations on the physiology of the cerebral cortex of the anthropoid apes. *Proceedings of the Royal Society, 72*, 152–155.

Grünthal, E. (1930). Die pathologische Anatomie der senilen Demenz und der ALZHEIMERschen Krankheit. (Mit besonderer Berücksichtigung der Beziehungen zur Klinik.) [The pathological anatomy of senile dementia and of ALZHEIMER's disease. (With special consideration of clinical questions.)]. In O. Bumke (Ed.), *Handbuch der Geisteskrankheiten, Vol. 7. Die Anatomie der Psychosen* (pp. 638–672). Berlin: Springer.

Grünthal, E. (1932). Zur Kenntnis der Psychopathologie des Korsakowschen Symptomenkomplexes [On our knowledge of the Korsakoff symptom complex]. *Monatsschrift für Psychiatrie und Neurologie, 53*, 89–132.

Grünthal, E. (1934). Der Zellbau im Thalamus der Säuger und des Menschen [The cytoarchitecture in the thalamus of mammals and of man]. *Journal für Psychologie und Neurologie, 46*, 41–112.

Grünthal, E. (1936 a). Über Unterschiede im Gehirnbau der Anthropoiden und des Menschen und das eigentlich Menschliche im Gehirn [On differences in brain architecture of anthropoids and the human and the particularly human elements in the brain]. *Fortschritte der Neurologie und Psychiatrie, 7*, 261–284.

Grünthal, E. (1936 b). *Über die Erkennung der traumatischen Hirnverletzung* [On the diagnosis of traumatic brain damage]. Berlin: Karger.

Grünthal, E. (1939). Ueber das Corpus mammillare und den Korsakowschen Symptomenkomplex [On the corpus callosum and the Korsakoff symptom complex]. *Confinia Neurologica, 2*, 64–95.

Grünthal, E. (1942). Über thalamische Demenz [On thalamic dementia]. *Monatsschrift für Psychiatrie und Neurologie, 106*, 114–128.

Grünthal, E. (1947). Über das klinische Bild nach umschriebenem beiderseitigem Ausfall der Ammonshornrinde. Ein Beitrag zur Kenntnis der Funktion des Ammonshorns [On the clinical picture of circumscribed bilateral loss of Ammon's horn's cortex. A contribution to the function of the Ammon's horn]. *Monatsschrift für Psychiatrie und Neurologie, 113*, 1–16.

Grünthal, E., & Störring, G.E. (1930). Über das Verhalten bei umschriebener, völliger Merkunfähigkeit [On behavior in the isolated, complete disability to memorize]. *Monatsschrift für Psychiatrie und Neurologie, 74*, 354–369.

Grünthal, E., & Störring, G.E. (1933). Ergänzende Beobachtungen und Bemerkungen zu dem in Band 74 (1930) dieser Zeitschrift beschriebenen Fall mit reiner Merkunfähigkeit [Supplementing observations und remarks to the case of pure loss of the ability to memorize, described in volume 74 of this journal]. *Monatsschrift für Psychiatrie und Neurologie, 77*, 374–382.

Gudden, B. von (1870 a). Anomalien des menschlichen Schädels [Anomalies of the human skull]. *Archiv für Psychiatrie und Nervenkrankheiten, 2*, 367–376.

Gudden, B. von (1870 b). Experimentaluntersuchungen über das peripherische und centrale Nervensystem [Experimental investigations on the peripheral and central nervous system]. *Archiv für Psychiatrie und Nervenkrankheiten, 2*, 693–723.

Gudden, B. von (1886). Ueber die Frage der Localisation der Functionen der Grosshirnrinde [On the question of localization of functions in the brain]. *Allgemeine Zeitschrift für Psychiatrie und ihre Grenzgebiete, 42*, 478–499.

Gudden, B. von (1896). Klinische und anatomische Beiträge zur Kenntnis der multiplen Alkoholneuritis nebst Bemerkungen über die Regenerationsvorgänge im peripheren Nervensystem [Clinical and anatomical contributions to an understanding of multiple alcohol neuritis together with remarks on the processes of regeneration in the peripheral nervous system]. *Archiv für Psychiatrie und Nervenkrankheiten, 28*, 643–741.

Guder, P. (1886). *Die Geistesstörungen nach Kopfverletzungen unter besonderer Berücksichtigung ihrer gerichtsärztlichen Beurteilung* [Mental disturbances after head injuries with special consideration of their evaluation by the forensic medical examiner]. Jena: Fischer.

Gussenbauer, K. (1894). Antrittsrede, anlässlich der Uebernahme der II. chirurgischen Klinik zu Wien [Inaugural lecture on the occasion of succeeding to director of the II. surgical clinic in Vienna]. *Wiener klinische Wochenschrift, 7*, 805–809.

Guthrie, M.B., & McMullen, R.B. (1978). Single case study. Cystic lesions after transorbital leukotomy. *Journal of Nervous and Mental Disease, 166*, 893–896.

Gürtler, K. (1923). Über Stirnhirnsyndrome [On prefrontal syndromes]. *Deutsche Zeitschrift für Nervenheilkunde, 76*, 221–235.

Häcker, V. (1914). *Ueber Gedächtnis, Vererbung und Pluripotenz* [On memory, heredity, and pluripotency]. Jean: G. Fischer.

Hadden, W.B. (1888). A case of tumour of the brain with a long history and with few symptoms. *Brain, 11*, 523–527.

Haddenbrock, S. (1949). Radikaltherapie durch Defrontalisation? Theoretisches und kritisches zur präfrontalen Leukotomie (*Moniz*) [Radical therapy by defrontalization? Theoretical and critical contributions on prefrontal leucotomy (*Moniz*)]. *Medizinische Klinik, Nr. 3*, 69–74.

Häfner, H. (1951). Amnestische Symptome nach Elektroschocktherapie. Ein Beitrag zur Psychopathologie des Organischen Schocksyndroms [Amnesic symptoms after electroshock therapy. A contribution to the psychopathology of the organic shock syndrom]. *Archiv für Psychiatrie und Zeitschrift Neurologie, 186*, 371–389.

Häfner, H. (1953). Psychopathologie der cerebralorganisch bedingten Zeitsinnesstörungen [Psychopathology of cerebral-organic disturbances of the sense of time]. *Archiv für Psychiatrie und Nervenkrankheiten, 190*, 530–545.

Häfner, H. (1954). Über Zeitdehnungs- und Zeitbeschleunigungsphänomene im Rahmen von Zwischenhirnstörungen [On phenomena of slowed-motion and speeded-up motion of the time-sense in disturbances of the diencephalon]. *Monatsschrift für Psychiatrie und Neurologie, 127*, 336–348.

Häfner, H. (1957). Psychopathologie des Stirnhirns 1939 bis 1955 [Psychopathology of the frontal lobe

1939 to 1955]. *Fortschritte der Neurologie und Psychiatrie, 25*, 205–252.

Hallervorden, J., & Spatz, H. (1922). Eigenartige Erkrankung im extrapyramidalen System mit besonderer Beteiligung des Globus pallidus and der Substantia nigra. Ein Beitrag zu den Beziehungen zwischen diesen beiden Zentren [Peculiar disease of the extrapyramidal system with special involvement of the globus pallidus and the substantia nigra, with an interpretation of their relationship]. *Zeitschrift für die gesamte Neurologie und Psychiatrie, 79*, 254–302.

Halpern, F. (1930). Kasuistischer Beitrag zur Funktion des Stirnhirns [Casuistic contribution to the function of the prefrontal cortex]. *Archiv für Psychiatrie und Nervenkranheiten, 90*, 446–456.

Halstead, W.C. (1947). *Brain and intelligence. A quantitative study of the frontal lobes.* Chicago: University of Chicago Press.

Halstead, W.C., Carmichael, H.T., & Bucy, P.C. (1946). Prefrontal lobotomy: A preliminary appraisal of the behavioral results. *American Journal of Psychiatry, 103*, 217–228.

Handmann, E. (1906). Ueber das Hirngewicht des Menschen auf Grund von 1414 im pathologischen Institut zu Leipzig vorgenommenen Hirnwägungen [Weight of the human brain on the basis of 1414 measurements, done at the pathological institute of Leipzig]. *Archiv für Anatomie und Physiologie, Anatomische Abteilung*, 1–40.

Hanfmann, E., Rickers-Ovsiankina, M., & Goldstein, K. (1944). Case lanuti: extreme concretization of behavior due to damage of the brain cortex. *Psychological Monographs, 57*, 1–72 (Whole No. 264).

Hansemann, D. (1899). Ueber das Gehirn von HERMANN V. HELMHOLTZ [On the brain of HERMANN V. HELMHOLTZ]. *Zeitschrift für Psychologie und Physiologie der Sinnesorgane, 20*, 1–12.

Hansemann, D. (1907). *Ueber die Hirngewichte von Th. Mommsen, R.W. Bunsen und Ad. v. Menzel* [On the brain weights of Th. Mommsen, R.W. Bunsen and Ad. v. Menzel]. Stuttgart: E. Schweizerbart'sche Verlagsbuchhandlung.

Harlow, J.M. (1848). Passage of an iron rod through the head. *Boston Medical and Surgical Journal, 39*, 389–393.

Harlow, J.M. (1869). *Recovery from the passage of an iron bar through the head.* Boston: D. Clapp and Son.

Harris, L.J. (1991). Cerebral control for speech in right-handers and left-handers: an analysis of the views of Paul Broca, his contemporaries, and his successors. *Brain and Language, 40*, 1–50.

Härtl, J. (1916). Fehlende Erinnerung des Verletzten für einen Schädelschuss. Verkannter Mordversuch [Lack of remembrance for a shot into the skull]. *Deutsche Medizinische Wochenschrift, 42*, 1352–1353.

Hartmann, F. (1907). Beiträge zur Apraxielehre [Contributions to the doctrine of aphasia]. *Monatsschrift für Psychiatrie und Neurologie, 21*, 97–118.

Hartmann, H. (1930). Gedächtnis und Lustprinzip. Untersuchungen an Korsakoffkranken [Memory and the principle of lust. Investigations on Korsakoff's patients]. *Zeitschrift für die gesamte Neurologie und Psychiatrie, 126*, 496–519.

Hartmann, K., & Simma, K. (1952). Untersuchungen über die Thalamusprojektion beim Menschen [Investigation on the thalamic projection in man]. *Monatsschrift für Psychiatrie und Neurologie, 123*, 329–353.

Harvey, G. (1846). Instance of fracture of the cranium, with depression, and subsequent hernia cerebri. *Lancet, ii*, 503–506.

Hassler, R. (1948). Über die Thalamus-Stirnhirn-Verbindungen beim Menschen [On thalamus-frontal lobe connections in man]. *Nervenarzt, 19*, 9–12.

Hassler, R. (1950). Über die anatomischen Grundlagen der Leukotomie [On the anatomical bases of leucotomy]. *Fortschritte der Neurologie und Psychiatrie, 18*, 351–367.

Hawton, K., Shepstone, B., Soper, N., & Reznek, L. (1990). Single-photon emission computerised tomography (SPECT) in schizophrenia. *British Journal of Psychiatry, 156*, 425–427.

Hay, W. (1875). Case of mania with traumatic hemiplegia. *Transactions of the American Neurological Association (New York), 1*, 180–184.

Heath, R.G., & Pool, J.L. (1948). Bilateral fractional resection of frontal cortex for the treatment of psychoses. *Journal of Nervous and Mental Disease, 107*, 411–429.

Hebb, D.O. (1939). Intelligence in man after large removals of cerebral tissue: Report of four left frontal lobe cases. *Journal of General Psychology, 21*, 73–87.

Hebb, D.O. (1941). Human intelligence after removal of cerebral tissue from the right frontal lobe. *Journal of General Psychology, 25*, 257–265.

Hebb, D.O. (1942). The effect of early and late brain injury upon test scores, and the nature of normal adult intelligence. *Proceedings of the American Philosophical Society, 85*, 275–292.

Hebb, D.O. (1945). Man's frontal lobes. A critical review. *A.M.A. Archives of Neurology and Psychiatry, 54*, 10–26.

Hebb, D.O., & Penfield, W. (1940). Human behavior after extensive bilateral removal from the frontal lobes. *A.M.A. Archives of Neurology and Psychiatry, 44*, 421–438.

Hechst, B. (1932). Über einen Fall von Mikroencephalie ohne geistigen Defekt [On a case with microencephalitis without mental defect]. *Archiv für Psychiatrie und Nervenkrankheiten, 97*, 64–76.

Hegglin, K. (1953). Über einen Fall von isolierter, linksseitiger Ammonshornerweichung bei präseniler Demenz [On a case of isolated, left-sided softening of Ammon's horn in presenile dementia]. *Monatsschrift für Psychiatrie und Neurologie, 125*, 170–186.

Heidenhain, L. (1901). Ueber Exstirpation von Hirngeschwülsten [On extirpation of brain tumors]. *Archiv für klinische Chirurgie, 64*, 849–890 (and 2 tables).

Heilbronner, K. (1901). Ueber die transcorticale motorische Aphasie und die als „Amnesie" bezeichnete Sprachstörung [On transcortical motoric aphasia and the language disturbance termed "amnesia"]. *Archiv für Psychiatrie und Nervenkrankheiten, 34*, 341–443.

Heilbronner, K. (1903). Ueber Fugues und fugueähnliche Zustände [On fugues and fugue-related states]. *Jahrbücher für Psychiatrie und Neurologie, 23*, 107–206.

Heilbronner, K. (1904/05). Zur klinisch-psychologischen Untersuchungstechnik [On the clinical-psychological technique of investigation]. *Monatsschrift für Psychiatrie und Neurologie, 17*, 115–132.

Heilbronner, K. (1905 a). Ueber Haftenbleiben und Stereotypie [On perseverating and stereotypy]. *Allgemeine Zeitschrift für Psychiatrie und psychisch-gerichtliche Medizin, 62*, 612–616.

Heilbronner, K. (1905 b). Ueber Haftenbleiben und Stereotypie [On persisting and stereotypy]. *Monatsschrift für Psychiatrie und Neurologie, 18 (Suppl.)*, 293–371.

Heilbronner, K. (1905 c). Studien über eine eklamptische Psychose [Studies on an eclampsic psychosis]. *Monatschrift für Psychologie, 17*, 277–287 and 367–460.

Heilbronner, K. (1908). Zur Symptomatologie der Aphasie mit besonderer Berücksichtigung der Beziehungen zwischen Sprachverständniss, Nachsprechen und Wortfindung [On the symptomatology of aphasia with special consideration of the relations between language comprehension, repeating, and word finding]. *Archiv für Psychiatrie und Nervenkrankheiten, 43*, 698–759.

Heilbronner, K. (1910). Zur Rückbildung der sensorischen Aphasie [On recovery from sensory aphasia]. *Archiv für Psychiatrie und Nervenkrankheiten, 46*, 766–804.

Heilbrunn, G., & Hletko, P. (1943). Disappointing results with bilateral prefrontal lobotomy in chronic schizophrenia. *American Journal of Psychiatry, 99*, 569–570.

Heimann, H. (1951). Erfahrungen mit der frontalen Lobotomie bei Schizophrenen [Experiences with frontal lobotomy in schizophrenics]. *Monatsschrift für Psychiatrie und Neurologie, 21*, 163–199.

Heimann, H. (1963). Psychochirurgie [Psychosurgery]. In H.W. Gruhle, R. Jung, W. Mayer-Gross & M. Müller (Eds.), *Psychiatrie der Gegenwart* (*Vol. I/2. Grundlagen und Methoden der Klinischen Psychiatrie*) (pp. 660–719). Göttingen: Springer.

Heine, R. (1911). Die forensische Bedeutung der Amnesie [The forensic significance of amnesia]. *Vierteljahresschrift für gerichtliche Medicin (3. Folge), 42*, 51–93.

Heine, R. (1914). Über Wiedererkennen und rückwirkende Hemmung [On recognition and backward inhibition]. *Zeitschrift für Psychologie, 68*, 161–236.

Henning, A. (1926). Über Stirnhirnsyndrome [On frontal lobe syndroms]. *Monatsschrift für Psychiatrie und Neurologie, 59*, 215–224.

Henschen, S.E. (1890–1908). *Klinische und anatomische Beiträge zur Pathologie des Gehirns (4 Vols.)* [Clinical and anatomical contributions on the pathology of the brain (4 vols)]. Upsala: Almquist & Wiksells.

Henschen, S.E. (1919). Über Sprach-, Musik- und Rechenmechanismen und ihre Lokalisationen im Grosshirn [On mechanisms of language, music, and calculation and their localization in the cerebrum]. *Zeitschrift für die gesamte Neurologie und Psychiatrie, 52*, 273–298.

Henschen, S.E. (1923). 40jähriger Kampf um das Sehzentrum und seine Bedeutung für die Hirnforschung [40 years' fighting for the visual center and its significance in brain research]. *Zeitschrift für die gesamte Neurologie und Psychiatrie, 87*, 505–535.

Hering, E. (1895). *Memory as a general function of organized matter*. Chicago: Open Court.

Hering, E. (1921). *Ueber das Gedächtnis als eine allgemeine Funktion der organisierten Materie. Vortrag gehalten in der feierlichen Sitzung der Kaiserlichen Akademie der Wissenschaften in Wien am XXX. Mai MDCCCLXX* [On memory as a general function of organized matter. Lecture given in the high session of the Imperial Academy of Sciences in Vienna on the 30th of May in 1870].

(3rd ed.). Leipzig: Akademische Verlagsgesellschaft.

Hermanides, S.R., & Köppen, M. (1903). Ueber die Furchen und über den Bau der Grosshirnrinde bei den Lissencephalen insbesondere über die Localisation des motorischen Centrums und der Sehregion [On the sulci and the construction of the cerebral cortex in lissencephalics, especially on the localization of the motor center and the visual region]. *Archiv für Psychiatrie und Nervenkrankheiten, 38*, 616–633 (and 1 Table).

Herner, T. (1961). *Treatment of mental disorders with frontal stereotaxic thermo-lesions*. Copenhagen: Ejnar Munksgaard.

Herter, P. (1916). Zur Symptomatologie der Stirnhirntumoren [On the symptomatology of frontal lobe tumors]. *Archiv für Psychiatrie und Nervenkrankheiten, 56*, 280–289.

Herzfeld, J. (1901). Rhinogener Stirnlappenabscess, durch Operation geheilt [Rhinogenic abscess of the frontal lobe, cured by surgery]. *Berliner klinische Wochenschrift, No. 47*, 1180–1183.

Herzog, (n.n.g.) (1842). Sieben Fälle von Geistesstörung durch Kopfverletzung [Seven cases of mental disturbance by head injuries]. *Vermischte Abhandlungen von einer Gesellschaft praktischer Aerzte zu St. Petersburg, 6*, 80–87.

Heveroch, A. (1914). Woher stammt unser Bewusstsein? Wie werden wir uns des Seins bewusst? [Where is the origin of consciousness? How do we become aware of our existence?]. *Archiv für Psychiatrie und Nervenheilkunde, 53*, 593–648.

Hey, J. (1904). *Das Gansersche Symptom und seine klinische und forense Bedeutung* [The Ganser symptom and its clinical and forensic importance]. Berlin: Hirschwald.

Heyck, H. (1954). Kritischer Beitrag zur Frage anatomischer Veränderungen im Thalamus bei Schizophrenie [Critical contribution to the question of anatomical changes in the thalamus of schizophrenics]. *Monatsschrift für Psychiatrie und Neurologie, 128*, 106–128.

Heymans, G. (1904). Eine Enquete über Depersonalisation und „Fausse Reconnaissance" [An inquiry on depersonalization and "fausse reconnaissance"]. *Zeitschrift für Psychologie, 36*, 321–343.

Heymans, G. (1906). Weitere Daten über Depersonalisation und „Fausse Reconnaissance" [Further data on depersonalization and "fausse reconnaissance"]. *Zeitschrift für Psychologie, 43*, 1–17.

Hill, A.L. (1975). An investigation of calendar calculating by an idiot savant. *American Journal of Psychiatry, 132*, 557–560.

Hinshelwood, J. (1895). Word-blindness and visual memory. *Lancet, ii*, 1564–1570.

Hirosawa, K., & Kato, K. (1935). Über die Fasern, insbesondere die corticalen extrapyramidalen aus den Areae 8 (alpha, beta, gamma, delta) und 9 (c, d) der Grosshirnrinde beim Affen [On the fibers, especially the cortical extrapyramidal ones, from areas 8 (alpha, beta, gamma, delta) and 9 (c, d) of the monkey's cerebral cortex]. *Folia Anatomica Japonica, 13*, 189–217.

Hirose, S. (1977). Psychiatric evaluation of psychosurgery. In W.H. Sweet, S. Obrador, & J.G. Martín-Rodríguez (Eds.), *Neurosurgical treatment in psychiatry, pain and epilepsy* (pp. 203–210). Baltimore: University Park Press.

Hirose, S. (1979). Past and present trends of psychiatric surgery in Japan. In. E.R. Hitchcock, H.T. Ballantine, Jr., & B.A. Meyerson (Eds.), *Modern concepts in psychiatric surgery* (pp. 349–357). New York: Elsevier/North-Holland Biomedical Press.

Hitchcock, E., Laitinen, L., & Vaernet, K. (Eds.). (1972). *Psychosurgery. Proceedings of the Second International Conference on Psychosurgery*. Springfield, IL: Charles C. Thomas.

Hitzig, E. (1874a). Ueber Localisation psychischer Centren in der Hirnrinde [On the localization of psychic centers in the cerebral cortex]. *Zeitschrift für Ethnologie, 6*, 42–47.

Hitzig, E. (1874b). *Untersuchungen über das Gehirn* [Investigations on the brain]. Berlin: Hirschwald.

Hitzig, E. (1874c). Ueber Localisation psychischer Centren in der Hirnrinde [On the localization of psychic centers in the cerebral cortex]. *Verhandlungen der Berliner Gesellschaft für Anthropologie, Ethnologie und Urgeschichte*, 42–47.

Hitzig, E. (1874d). Ueber den relativen Werth einiger Electrisations-Methoden [On the comparative value of some methods of electrization]. *Archiv für Psychiatrie und Nervenkrankheiten, 4*, 139–158.

Hitzig, E. (1876). Untersuchungen über das Gehirn [Investigations on the brain]. *Archiv für Anatomie, Physiologie und wissenschaftliche Medicin*, 692–711.

Hitzig, E. (1884). Zur Physiologie des Grosshirns [On the physiology of the cerebrum]. *Archiv für Psychiatrie und Nervenkrankheiten, 15*, 270–275.

Hitzig, E. (1887). Erwiderung dem Herrn Professor Zuntz [Reply to Professor Zuntz]. *Pflüger's Archiv für die gesammte Physiologie des Menschen und der Thiere, 40*, 129–136.

Hitzig, E. (1900a). Hughlings Jackson and the cortical motor centres in the light of physiological research. *Brain, 23*, 545–581.

Hitzig, E. (1900b). Ueber das corticale Sehen des Hundes [On cortical vision in the dog]. *Archiv für*

Psychiatrie und Nervenkrankheiten, 33, 700–720 (and 2 tables).
Hitzig, E. (1900 c). Ueber den Mechanismus gewisser cortikaler Sehstörungen des Hundes [On the mechanism of certain cortical visual disturbances in the dog]. *Berliner klinische Wochenschrift, 37*, 1001–1003.
Hitzig, E. (1901 a). Alte und neue Untersuchungen über das Gehirn [Old and recent investigations on the brain]. *Archiv für Psychiatrie und Nervenkrankheiten, 33*, 1–38.
Hitzig, E. (1901 b). Aufklärung über einige Streitpunkte in der Localisationslehre [Clarifying some controversies in the doctrine of localization]. *Monatsschrift für Psychiatrie und Neurologie, 10*, 457–458.
Hitzig, E. (1903 a). Alte und neue Untersuchungen über das Gehirn [Old and recent investigations on the brain]. *Archiv für Psychiatrie und Nervenkrankheiten, 37*, 299–467 and 849–1013.
Hitzig, E. (1903 b). Ueber die Function der motorischen Region des Hundehirns und über die Polemik des Herrn H. Munk [On the function of the motor region of the dog brain and on the polemics of Mr. H. Munk]. *Archiv für Psychiatrie und Nervenkrankheiten, 36*, 605–629.
Hitzig, E. (1903 c). Einige Bemerkungen zu der Arbeit C. von Monakow's „Ueber den gegenwärtigen Stand der Frage nach der Localisation im Grosshirn." [Some remarks on the publication of C. von Monakow "On the present state of the question on the localization in the cerebrum]. *Archiv für Psychiatrie und Nervenkrankheiten, 36*, 907–913.
Hoch, E. (1949). Die Persönlichkeitsveränderungen nach präfrontaler Leukotomie [On personality disturbances after prefrontal leucotomy]. *Schweizer Archiv für Neurologie und Psychiatrie, 64*, 119–174.
Hoche, A.E. (1933). *Die Wunder der Therese Neumann von Konnersreuth* [The wonders of Therese Neumann von Konnersreuth]. München: Lehmanns Verlag.
Hoff, H., & Pötzl, O. (1932). Über die Wirkungen des Wärmestichs bei vorgeschrittener Schizophrenie. *Psychiatrisch-neurologische Wochenschrift, 34*, 110–113.
Hoff, H., & Pötzl, O. (1938). Anatomischer Befund eines Falles mit Zeitrafferphänomen [Anatomical proof of a case with a speeded-up motion phenomenon]. *Deutsche Zeitschrift für Nervenheilkunde, 145*, 150–178.
Hoff, P., & Hippius, H. (1989). Alois Alzheimer 1864–1915. Ein Überblick über Leben und Werk anlässlich seines 125. Geburtstages [Alois Alzheimer 1864–1915. A survey on his life and work on the occasion of his 125th birthday]. *Der Nervenarzt, 60*, 332–337.
Höffding, H. (1889). Über Wiedererkennnen, Association und psychische Aktivität [On recognition, association, and psychic activity]. *Vierteljahresschrift für wissenschaftliche Philosophie, 13*, 420–458.
Höffding, H. (1890). Über Wiedererkennen, Association und psychische Aktivität [On recognition, association, and psychic activity]. *Vierteljahresschrift für wissenschaftliche Philosophie, 14*, 27–54, 167–205, 293–316.
Hofmann, F.B. (1921). Die physiologischen Grundlagen der Bewusstseinsvorgänge [The physiological bases of conscious acts]. *Die Naturwissenschaften 9*, 165–172.
Hofstatter, L., Smolik, E.A., & Busch, A.K. (1945). Prefrontal lobotomy in treatment of chronic psychoses. *A.M.A. Archives of Neurology and Psychiatry, 53*, 125–130.
Högner, P. (1927). Die klinischen Erscheinungen bei Erkrankungen des 3. Gehirnventrikels und seiner Wandungen [Clinical symptoms after diseases involving the third ventricle and its walls]. *Deutsche Zeitschrift für Nervenheilkunde, 97*, 238–266.
Hoheisel, H.P. (1954). Kriminalität bei Hirnverletzten unter Bezugnahme auf den Ort der Verletzung [Criminal behavior in brain injured persons with consideration of the locus of the injury]. *Deutsche Zeitschrift für gerichtliche Medizin, 43*, 59–73.
Hohne, H.H., & Walsh, K.W. (1970). *Surgical modification of the personality (Mental Health Authority, Victoria, Special publication no. 2)*. Melbourne: Victoria Government Printer.
Holländer, B. (1900). *Die Localisation der psychischen Thätigkeiten im Gehirn. Ergebnisse der Experimental-Physiologie, von Sectionsbefunden, von anatomischen und klinischen Beobachtungen, verwerthet für die Localisationslehre und Psychiatrie* [The localization of psychic functions in the brain. Results of experimental physiology, observations from sections, and anatomical and clinical observations, evaluated for the theory of localization and psychiatry]. Berlin: August Hirschwald.
Holmes, G. (1901). Discussion of the mental symptoms associated with cerebral tumours. *Proceedings of the Royal Society of Medicine, 24*, 997–1000.
Höniger, (n.n.g.) (1901). Zur Diagnose der Geschwülste des Stirnhirns [On the diagnosis of tumors of the frontal lobe]. *Muenchener medicinische Wochenschrift, No. 19*, 740–743.
Hoppe, F. (1908). Befunde von Tumoren oder Zystizerken im Gehirne Geisteskranker [Findings on tumors or cysticerks in the brains of mental pa-

tients]. *Monatsschrift für Psychiatrie und Neurologie, 25*, 32–54.

Horel, J.A. (1978). The neuroanatomy of amnesia. A critique of the hippocampal memory hypothesis. *Brain, 101*, 403–445.

Horrax, G. (1923). Visual hallucinations as a cerebral localizing phenomenon. *A.M.A. Archives of Neurology and Psychiatry, 10*, 532–547.

Horrax, G., & Bailey, P. (1928). Pineal pathology. Further studies. *A.M.A. Archives of Neurology and Psychiatry, 19*, 394–414.

Horsley, V. (1887). *Brain surgery*. London: John Bale and Sons.

Horsley, V., & Schaefer, E.A. (1888). A record of experiments upon the functions of the cerebral cortex. *Philosophical Transactions of the Royal Society (London), 179 b*, 1–45.

Horwitz, W.A., Kestenbaum, C., Person, E., & Jarvik, L. (1965). Identical twins "idiot savants" calendar calculators. *American Journal of Psychiatry, 132*, 1075–1079.

Hrdlicka, A. (1903). An Eskimo brain. *American Anthropologist, 3*, 454–500.

Hübner, A.H. (1910). Zur Histopathologie der senilen Hirnrinde [On the histopathology of the senile cortex]. *Archiv für Psychatrie und Nervenkrankheiten, 46*, 598–609.

Hüffer, H. (1911). *Annette von Droste-Hülshoff und ihre Werke* [Annette von Droste-Hülshoff and her works]. Gotha: F.A. Perthes.

Hughlings-Jackson, J. (1876). Case of large cerebral tumour without optic neuritis, and with left hemiplegia and imperception. *Royal London Ophthalmic Hospital Reports, 8*, 434–444.

Hughlings-Jackson, J. (1879). On affections of speech from disease of the brain. *Brain, 1*, 304–330.

Hughlings-Jackson, J. (1884). Croonian lectures on the evolution and dissolution of the nervous system. *Lancet, i*, 555–558, 649–652, 739–744.

Hughlings-Jackson, J. (1932). On some implications of dissolution of the nervous system. In J. Taylor (Ed.), *Selected writings of John Hughlings-Jackson (Vol. 2)* (pp. 29–44). London: Hodder & Straughton.

Humphreys, M.S., Bain, J.D. & Pike, R. (1989). Different ways to cue a coherent memory system: A theory for episodic, semantic, and procedural tasks. *Psychological Review, 96*, 208–233.

Hunt, J.W. (1879). Case of cerebral tumour. *Brain, 1*, 574–576.

Hunt, T. (1942). Intelligence and personality profiles. In W. Freeman and J.W. Watts (Eds.), *Psychosurgery* (pp. 153–181). Springfield, IL: C.C. Thomas.

Huppert, F.A., & Piercy, M. (1977). Recognition memory in amnesic patients: a defect of acquisition? *Neuropsychologia, 15*, 643–652.

Huppert, F.A., & Piercy, M. (1978). Dissociation between learning and remembering in organic amnesia. *Nature, 275*, 317–318.

Huppert, F.A., & Piercy, M. (1979). Normal and abnormal forgetting in organic amnesia: effect of locus of lesion. *Cortex, 15*, 385–390

Huppert, F.A. & Piercy, M. (1982). In search of the functional locus of amnesic syndromes. In L.S. Cermak (Eds.) *Human memory and amnesia* (pp. 123–137). Hillsdale, NJ: Erlbaum.

Hurd, A.W. (1905). Korsakoff psychosis – report of cases. *American Journal of Insanity. 62*, 63–76.

Huschke, E. (1854). *Schaedel, Hirn und Seele des Menschen und der Thiere nach Alter, Geschlecht und Race* [Skull, brain, and soul of man and animals separated according to age, sex, and race]. Jena: F. Mauke.

Huss, M. (1852). *Alcoholismus chronicus*. Stockholm and Leipzig: Fritze.

Hussain, E.S., Freeman, H., & Jones, R.A.C. (1988). A cohort study of psychosurgery cases from a defined population. *Journal of Neurology, Neurosurgery, and Psychiatry, 51*, 345–352.

Hutton, E.L. (1943). Results of prefrontal leucotomy. *Lancet, i*, 362–366.

Hutton, E.L. (1947). Personality changes after leucotomy. *Journal of Mental Science, 93*, 31–42.

Irle, E., & Markowitsch, H.J. (1982). Thiamine deficiency in the cat leads to severe learning deficits and to widespread neuroanatomical damage. *Experimental Brain Research, 48*, 199–208

Irle, E., & Markowitsch, H.J. (1983). Differential effects of double and triple lesions of the cat's limbic system on subsequent learning behavior. *Behavioral Neuroscience, 97*, 908–910.

Isserlin, M. (1905). Assoziationsstörungen bei einem forensisch begutachteten Falle von epileptischer Geistesstörung [Problems in associating in a case with epilepsy-caused mental disturbance examined for forensic reasons]. *Monatsschrift für Psychiatrie und Neurologie, 18 (Suppl.)*, 419–446.

Isserlin, M. (1923). Über Störungen des Gedächtnisses bei Hirngeschädigten [On disturbances of memory in brain injured persons]. *Zeitschrift für die gesamte Neurologie und Psychiatrie, 85*, 84–97.

Jacob, H., & Pyrkosch, W. (1951). Frühe Hirnschäden bei Strangtod und in der Agonie [Early brain damage after death by strangulation and during agony]. *Archiv für Psychiatrie und Zeitschrift Neurologie, 187*, 177–186.

Jacobsen, C.F. (1935). Functions of the frontal association area in primates. *A.M.A. Archives of Neurology and Psychiatry, 33*, 558–569.

Jacobsen, C.F. (1936). Studies of cerebral function in primates: I. The functions of the frontal association area in monkeys. *Comparative Psychology Monographs, 13*, 3–60.

Jacobsen, C.F., & Nissen, H.W. (1937). Studies of cerebral function in primates: IV. The effects of frontal lobe lesions on the delayed alternation habit in monkeys. *Journal of Comparative and Physiological Psychology, 23*, 101–112.

Jacobsen, C.F., Wolfe, J.B., & Jackson, T.A. (1935). An experimental analysis of the functions of the frontal association areas in primates. *Journal of Nervous and Mental Disease, 82*, 1–14.

Jacobsohn, L. (1904). Anatomie des Nervensystems [Anatomy of the nervous system]. *Jahresbericht über die Leistungen und Fortschritte auf dem Gebiete der Neurologie und Psychiatrie, 7*, 10–85.

Jacoby, L.L., Baker, J.G., & Brooks, L.R. (1989). Episodic effects on picture identification: Implications for theories of concept learning and theories of memory. *Journal of Experimental Psychology: Learning, Memory and Cognition, 15*, 275–281.

Jaeger, G. (1880). *Die Entdeckung der Seele* [The discovery of the soul]. (2nd ed.). Leipzig: E. Günther.

Jaensch, E.R., & Mehmel, H. (1928). Gedächtnisleistungen eines schwachsinnigen Eidetikers [Memory performance of a feeble-minded eidetic]. *Psychiatrisch-Neurologische Wochenschrift, 30*, 101–103.

Jahrreiss, W. (1928 a). Störungen des Denkens [Disturbances of thought]. In O. Bumke (Ed.), *Handbuch der Geisteskrankheiten (Vol 1)* (pp. 530–599). Berlin: Springer.

Jahrreiss, W. (1928 b). Störungen des Bewusstseins [Disturbances of consciousness]. In O. Bumke (Ed.), *Handbuch der Geisteskrankheiten (Vol 1)* (pp. 601–661). Berlin: Springer.

Jakob, A. (1931). Über ein dreieinhalb Monate altes Kind mit totaler Erweichung beider Grosshirnhemisphären („Kind ohne Grosshirn") [On a child, aged three and a half months, with total softening of both cerebral hemispheres ("child without cerebrum")]. *Deutsche Zeitschrift für Nervenheilkunde, 117/19*, 240–265.

James, W. (1890). *The principles of psychology* (2 vols.). New York: Holt.

James, W. (1892). *Psychology*. New York: H. Holt.

James, W. (1909). *Psychologie* [Psychology]. Leipzig: Quelle & Meyer.

Jancke, H. (1953). Vom Sinn und Unsinn des Psychisch-Unbewussten [On the sense and non-sense of the psychic-unconsciousness]. *Monatsschrift für Psychiatrie und Neurologie, 125*, 494–514.

Janet, P. (1894). *Der Geisteszustand der Hysteriker (Die psychischen Stigmata)* [The mental state of hysterics (The psychic stigmata]. Leipzig and Wien: Deuticke.

Janet, P. (1907). *The major symptoms of hysteria*. New York: Macmillan.

Janus, (n.n.g.) (1911). *Zur Kasuistik der Schläfenlappentumoren* [On the casuistry of temporal lobe tumors]. Unpublished doctoral dissertation, Königliche Christian-Albrechts-Universität, Kiel. (Cited after Artom, 1923.)

Janzen, R. (1948). Zur Lehre von der Lokalisation im Zentralnervensystem [Localization in the central nervous system]. *Deutsche Zeitschrift für Nervenheilkunde, 158*, 525–542.

Jarho, L. (1973). Korsakoff-like amnesic syndrome in penetrating brain injury. A study of English war veterans. *Acta Neurologica Scandinavica, 49, (Suppl. 54)*, 1–156.

Jarvie, H.F. (1954). Frontal lobe wounds causing disinhibition. A study of six cases. *Journal of Neurology, Neurosurgery, and Psychiatry, 17*, 14–32.

Jaspers, K. (1910). Die Methoden der Intelligenzprüfung und der Begriff der Demenz [Methods for testing intelligence and the concept of dementia]. *Zeitschrift für die gesamte Neurologie und Psychiatrie/Referate, 1*, 401–452.

Jastrowitz, M. (1885). Demonstration eines Cerebraltumors am Fusse der mittleren, rechten Stirnwindung [Documentation of a cerebral tumor at the bottom of the medial, right frontal gyrus]. *Deutsche medicinische Wochenschrift, 11*, 457–458.

Jastrowitz, M. (1888). Beiträge zur Localisation im Grosshirn und über deren praktische Verwerthung [Contributions to localization in the cerebrum and to their practical evaluation]. *Deutsche medicinische Wochenschrift, 14*, 81–83 and 108–112.

Jeeves, M.A. (1990). Agenesis of the corpus callosum. In F. Boller & J. Grafman (Eds.), *Handbook of neuropsychology (Vol. 4)* (pp. 99–114). Amsterdam: Elsevier Science Publ.

Jefferson, G. (1937). Removal of right or left frontal lobes in man. *British Medical Journal, 2*, 199–206.

Jefferson, G. (1950). Tumours of the frontal lobe. *Postgraduate Medical Journal, 26*, 133–140.

Jelliffe, S.E. (1908). The alcoholic psychoses. Chronic alcoholic delirium (Korsakoff's psychosis). *New York Medical Journal, 88*, 769–777.

Jenkins, R.L., Holsopple, J.Q., & Lorr, M. (1954). Effects of prefrontal lobotomy on patients with severe chronic schizophrenia. *American Journal of Psychiatry, 111*, 84–90.

Jennings, H.S. (1931). *Behavior of the lower organisms*. New York: Columbia University Press.

Jensen, J. (1875). Untersuchungen über die Beziehungen zwischen Grosshirn und Geistesstörung an sechs Gehirnen geisteskranker Individuen [Investigations on the relations between cerebrum and mental illness in six brains of mentally ill individuals]. *Archiv für Psychiatrie und Nervenkrankheiten, 5*, 587–757 (and tables).

Jensen, J. (1880). Schädel und Hirn einer Microencephalin [Skull and brain of a female microencephalic]. *Archiv für Physiologie, 10*, 735–759 (and Table IX).

Jensen, J. (1889). Untersuchungen über 453 nach Meynert's Methode getheilten und gewogenen Gehirnen von geisteskranken Ostpreussen [Investigations on 453 brains of mentally ill East Prussians, sectioned and weighted according to Meynert's method]. *Archiv für Psychiatrie und Nervenkrankheiten, 20*, 170–221.

Jodl, F. (1903). *Lehrbuch der Psychologie* [Textbook of psychology]. (2nd ed.). Stuttgart: Cottas Nachfahren.

John, E.R. (1972). Switchboard versus statistical theories of learning and memory. *Science, 177*, 850–864.

Jolliffe, N., Wortis, H., & Fein, H.D. (1941). The Wernicke syndrome. *A.M.A. Archives of Neurology and Psychiatry, 46*, 569–597.

Jolly, P. (1872). Ueber multiple Hirnsklerose [On multiple brain sclerosis]. *Archiv für Psychiatrie und Nervenkrankheiten, 3*, 711–730.

Jolly, P. (1897). Die psychischen Störungen bei Polyneuritis [Psychic disturbances in polyneuritis]. *Neurologisches Centralblatt, 16*, 916–917.

Jolly, P. (1913). Die Heredität der Psychosen [The heredity of psychoses]. *Archiv für Psychiatrie und Nervenkrankheiten, 52*, 377–436.

Jones, G.N., & McCowan, P.K. (1949). Leucotomy in the periodic psychoses. *Journal of Mental Science, 95*, 101–114.

Jones, G.N., & Shanklin, J. (1950). Transorbital leucotomy in institutional practice. *American Journal of Psychiatry, 107*, 120–127.

Jones, R.E. (1949). Personality changes in psychotics following prefrontal lobotomy. *Journal of Abnormal and Social Psychology, 44*, 315–328.

Joschko, M. (1979). Bilateral prefrontal leucotomy: An ex post facto archival study of a complete hospital sample. *Journal of Clinical Neuropsychology, 1*, 167–182.

Jost, A. (1897). Die Assoziationsfestigkeit in ihrer Abhängigkeit von der Verteilung der Wiederholungen [Strength of association as dependent on the distribution of repetitions]. *Zeitschrift für Psychologie, 14*, 436–472.

Jung, C.G. (1902). Ein Fall von hysterischem Stupor bei einer Untersuchungsgefangenen [A case of hysteric stupor in a prisoner on trial]. *Journal für Psychologie und Neurologie, 1*, 110–122.

Jung, C.G. (1905 a). Experimentelle Beobachtungen über das Erinnerungsvermögen [Experimental observations on remembrance]. *Centralblatt für Nervenheilkunde und Psychiatrie, 28*, 653–666.

Jung, C.G. (1905 b). *Ueber das Verhalten der Reaktionszeit beim Assoziationsexperiment* [On the behavior of reaction time in an association experiment]. Leipzig: Barth.

Jung, C.G. (1905 c). Diagnostische Assoziationsstudien. III. Beitrag: Analyse der Assoziationen eines Epileptikers [Diagnostic association studies. III. Contribution: Analysis of the associations of an epileptic]. *Journal für Psychologie und Neurologie, 5*, 73–90.

Jung, C.G. (1905d). Diagnostische Assoziationsstudien. IV. Beitrag: Über das Verhalten der Reaktionszeit beim Assoziationsexperimente [Diagnostic association studies. IV. Contribution: On the behavior of reaction time in an association experiment] *Journal für Psychologie und Neurologie, 6*, 1–36.

Jung, C.G. (1905e). Kryptomnesie [Cryptomnesia]. *Die Zukunft, 13*, 103–115.

Jung, C.G. (1966). *Psychiatrische Studien* [Psychiatric studies]. Zürich: Rascher.

Jung, C.G., & Riklin, F. (1904). Diagnostische Assoziationsstudien. I. Beitrag: Experimentelle Untersuchungen über Assoziationen Gesunder [Diagnostic association studies. I. Contribution: Experimental investigations on associations of healthy people]. *Journal für Psychologie und Neurologie, 4*, 24–67.

Jung, R. (1963). Hans Berger und die Entdeckung des EEG nach seinen Tagebüchern und Protokollen [Hans Berger and the discovery of the EEG according to his diary and protocols]. In R. Werner (Ed.), *Jenenser EEG-Symposion. 30 Jahre Elektroenzephalographie* (pp. 20–53). Berlin: VEB Verlag.

Kaes, T. (1905). Die Rindenbreite als wesentlicher Factor zur Beurtheilung der Entwicklung des Gehirns und namentlich der Intelligenz [Cortical width as a prominent factor for the determination of the development of the brain and especially of intelligence]. *Neurologisches Zentralblatt, 22*, 1026–1047.

Kaes, T. (1909 a). Replik [Reply]. *Neurologisches Centralblatt, 28*, 639–641.

Kaes, T. (1909 b). Ueber Rindenmessungen. Eine Erwiderung an Dr. K. Brodmann [On cortical measurements. A reply to Dr. K. Brodmann]. *Neurologisches Centralblatt, 28*, 178–182.

Kalberlah, F. (1904). Ueber die acute Commotionspsychose, zugleich ein Beitrag zur Aetiologie des Korsakow'schen Symptomencomplexes [On acute psychosis after concussion, at the same time a contribution on the etiology of Korsakoff's symptom complex]. *Archiv für Psychiatrie und Nervenkrankheiten, 38*, 402–438.

Kalinowsky, L.B. (1952). Quantitatives Prinzip und Stirnhirnfunktion bei den psychochirurgischen Methoden [Quantitative principle and frontal lobe function in psychosurgical methods]. *Archiv für Psychiatrie und Zeitschrift Neurologie, 187*, 435–440.

Kandinsky, V. (1885). *Kritische und klinische Betrachtungen im Gebiete der Sinnestäuschungen* [Critical and clinical considerations in sensory illusions]. Berlin: Friedländer & Sohn.

Kant, F. (1932). Die Pseudoencephalitis Wernicke der Alkoholiker. (Polioencephalitis haemorrhagica superior acuta.) [Pseudoencephalitis of Wernicke in alcoholics. (Polioencephalitis haemorrhagica superior acuta.)]. *Archiv für Psychiatrie und Nervenkrankheiten, 98*, 702–768.

Kaplan, L. (1898). Ueber psychische Erscheinungen bei einem Falle von Tumor des Schläfenlappens [On psychic phenomena in a case of tumor of the temporal lobe]. *Allgemeine Zeitschrift für Psychiatrie und psychisch-gerichtliche Medicin, 54*, 957–978.

Kapur, N., Young, A., Bateman, D., & Kennedy, P. (1989). Focal retrograde amnesia: a long term clinical and neuropsychological follow-up. *Cortex, 25*, 387- 402.

Karbowski, K. (1990). Sixty years of clinical electroencephalography. *European Neurology, 30*, 170–175.

Karplus, J.P. (1902). Ueber ein Australiergehirn nebst Bemerkungen über einige Negergehirne [On the brain of an Australian with remarks on some Negro brains]. *Arbeiten aus dem Neurologischen Institut an der Wiener Universität, 9*, 26–27.

Karplus, J.P. (1905). *Ueber Familienähnlichkeiten an den Grosshirnfurchen des Menschen* [On family-dependent similarities in the cerebral cortical sulci of the human]. Leipzig: Urban & Schwarzenberg.

Karplus, J.P., & Kreidl, A. (1912). Affen ohne Grosshirn [Monkeys without cerebral cortex]. *Wiener klinische Wochenschrift, 25*, 107–108.

Karyofilis, A. (1974). *Hans Berger. Eine biographische Studie* [Hans Berger. A biographical study]. Hildesheim: Karyofilis.

Kaufmann, E. (1887). Ueber Mangel des Balkens im menschlichen Gehirn (I. Theil) [On callosal lack in the human brain (First part)]. *Archiv für Psychiatrie und Nervenkrankheiten, 18*, 769–781 (and 1 table).

Kaufmann, E. (1888). Ueber Mangel des Balkens im menschlichen Gehirn (II. Theil) [On callosal lack in the human brain (2nd part)]. *Archiv für Psychiatrie und Nervenkrankheiten, 19*, 229–243 (and 1 table).

Kehrer, F.A. (1913). Beiträge zur Aphasielehre mit besonderer Berücksichtigung der amnestischen Aphasie [Contributions on aphasia with special consideration of amnesic aphasia]. *Archiv für Psychiatrie und Nervenkrankheiten, 52*, 103–299.

Kellner, (n.n.g.) (1898). Ueber transitorische postepileptische Geistesstörungen [On transitory postepileptic mental disturbances]. *Allgemeine Zeitschrift für Psychiatrie und ihre Grenzgebiete, 58*, 863–870.

Kennedy, F. (1898). On the experimental investigation of memory. *Psychological Review, 5*, 477–499.

Kern, B. (1907). Das Wesen des menschlichen Seelen- und Geisteslebens als Grundriss einer Philosophie des Denkens [The nature of human mental life as basis of a philosophy of cognition]. Berlin: Hirschwald.

Kessler, J., Huber, M., Markowitsch, H.J., Pawlik, G., & Heiss, W.-D. (1991) Complex sensory cross integration deficits in a case of corpus callosum agenesis with bilateral language representation: positron-emission-tomography and neuropsychological findings. *International Journal of Neuroscience, 58*, 275–282.

Kiloh, L.G., Smith, J.S., & Johnson, G.F. (1988). *Physical treatments in psychiatry*. Melbourne: Blackwell Scientific Publications.

King, H.E., Clausen, J., & Scarff, J.E. (1950). Cutaneous thresholds for pain before and after unilateral prefrontal lobotomy. A preliminary report. *Journal of Nervous and Mental Disease, 112*, 93–96.

Kinnaman, A.J. (1902 a). Mental life of two *Macacus rhesus* monkeys in captivity.-I. *American Journal of Psychology, 13*, 98–172.

Kinnaman, A.J. (1902 b). Mental life of two *Macacus rhesus* monkeys in captivity.-II. *American Journal of Psychology, 13*, 173–218.

Kirkpatrick, E.A. (1894). An experimental study of memory. *Psychological Review, 1*, 602–629.

Klebanoff, S.G. (1945). Psychological changes in organic brain lesions and ablations. *Psychological Bulletin, 42*, 585–623.

Kleist, K. (1923). Wesen und Lokalisation der Paralogie [Nature and localization of paralogy]. *Zen-*

tralblatt für die gesamte Neurologie und Psychiatrie, 33, 82–83.

Kleist, K. (1934 a). Kriegsverletzungen des Gehirns in ihrer Bedeutung für die Hirnlokalisation und Hirnpathologie [War-related injuries of the brain and their significance for brain localization and brain pathology]. In K. Bonhoeffer (Ed.), *Handbuch der Aerztlichen Erfahrungen im Weltkriege 1914/18, Vo. 4: Geistes- und Nervenkrankheiten* (pp. 343–1360). Leipzig: Barth.

Kleist, K. (1934 b). *Gehirnpathologie. Vornehmlich auf Grund der Kriegserfahrungen* [Brain pathology. Based on war experiences]. Leipzig: Barth.

Kleist, K. (1936). Bericht über die Gehirnpathologie in ihrer Bedeutung für Neurologie und Psychiatrie [Report on brain pathology in its significance for neurology and psychiatry]. *Zeitschrift für die gesamte Neurologie und Psychiatrie, 158*, 159–193.

Kleist, K., & Gonzalo, J. (1938). Über Thalamus- und Subthalamussyndrome und die Störungen einzelner Thalamuskerne [On thalamic and subthalamic syndromes and the disturbances of single thalamic nuclei]. *Monatsschrift für Psychiatrie, 99*, 87–130.

Klinger, M. (1967). Zur cerebralen Lokalisationslehre. Betrachtungen zur Geschichte einer Hypothese [On cerebral localization. Considerations on the history of a hypothesis]. *Schweizerische Medizinische Wochenschrift, 97*, 725–731.

Klüver, H. (1958). "The temporal lobe syndrome" produced by bilateral ablations. In G.E.W. Wolstenholme and C. M. O'Connor, (Eds.), *Ciba foundation symposium on the neurological basis of behaviour* (pp. 175–186), Boston: Little, Brown and Co.

Klüver, H., & Bucy, P.C. (1937). "Psychic blindness" and other symptoms following bilateral lobectomy in rhesus monkeys. *American Journal of Physiology, 119*, 352–353.

Klüver, H., & Bucy, P.C. (1939). Preliminary analysis of functions of the temporal lobes. *A.M.A. Archives of Neurology and Psychiatry, 42*, 979–1000.

Knapp, A. (1905). *Die Geschwülste des rechten und linken Schläfenlappens. Eine klinische Studie* [Tumors of the right and left temporal lobe. A clinical study]. Wiesbaden: J.F. Bergmann.

Knapp, A. (1906). *Die polyneuritischen Psychosen* [Polyneuritic psychoses]. Wiesbaden: J.F. Bergmann.

Knapp, A. (1918 a). Epilepsie und Korsakowscher Symptomenkomplex [Epilepsy and Korsakoff's symptom complex]. *Monatsschrift für Psychiatrie und Neurologie, 44*, 74–79.

Knapp, A. (1918 b). Die Tumoren des Schläfenlappens [Tumors of the temporal lobe]. *Zeitschrift für die gesamte Neurologie und Psychiatrie/ Originalien, 17*, 226–289.

Knapp, P.C. (1906). The mental symptoms of cerebral tumour. *Brain, 29*, 35–56.

Knauer, A. (1909). Zur Pathologie des linken Schläfenlappens [On the pathology of the left temporal lobe]. *Klinik für psychische und nervöse Krankheiten, 4*, 115–194.

Knight, G.G. (1964). The orbital cortex as an objective in the surgical treatment of mental illness. The results of 450 cases of open operation and the development of the stereotactic approach. *British Journal of Surgery, 51*, 114–123.

Knight, G.G. (1972). Bifrontal stereotaxic tractotomy in the substantia innominata. In E. Hitchcock, L. Laitinen, & K. Vaernet (Eds.), *Psychosurgery. Proceedings of the Second International Conference on Psychosurgery* (pp. 267–277). Springfield: Charles C. Thomas.

Knörlein, (n.n.g.) (1865). Krankengeschichte und Sectionsbefund eines basalen Hirntumors [Case history and post-mortem findings of a basal brain tumor]. *Allgemeine Wiener medicinische Zeitschrift, 15*, 250–252.

Köbcke, H. (1947). Psychochirugie – „die präfrontale Leukotomie" [Psychosurgery – "the prefrontal leucotomy"]. *Deutsche medizinische Wochenschrift, 35/36*, 515–517.

Kodis, J. (1893). *Zur Analyse des Apperceptionsbegriffes* [Analysis of the concept of apperception]. Berlin: S. Calvery & Co.

Kogerer, H. (1920/21). Beitrag zur Psychologie der Gedächtnisstörungen [Contribution to the psychology of memory disturbances]. *Allgemeine Zeitschrift für Psychiatrie und psychisch-gerichtliche Medizin, 76*, 774–790.

Kohlbrugge, J.H.F. (1901). Gehirnwägungen [Brain weights]. *Monatsschrift für Psychiatrie und Neurologie, 10*, 212–213.

Köhler, F. (1897). Experimentelle Studien auf dem Gebiete des hypnotischen Somnambulismus [Experimental studies in hypnotic somnambulism]. *Zeitschrift für Hypnotismus, Psychotherapie sowie andere psychophysiologische und psychopathologische Forschungen, 6*, 357–374.

Kohnstamm, O. (1917). Über das Krankheitsbild der retro-anterograden Amnesie und die Unterscheidung des spontanen und lernenden Merkens [On case aspects of retro-anterograde amnesia and the differentiation of spontaneous and learned remembrance]. *Monatsschrift für Psychiatrie und Neurologie, 41*, 373–382.

Kolb, L.C. (1953). Clinical evaluation of prefrontal lobotomy. *Journal of the American Medical Association, 152*, 1085–1089.

Kolbe, H.J. (1903). Ueber die psychischen Funktionen der Tiere [On the psychic functions of animals]. *Naturwissenschaftliche Wochenschrift (N.F.), 3*, 1–7.

Kolle, K. (1970). *Grosse Nervenärzte (Vols. 1–3)* [Great neurologists (Vols. 1–3)]. Stuttgart: Georg Thieme.

Kolodny, A. (1928). The symptomathology of tumours of the temporal lobe. *Brain, 51*, 385–417.

Konrád, E. (1907). Ueber einen Fall von retrograder Amnesie [On a case of retrograde amnesia]. *Archiv für Psychiatrie und Nervenkrankheiten, 42*, 949–959.

König, (n.n.g.) (1886). Demonstration eines Idioten-Gehirns [Demonstration of the brain of an idiot]. *Allgemeine Zeitschrift für Psychisch-gerichtliche Medicin, 42*, 138–142.

Kopelman, M.D. (1989). Remote and autobiographical memory, temporal context memory and frontal atrophy in Korsakoff and Alzheimer patients. *Neuropsychologia, 27*, 437–460.

Köppen, M. (1896). Beiträge zum Studium der Hirnrindenerkrankungen [Contribution to the study of cortical diseases]. *Archiv für Psychiatrie und Nervenkrankheiten, 28*, 931–963 (and 3 tables).

Kornmüller, A.E. (1937). Lokalisationslehre oder Ganzheit des Zentralnervensystems? [Localization vs. holistic views of the central nervous system]. *Zeitschrift für die gesamte Neurologie und Psychiatrie, 158*, 245–246.

Környey, S. (1931). Über den Hirnbefund in zwei Fällen von akutem katatonem Erregungszustand bei Bleischädigung [On the brain examination in two cases of acute catatonic states of excitement after lead intoxication]. *Deutsche Zeitschrift für Nervenheilkunde, 122*, 18–35.

Korsakoff, S.S. (1889). Etude mèdico-psychologique sur une forme des maladies de la memoire [Medico-psychological study on a form of memory disease]. *Revue Philosophique, 5*, 501–530.

Korsakoff, S.S. (1890). Eine psychische Störung combiniert mit multipler Neuritis (psychosis polyneuritica seu Cerebropathia psychia toxaemica) [A psychic disturbance combined with multiple neuritis (psychosis polyneuritica seu cerebropathia psychia toxaemica)]. *Allgemeine Zeitschrift für Psychiatrie, 46*, 475–485.

Korsakow, S.S. (1890). Ueber eine besondere Form psychischer Störung combiniert mit multipler Neuritis [On a special case of psychic disturbance combined with multiple neuritis]. *Archiv für Psychiatrie und Nervenkrankheiten, 21*, 669–704.

Korsakow, S.S. (1891). Erinnerungstäuschungen (Pseudoreminiscenzen) bei polyneuritischer Psychose [Delusions of memory (pseudoreminiscences) in polyneuritic psychosis]. *Allgemeine Zeitschrift für Psychiatrie, 47*, 390–410.

Korsakow, S.S., & Serbski, W. (1892). Ein Fall von polyneuritischer Psychose mit Autopsie [A case of polyneuritic psychosis with autopsy]. *Archiv für Psychiatrie und Nervenkrankheiten, 23*, 112–134.

Koskoff, Y.D., Dennis, W., Lazovik, D. & Wheeler, E.T. (1948). The psychological effects of frontal lobotomy performed for the alleviation of pain. In J.F. Fulton, W.C. Aring, & S.B. Wortis (Eds.), *The frontal lobes. (Research publications of the association for research in nervous and mental disease, Vol. 27)* (pp. 741–753). Baltimore: Williams & Wilkins.

Kotschetkowa, L. (1901). Beiträge zur pathologischen Anatomie der Mikrogyrie und der Mikrocephalie [Contributions to the pathological anatomy of microgyri and microencephaly]. *Archiv für Psychiatrie und Nervenkrankheiten, 33*, 39–106 (and 2 tables).

Kraepelin, E. (1882). Ueber die Einwirkung einiger medicamentöser Stoffe auf die Dauer einfacher psychischer Vorgänge [The influence of some medical drugs on the duration of simple psychic actions]. *Philosophische Studien, 1*, 573–605.

Kraepelin, E. (1886 a). Ueber Erinnerungsfälschungen [On delusions of remembrance]. *Archiv für Psychiatrie und Nervenkrankheiten, 17*, 830–843.

Kraepelin, E. (1886 b). Psychiatrie [Psychiatry]. *Allgemeine Zeitschrift für Psychiatrie und psychisch-gerichtliche Medicin, 42*, 162–185.

Kraepelin, E. (1887 a). Ueber Erinnerungsfälschungen [On delusions of remembrance]. *Archiv für Psychiatrie und Nervenkrankheiten, 18*, 199–239.

Kraepelin, E. (1887 b). Ueber Erinnerungsfälschungen [On delusions of remembrance]. *Archiv für Psychiatrie und Nervenkrankheiten, 18*, 395–436.

Kraepelin, E. (1889). Ueber den Einfluss der Uebung auf die Dauer von Associationen [The influence of practice on the duration of associations]. *St. Petersburger Medicinische Wochenschrift, 14*, 9–10.

Kraepelin, E. (1892). *Ueber die Beeinflussung einfacher psychischer Vorgänge durch einige Arzneimittel* [The influence of some drugs on simple psychic actions]. Jena: Gustav Fischer.

Kraepelin, E. (1896). *Psychiatrie* [Psychiatry]. (5th ed.). Leipzig: Barth.

Kraepelin, E. (1900). Ueber die Merkfähigkeit [On remembrance]. *Monatsschrift für Psychiatrie und Neurologie, 8*, 245–250.

Kraepelin, E. (1918). *Hundert Jahre Psychiatrie* [One hundred years of psychiatry]. Berlin: Springer.

Kraemer, N. (1912). *Experimentelle Untersuchungen zur Erkenntnis des Lernprozesses* [Experimental investigations on the recognition of the process of learning]. Leipzig: Quelle & Meyer.

Krafft-Ebing, R. von (1898). Über retrograde allgemeine Amnesie [On retrograde general amnesia]. *Arbeiten aus dem Gesammt-Gebiet der Psychiatrie und Neuropathologie, 3*, 213–224.

Kramer, F. (1915). Schussverletzung des Stirnhirns mit akinetischem Symptombild [A gunshot wound of the frontal lobe with an akinetic symptom]. *Neurologisches Zentralblatt, 34*, 781.

Krauss, R. (1904). Ueber Auffassungs- und Merkversuche bei einem Falle von polyneuritischer Psychose [On experiments of conception and remembrance in a case of polyneuritic psychosis]. *Psychologische Arbeiten, 4*, 523–537.

Krauss, S. (1930). Untersuchungen über Aufbau und Störung der menschlichen Handlung. I. Teil: Die Korsakowsche Störung [Investigations on the construction and disturbance of human action. I. Part: Korsakoff's disturbance]. *Archiv für die gesamte Psychologie, 77*, 649–692.

Kretschmer, E. (1928). Störungen des Gefühlslebens, Temperamente [Disturbances of emotional life, temperaments]. In O. Bumke (Ed.), *Handbuch der Geisteskrankheiten (Vol. 1)* (pp. 662–688). Berlin: Springer.

Kretschmer, E. (1949). Die Orbitalhirn- und Zwischenhirnsyndrome nach Schädelbasisfrakturen [The orbital brain and diencephalic syndroms after fractures of the basis of the skull]. *Allgemeine Zeitschrift für Psychiatrie und ihre Grenzgebiete, 124*, 358–360.

Kretschmer, E. (1954). Verletzungen der Schädelbasis und ihre psychiatrisch-neurologischen Folgen [Injuries of the basis of the skull and their psychiatric-neurological consequences]. *Deutsche Medizinische Wochenschrift, 79*, 1709–1713.

Kriworotow, W. (1883). *Ueber die Functionen des Stirnlappens des Grosshirns* [On the functions of the frontal lobe of the cerebral cortex]. Dissertation of the Medical Faculty of the Kaiser Wilhelm-University Strassburg. Strassburg: Kayser.

Kroh, O., Götz, W., Scholl, R., & Ziegler, W. (1927). Weitere Beiträge zur Psychologie des Haushuhns [Further contributions on the psychology of the domestic hen]. *Zeitschrift für Psychologie und Physiologie der Sinnesorgane, 103*, 203–227.

Kronthal, P. (1916). Ueber den Seelensitz [On the seat of the soul]. *Archiv für Psychiatrie und Nervenkrankheiten, 56*, 219–227.

Krüger, D.W. (1953). Ist die Leukotomie als Eingriff zur Schmerzbekämpfung zu verantworten? [Can leucotomy be justified as a treatment for pain control?] *Wiener medizinische Wochenschrift, 113*, 613–615.

Krücke, W. (1963). Ludwig Edinger. In K. Kolle (Ed.), *Grosse Nervenärzte (Vol. 3)* (pp. 9–29). Stuttgart: Thieme.

Kühlmann, A. (1908). Beitrag zur Frage der Ammonshornveränderungen bei Epilepsie [Contribution to the question of changes in Ammon's horn in epilepsy]. *Archiv für Psychiatrie und Nervenkrankheiten, 44*, 945–958.

Kühn, A. (1914). Über Einprägung durch Lesen und Rezitieren [On memorizing by reading and reciting]. *Zeitschrift für Psychologie, 68*, 396–481.

Külpe, O. (1893). *Grundriss der Psychologie* [Compendium of psychology]. Leipzig: W. Engelmann.

Kussmaul, A. (1859). *Untersuchungen über das Seelenleben des neugeborenen Menschen* [Investigations of the psychology of infants]. Tübingen: F. Pietzcker.

Kussmaul, A. (1910). *Die Störungen der Sprache. Versuch einer Pathologie der Sprache* [Disturbances of language. Attempting a psychology of language]. (4th ed.). Leipzig: F.C.W. Vogel.

Kussmaul, (n.n.g.), & Nothnagel, H. (1873). Krankheiten des Nervensystems [Illnesses of the nervous system]. In R. Virchow & A. Hirsch (Eds.), *Jahresbericht über die Leistungen und Fortschritte in der gesamten Medicin* (pp. 21–86). Berlin: Hirschwald.

Kürz, E., & Kraepelin, E. (1901). Ueber die Beeinflussung psychischer Vorgänge durch regelmässigen Alkoholgenuss [The influence of regular consumption of alcohol on psychic actions]. In E. Kraepelin (Ed.), *Psychologische Arbeiten (Vol. 3)* (pp.417–457). Leipzig: Engelmann.

Kutner, R. (1906). Ueber corticale Herderscheinungen in der amnestischen Phase polyneuritischer Psychosen [On focal cortical phenomena in the amnesic phase of polyneuritic psychoses]. *Archiv für Psychiatrie und Nervenkrankheiten, 41*, 134–157.

Laitinen, L.V., & Livingston, K.E. (Eds.). (1973). *Surgical approaches in psychiatry.* Lancaster, UK: Medical and Technical Publ. Comp.

Landis, C., Zubin, J., & Mettler, F.A. (1950). The functions of the human frontal lobe. *Journal of Psychology 30*, 123–128.

Lange, C. (1887). *Über Gemüthsbewegungen* [On emotions]. Leipzig: Theodor Thomas.

Lange, J. (1937). Grundsätzliche Erörterungen zu Kleists hirnpathologischen Lehren [Basic discussions on Kleist's brain pathological studies]. *Zeitschrift für die gesamte Neurologie und Psychiatrie, 158*, 247–251.

Lange, J. (1938). Hirnchirurgie und Lokalisationslehre. (Hirnlappen- und Hemisphärenausschneidungen) [Brain surgery and the theory of localization. (Sectioning the brain lobes and hemispheres)]. *Monatsschrift für Psychiatrie und Neurologie, 99*, 130–144.

Langworthy, O.R., & Fox, H.M. (1937). Thalamic syndrome. Syndrome of the posterior cerebral artery; a review. *Archives of Internal Medicine, 60*, 203–227.

Lannois, (n.n.g.), & Paviot, (n.n.g.) (1902). Un cas de tumeur cèrèbrale a forme psycho-paralytique et evolution fèbrile [A case with a cerebral tumor of psycho-paralytic form and the fevrile evolution]. *Lyon medicale, 99*, 561.

Lashley, K.S. (1929). *Brain mechanisms and intelligence*. Chicago: University of Chicago Press.

Lashley, K.S. (1937). Factors limiting recovery after central nervous lesions. *Journal of Nervous and Mental Disease, 88*, 733–755.

Lashley, K.S., & Clark, G. (1946). The cytoarchitecture of the cerebral cortex of Ateles: A critical examination of architectonic studies. *Journal of Comparative Neurology, 85*, 233–305.

Laubenthal, F. (1953). Hirn und Seele [Brain and soul]. Salzburg: O. Müller.

Lauber, H.L. (1958). Sexuelle Enthemmung und Exhibitionsmus bei Frontalhirnverletzten [Sexual disinhibition and exhibitionism in the frontal lobe injured]. *Archiv für Psychiatrie und Zeitschrift für die gesamte Neurologie, 197*, 293–306.

Laughlin, H.P. (1956). *The neuroses in clinical practice*. Philadelphia: Saunders.

Lawson, R. (1878). On the symptomatology of alcoholic brain disorders. *Brain, 1*, 182–194.

Lazarus, M. (1876). *Das Leben der Seele in Monographieen über seine Erscheinungen. (Vol. 1)* [The life of the soul in monographs on its phenomena. (Vol. 1)]. Berlin: F. Dümmler.

Lazarus, M. (1878). *Das Leben der Seele in Monographien über seine Erscheinungen. (Vol. 2)* [The life of the soul in monographs on its phenomena. (Vol. 2)]. (2nd ed.). Berlin: F. Dümmler.

Lazarus, M. (1882). *Das Leben der Seele in Monographien über seine Erscheinungen. (Vol. 3)* [The life of the soul in monographs on its phenomena. (Vol. 3)]. (2nd ed.). Berlin: F. Dümmler.

Leavitt, F.H. (1935). The etiology of temporary amnesia. *American Journal of Psychiatry, 91*, 1079–1088.

Le Beau, J. (1951). The surgical uncertainties of prefrontal topectomy and leucotomy (observations on 100 cases). *Journal of Mental Science, 97*, 480–504.

Le Beau, J., & Petrie, A. (1953). A comparison of the personality changes after (1) prefrontal selective surgery for the relief of intract-cingulectomy and topectomy. *Journal of Mental Science, 99*, 53–61.

Le Beau, J., & Choppy, M. (1956). Sur les variations du lobe frontal et de certaines fonctions mentales [On the variations of the frontal lobe and certain mental functions]. *Encéphale, 45*, 242–255.

Leichtenstern, (n.n.g.) (1892). Ueber primäre acute haemorrhagische Encephalitis (mit Demonstration) [On primary acute hemorrhagic encephalitis (with demonstration)]. *Deutsche medizinische Wochenschrift, 18*, 39–40.

Leidesdorf, M. (1865). *Lehrbuch der psychischen Krankheiten* [Textbook of psychic illnesses]. (2nd ed.). Erlangen: F. Enke.

Lemke, R. (1937). Über doppelseitige Stirnhirntumoren [On bilateral frontal lobe tumors]. *Archiv für Psychiatrie und Nervenkrankheiten, 106*, 54–70.

Leonhard, K. (1959). Die biologische Aufgabe des Stirnhirns gemäss den Ausfällen durch Verletzungen. Eine klinische Untersuchung [The biological task of the frontal lobe according to deficits after injury. A clinical investigation]. *Deutsche Zeitschrift für Nervenheilkunde, 179*, 75–101.

Leszynsky, W.M. (1909). A case of gunshot wound of the brain without focal symptoms. *Journal of Nervous and Mental Disease, 36*, 714–715.

Levin, H.S. (1991). Pioneers in research on the behavioral sequelae of head injury. *Journal of Clinical and Experimental Neuropsychology, 13*, 133–154.

Levin, H.S., Eisenberg, H.M., & Benton, A.L. (Eds.) (1991). *Frontal lobe function and dysfunction*. New York: Oxford University Press.

Levin, H.S., Peters, H.B. & Hulkonen, D.A. (1983). Early oncepts of anterograde and retrograde amnesia. *Cortex, 19*, 427–440.

Levin, S., Greenblatt, M., Healey, M.M., & Solomon, H.C. (1950). Electroencephalographic and clinical effects of prefrontal lobotomy, with consideration of post-lobotomy convulsive seizures. In M. Greenblatt, R. Arnot, & H.C. Solomon (Eds.), *Studies in lobotomy* (pp. 400–427). New York: Grune & Stratton.

Lewandowsky, M., & Stadelmann, E. (1908). Über einen bemerkenswerten Fall von Hirnblutung und über Rechenstörungen bei Herderkrankung des Gehirns [On a remarkable case of brain bleeding and on calculation disturbances in focal disease of the brain]. *Journal für Psychologie und Neurologie, 11*, 249–265.

Lewin, K. (1922 a). Das Problem der Willensmessung und das Gesetz der Assoziation. I. [The problem of the measurement of will and the law of association. I.]. *Psychologische Forschung, 1*, 191–302.

Lewin, K. (1922 b). Das Problem der Willensmessung und das Gesetz der Assoziation. II. [The problem of the measurement of will and the law of association. II.]. *Psychologische Forschung,* 2, 65–140.

Lewis, S.W. (1990). Computerised tomography in schizophrenia 15 years on. *British Journal of Psychiatry, 157 (Suppl. 9)*, 16–24.

Lewy, F.H. (1908). Ein ungewöhnlicher Fall von Sprachstörung als Beitrag zur Lehre von der sogenannten amnestischen und Leitungsaphasie [An unusual case of language disturbance as a contribution to the theory of socalled amnesic and conduction aphasia]. *Neurologisches Zentralblatt, 27*, 802–814 and 850–862.

Leyden, E., & Jastrowitz, M. (1888). *Beiträge zur Lehre von der Localisation im Gehirn und über deren praktische Verwerthung* [Contributions to the theory on localization in the brain and on its practical use] . Leipzig: Thieme.

Lhermitte, J. (1922). Syndrome de la calotte du péduncole cérébral. Les troubles psycho-sensoriels dans les lésions du mésocéphale [Syndrome of the calotte of the cerebral peduncule. Psychosensory disturbances in mesocephalic lesions]. *Revue neurologique, 29*, 1359–1365.

Lhermitte, J., Doussinet (n.n.g.), & de Ajuriaguerra (n.n.g.). (1937). Une observation de la forme korsakowienne des tumeurs du 3ᵉ ventricule [An observation of Korsakoff-like symptomatology in tumors of the third ventricle]. *Revue neurologique, 68*, 709–727.

Liberson, W.T., Scoville, W.B., & Dunsmore, R.H. (1951). Stimulation studies of the prefrontal lobe and uncus in man. *Electroencephalography and Clinical Neurophysiology, 3*, 1–8.

Lichtenthaeler, C. (1974). *Geschichte der Medizin (2 Bände)* [History of medicine (2 vols.)]. Köln: Deutscher Ärzte-Verlag.

Lichtheim, L. (1885). On aphasia. *Brain, 7*, 433–484.

Lidz, T. (1949). Analysis of a prefrontal lobe syndrome and its theoretic implications. *A.M.A. Archives of Neurology and Psychiatry, 62*, 1–26.

Liebaldt, G.P., & Scheller, H. (1971). Amnestisches Syndrom and Korsakow-Syndrom – Zwei auch anatomisch-lokalisatorisch unterscheidbare Syndrome? [Amnesic syndrome and Korsakoff's syndrome – Two syndromes which can be differentiated on the basis of anatomical localization?] *Nervenarzt, 42*, 402–413.

Liepmann, H. (1898). [On the case of a Korsakoff amnesic.] *Verhandlungen der Schlesischen Gesellschaft für Vaterländische Kultur*. (Cited after Liepmann, 1910.)

Liepmann, H. (1907 a). Zwei Fälle von Zerstörung der unteren hinteren Stirnhirnwindung [Two cases of destruction in the lower posterior frontal lobe gyrus]. *Journal für Psychologie und Neurologie, 9*, 279–285 (and 1 Table).

Liepmann, H. (1907 b). Ueber die Rolle des Balkens beim Handeln und das Verhältnis der aphasischen und apraktischen Störungen zu Intelligenz [On the role of the corpus callosum in behavior and the relation of aphasic and apraxic disturbances to intelligence]. *Berliner Klinische Wochenschrift, No. 28*, 901.

Liepmann, H. (1910). Beitrag zur Kenntnis des amnestischen Symptomenkomplexes [Contribution to the knowledge of the amnesic symptom complex]. *Neurologisches Zentralblatt, 29*, 1147–1161.

Liepmann, H. (1913). Zur Lokalisation der Hirnfunktionen mit besonderer Berücksichtigung der Beteiligung der beiden Hemisphären an den Gedächtnisleistungen [On the localization of brain functions with special consideration of the contribution of both hemispheres in memory performance]. *Zeitschrift für Psychologie, 63*, 1–18.

Liepmann, H., & Maas, O. (1907). Fall von linksseitiger Agraphie und Apraxie bei rechtsseitiger Lähmung [A case of left-sided agraphia and apraxia with right-sided paralysis]. *Journal für Psychologie und Neurologie, 10*, 214–227 (and 2 tables).

Liepmann, H., & Quensel, F. (1909). Ein neuer Fall von motorischer Aphasie mit anatomischem Befund [A new case of motoric aphasia with anatomical evidence]. *Monatsschrift für Psychiatrie und Neurologie, 23*, 189–216 (und 2 Tafeln).

Lilly, R., Cummings, J.L., Benson, D.F., & Frankel, M. (1983). The human Klüver-Bucy syndrome. *Neurology, 33*, 1141–1145.

Lindsay, W.S. (1904). Perforating wound of both cerebral hemispheres. *Medical Record (N.Y.)*, 186–187.

Lipmann, O. (1903). Praktische Ergebnisse der experimentellen Untersuchung des Gedächtnisses [Practical results of the experimental investigation of memory]. *Journal für Psychologie und Neurologie, Bd. II*, 108–118.

Lipmann, O. (1904). Die Wirkung der einzelnen Wiederholungen auf verschieden starke und verschieden alte Assoziationen [The effect of single repetitions on differences in strong and differentially old associations]. *Zeitschrift für Psychologie, 35*, 195–233.

Lipmann, O. (1908). Ein neuer Expositionsapparat mit ruckweiser Rotation für Gedächtnis- und Lernversuche. [A new exposition apparatus with interrupted rotation for experiments on memory and learning]. *Zeitschrift für Psychologie, 49*, 270–277.

Lipmann, O. (1911). *Die Spuren interessebetonter Erlebnisse und ihre Symptome (Theorie, Methoden und Ergebnisse der „Tatbestandsdiagnostik")* [The traces of interest-aroused experiences and their symptoms (theory, methods, and results of the diagnosis based on factual findings]. Leipzig: Barth.

Lipps, T. (1903). *Leitfaden der Psychologie* [Textbook of psychology]. Leipzig: W. Engelmann.

Lisowski, F.P. (1967). Prehistoric and early historic trepanation. In D. Brothwell & A.T. Sandison (Eds.), *Diseases in antiquity* (pp. 651–672). Springfield, IL: C.C. Thomas.

Lissauer, H. (1890a). Ein Fall von Seelenblindheit nebst einem Beitrage zur Theorie derselben [A case of optic agnosia with a contribution on its theory]. *Archiv für Psychiatrie und Nervenkrankheiten, 21*, 222–270.

Lissauer, H. (1890b). Sehhügelveränderungen bei progressiver Paralyse [Changes in the optic thalamus in progressive paralysis]. *Deutsche Medicinische Wochenschrift, 16*, 561–564.

Livingston, R.B., Chapman, W.P., Livingston, K.E., & Kraintz, L. (1948). Stimulation of orbital surface of man prior to frontal lobotomy. In J.F. Fulton, W.C. Aring & S.B. Wortis (Eds.), *The frontal lobes. (Research publications of the association for research in nervous and mental disease, Vol. 27)* (pp. 421–432). Baltimore: Williams & Wilkins.

Livingston, R.B., Fulton, J.F., Delgado, J.M.R., Sachs, E., Brendler, S.J., Jr., & Davis, G.D. (1948). Stimulation and regional ablation of orbital surface of frontal lobes. In J.F. Fulton, W.C. Aring & S.B. Wortis (Eds.), *The frontal lobes. (Research publications of the association for research in nervous and mental disease, Vol. 27)* (pp. 405–420). Baltimore: Williams & Wilkins.

Lobosky, J.M., Van Gilder, J.C., & Damasio, A.R. (1984). Behavioural manifestations of third ventricular colloid cyst. *Journal of Neurology, Neurosurgery, and Psychiatry, 47*, 1075–1080.

Loeb, J. (1884). Die Sehstörungen nach Verletzung der Grosshirnrinde. Nach Versuchen am Hunde [Visual disturbances after injury of the cerebral cortex. Experiments on the dog]. *Archiv für die Gesammte Physiologie des Menschen und der Thiere, 34*, 76–172.

Loeb, J. (1885). Die elementaren Störungen einfacher Functionen nach oberflächlicher, umschriebener Verletzungen des Grosshirns [Elementary disturbances of simple functions following superficial, circumscribed injuries of the cerebrum]. *Pflügers Archiv für die gesammte Physiologie des Menschen und der Thiere, 37*, 51–56.

Loeb, J. (1886). Beiträge zur Physiologie des Grosshirns [Contributions to the physiology of the cerebrum]. *Pflüger's Archiv für die gesammte Physiologie des Menschen und der Thiere, 39*, 265–346.

Loeb, J. (1899). *Einleitung in die vergleichende Gehirnphysiologie und vergleichende Psychologie. Mit besonderer Berücksichtigung der wirbellosen Thiere* [Introduction to comparative brain physiology and comparative psychology. With special emphasis on invertebrates]. Leipzig: Barth.

Loftus, E.F. (1974). On reading the fine print. *Quarterly Journal of Experimental Psychology, 27*, 324.

Lomer, G. (1905). Beobachtungen über farbiges Hören (auditio colorata) [Observations on colored hearing (auditio colorata)]. *Archiv für Psychiatrie und Nervenkrankheiten, 40*, 593–601.

Lorente de Nó, R. (1933). Studies on the structure of the cerebral cortex. I. The area entorhinalis. *Journal für Psychologie und Neurologie, 45*, 381–437.

Lorente de Nó, R. (1934). Studies on the structure of the cerebral cortex. II. Continuation of the study of the ammonic system. *Journal für Psychologie und Neurologie, 46*, 113–177.

Losskij, N. (1904). *Die Grundlehren der Psychologie vom Standpunkte des Voluntarismus* [Basic theories of the psychology of voluntarism]. Leipzig: J.A. Barth.

Lubbock, J. (1889). *Die Sinne und das geistige Leben der Tiere, insbesondere der Insekten* [The senses and mental life of animals, espcially of insects]. (transl. by W. Marshall). Leipzig: F.A. Brockhaus.

Luchins, D.J. (1990). A possible role of hippocampal dysfunction in schizophrenic symptomatology. *Biological Psychiatry, 28*, 87–91.

Luciani, L. (1884). On the sensorial localisations in the cortex cerebri. *Brain, 7*, 145–160.

Luciani, L., & Seppilli, G. (1886). *Die Functions-Localisation auf der Grosshirnrinde an Thierexperimenten und Klinischen Fällen nachgewiesen* [Functional localization in the cerebral cortex based on animal experiments and clinical cases]. (transl. by M.O. Fraenkel). Leipzig: Denicke's Verlag.

Luciani, L., & Tamburini, A. (1878). Ricerche sperimentali sulle funzioni del cervello [Experimental investigations on the functions of the cerebrum]. *Rivista Sperimentale di Freniatria e di Medicina Legale, 4*, 69–89, and 225–280.

Lücke, (n.n.g.) (1903). Ueber das Ganser'sche Symptom mit Berücksichtigung seiner forensischen Bedeutung [On the Ganser symptom with consideration of its forensic importance]. *Allgemeine Zeitschrift für Psychiatrie, 60*, 1–35.

Lücken, (n.n.g.) (1909). *Zur Diagnose und Symptomatologie der Tumoren des rechten Schläfenlappens* [On the diagnosis and symptomatology of tumors of the right temporal lobe]. Unpublished doctoral dissertation, Königliche Christian-Albrechts-Universität, Kiel. (cited after Artom, 1923).

Lückerath, M. (1900). Beitrag zu der Lehre von der Korsakowschen Psychose [Contribution to the theory of Korsakoff's psychosis]. *Neurologisches Zentralblatt, 19*, 341–347.

Lüers, T. (1950). Über fronto-thalamische Syndrome bei der Pick'schen Krankheit [On fronto-thalamic syndroms in Pick's disease]. *Deutsche Zeitschrift für Nervenheilkunde, 164*, 179–198.

Lüers, T., & Spatz, H. (1957). Picksche Krankheit. (Progressive umschriebene Grosshirnatrophie) [Pick's disease. (Progressive circumscribed atrophy of the cerebrum)]. In O. Lubarsch, F. Henke & R. Rössle (Eds.), *Handbuch der speziellen pathologischen Anatomie und Histologie, Vol. 13/Part A. Nervensystem* (pp. 614–715). Berlin: Springer.

Lührmann, F. (1896). Über Krämpfe und Amnesie nach Wiederbelebung Erhängter [On spasms and amnesia after resuscitation of hanged persons]. *Allgemeine Zeitschrift für Psychiatrie und ihre Grenzgebiete, 52*, 185–195.

Lundholm, H. (1932). The riddle of functional amnesia. *Journal of Abnormal and Social Psychology, 26*, 355–366.

Luria, A.R. (1968). *The mind of a mnemonist: A little book about a vast memory*. New York: Basic Books.

Mabille, H., & Pitres, A. (1913). Sur un cas d'amnesie de fixation post-apoplectique ayant persiste pendant vingt-trois ans [On a case of post-apoplexic amnesia persisting for twenty-five years]. *Revue de Medicine, 33*, 257–279.

MacKinnon, D.F., & Squire, L.R. (1989). Autobiographical memory and amnesia. *Psychobiology, 17*, 247–256.

Macmillan, M.B. (1986). A wonderful journey through skull and brains: The travels of Mr. Gage's tamping iron. *Brain and Cognition, 5*, 67–107.

MacPhail, E.M. (1982). *Brain and intelligence in vertebrates*. Oxford: Clarendon Press.

Mair, W.G.P., Warrington, E.K., & Weiskrantz, L. (1979). Memory disorder in Korsakoff psychosis. A neuropathological and neuropsychological investigation of two cases. *Brain, 102*, 749–783.

Malmo, R.B. (1948). Psychological aspects of frontal gyrectomy and frontal-lobotomy in mental patients. In J.F. Fulton, W.C. Aring, & S.B. Wortis (Eds.), *The frontal lobes. (Research publications of the association for research in nervous and mental disease, Vol. 27)* (pp. 537–564). Baltimore: Williams & Wilkins.

Mann, L. (1898). Casuistische Beiträge zur Hirnchirurgie und Hirnlocalisation [Casuistric contributions on brain surgery and brain localization]. *Monatsschrift für Psychiatrie und Neurologie, 4*, 369–378.

Marburg, O. (1906). Die sogenannte „akute multiple Sklerose" (Encephalomyelitis periaxialis scleroticans) [The socalled "acute multiple sclerosis" (encephalomyelitis periaxialis scleroticans)]. *Jahrbücher für Psychiatrie und Neurologie, 27*, 211–312 (and 3 tables).

Marchan, L., & Courtois, A. (1934). Le psychose aigue de Korsakoff des alcooliques [The acute Korsakoff psychosis of alcoholics]. *Revue neurologique, 41*, 425–453.

Marchiafava, E., & Bignami, A. (1903). Sopra un'alterazione del corpo calloso osservata in soggetti alcoolisti [On alterations in the corpus callosum observed in alcoholics]. *Rivista di Patologia Nervosa e Mentali, 8*, 544–549.

Marcus, H. (1926). Gedächtnisstörungen bei krankhaften Veränderungen im Frontalhirn und in der Insula [Memory disturbances after disease-based changes of the frontal lobe and the insula]. *Zeitschrift für die gesamte Neurologie und Psychiatrie, 101*, 330–349.

Markowitsch, H.J. (1982). Thalamic mediodorsal nucleus and memory. A critical evaluation of studies in animals and man. *Neuroscience and Biobehavioral Reviews, 6*, 351–380.

Markowitsch, H.J. (1984). Can amnesia be caused by damage of a single brain region? *Cortex, 20*, 27–45.

Markowitsch, H.J. (1985).Der Fall H.M. im Dienste der Hirnforschung [Case H.M. serving brain research]. *Naturwissenschaftliche Rundschau, 38*, 410–416.

Markowitsch, H.J. (1986). Physiological and comparative psychology: Current research interests. *American Psychologist, 41*, 1301–1305.

Markowitsch, H.J. (1987). Demenz im Alter. [Dementia in the aged]. *Psychologische Rundschau, 38*, 145–154.

Markowitsch, H.J. (1988 a). Anatomical and functional organization of the primate prefrontal cortical system. In H.D. Steklis & J. Erwin (Eds.), *Comparative primate biology, Vol. IV. Neurosciences* (pp. 99–153). New York: Alan R. Liss.

Markowitsch, H.J. (1988 b). Long term memory processing in the human brain: On the influence of individual variations. In J. Delacour & J.C.S. Levy (Eds.), *Systems with learning and memory abilities* (pp. 153–176). Amsterdam: North-Holland Publ. Comp.

Markowitsch, H.J. (1988 c). Individual differences in memory performance and the brain. In H.J. Markowitsch (Ed.), *Information processing by the brain* (pp. 125–148). Toronto: Huber.

Markowitsch, H.J. (1988d). Transient psychogenic amnesias. *Italian Journal of Neurological Sciences, Suppl. 9*, 49–51.

Markowitsch, H.J. (1988e). Problems in the differential diagnosis of various forms of transient amnesias. *Italian Journal of Neurological Sciences, Suppl. 9*, 53–56.

Markowitsch, H.J. (1990a). Early concepts of transient disorders with symptoms of amnesia. In H.J. Markowitsch (Ed.), *Transient global amnesia and related disorders* (pp. 4–14). Toronto: Hogrefe & Huber Publs.

Markowitsch, H.J. (1990b). Transient psychogenic amnesic states. In H.J. Markowitsch (Ed.), *Transient global amnesia and related disorders* (pp. 181–190). Toronto: Hogrefe & Huber Publs.

Markowitsch, H.J. (Ed.). (1990c). *Transient global amnesia and related disorders*. Toronto: Hogrefe & Huber Publs.

Markowitsch, H.J. (1991a). Memory disorders after diencephalic damage: Heterogeneity of findings. In W.C. Abraham, M.C. Corballis & K.G. White (Eds.), *Memory mechanisms: A tribute to G.V. Goddard* (pp. 175–194). Hillsdale, NJ: LEA.

Markowitsch, H.J. (1991b). Das gestörte Altgedächtnis: Diagnoseverfahren bei Hirngeschädigten [Disturbed remote memory: Methods of diagnosis in the brain damaged]. *Die Rehabilitation, in press.*

Markowitsch, H.J., von Cramon, D.Y., & Schuri, U. (in subm.). The mnestic performance profile of a bilateral diencephalic infarct patient with preserved intelligence and severe amnesic disturbances.

Markowitsch, H.J., Kessler, J., Bast-Kessler, C., & Riess, R. (1984). Different emotional tones significantly affect recognition performance in patients with Korsakoff psychosis. *International Journal of Neuroscience, 25*, 145–159.

Markowitsch, H.J., Kessler, J., & Denzler, P. (1986). Recognition memory and psychophysiological responses towards stimuli with neutral and emotional content. A study with Korsakoff patients and recently detoxified and longterm abstinent alcoholics. *International Journal of Neuroscience, 29*, 1–35.

Markowitsch, H.J., & Pritzel, M. (1977). Comparative analysis of prefrontal learning in rats, cats, and monkeys. *Psychological Bulletin, 84*, 817–837.

Markowitsch, H.J., & Pritzel, M. (1979). The prefrontal cortex: Projection area of the thalamic mediodorsal nucleus? *Physiological Psychology, 7*, 1–6.

Markowitsch, H.J., & Pritzel, M. (1985). The neuropathology of amnesia. *Progress in Neurobiology, 25*, 189–287.

Markowitsch, H.J., & Pritzel, M. (1987). Single unit activity in cat prefrontal and parietal cortex during performance of a symmetrically reinforced go-no go task. *International Journal of Neuroscience, 32*, 719–746.

Markowitsch, H.J., Pritzel, M., Wilson, M., & Divac, I. (1984). The prefrontal cortex of a prosimian (*Galago senegalensis*) defined as the cortical projection area of the thalamic mediodorsal nucleus. *Neuroscience, 5*, 1771–1779.

Marlowe, W.B., Mancall, E.L., & Thomas, J.J. (1975). Complete Klüver-Bucy syndrome in man. *Cortex, 11*, 53–59.

Marshall, J. (1864). On the brain of a bushwoman and on the brains of two idiots of European descent. *Philosophical Transactions of the Royal Society, London, 154*, 501–558.

Marshall, J. (1892/93). On the brain of the late George Grote, F.R.S., with comments and observations on the human brain and its parts generally. *Journal of Anatomy and Physiology (N.S.), 7*, 21–65 (and 3 Plates).

Marshall, R.M. (1909). Four cases of intracranial tumour with mental symptoms. *Journal of Mental Science, 55*, 310–321.

Martin, J.J., Yap, M., Nei, I.P., & Tan, T.E. (1983). Selective thalamic degeneration – Report of a case with memory and mental disturbances. *Clinical Neuropathology, 2*, 156–162.

Marx, E.J. (1921). Über einen seltenen Fall von Korsakoffschem Symptomenkomplex bei Hirnarteriosklerose [On a rare case of Korsakoff's symptom complex in arterio-sclerosis of the brain]. *Neurobiologisches Zentralblatt, Suppl. 40*, 87–90.

Matell, M. (1893). Ein Fall von Heterotopie der grauen Substanz in den beiden Hemisphären des Grosshirns [A case of heterotopy of the gray matter in both hemispheres of the cerebrum]. *Archiv für Psychiatrie und Nervenkrankheiten, 25*, 124–136 (and 1 Table).

Matiegka, H. (1902). Ueber das Hirngewicht, die Schädelkapacität und die Kopfform, sowie deren Beziehungen zur psychischen Thätigkeit des Menschen [On brain weight, cranial capacity and head shape, as well as on their relations to the psychic activity of man]. *Sitzungsbericht der königlich böhmischen Gesellschaft der Wissenschaften, Mathematisch-naturwissenschaftliche Classe, Article 20*, 1–75.

Matthies, (n.n.g.) (1908). Über einen Fall von hysterischem Dämmerzustand mit retrograder Amnesie [On a case of hysterical somnolence with retrograde amnesia]. *Allgemeine Zeitschrift für Psychiatrie und ihre Grenzgebiete, 65*, 188- 206.

Maudsley, H. (1873). *Body and mind: An inquiry into their connection and mutual influence, specially in reference to mental disorders*. London: Macmillan.

Mayberg, H.S., Starkstein, S.E., Robinson, R.G., & Wagner, H. (1989). The role of the right basotemporal cortex in the production of secondary mania. *Society for Neuroscience Abstracts, 15*, 1223 (Abstr. No. 449.8).

Mayer, (n.n.g.) (1929). Die Commotio cerebri und ihre Bewertung [Cerebral concussion and its evaluation]. *Münchener medizinische Wochenschrift, 76*, 2135–2136.

Mayer-Gross, W., Slater, E., & Roth, M. (1969). *Clinical psychiatry*. (3rd ed.). London: Balliere, Tindall, & Cassell.

Mayes, A.R. (1988). *Human organic memory disorders*. Cambridge: Cambridge Univ. Press.

Mayes, A.R., Meudell, P.R., Mann, D., & Pickering, A. (1988). Location of lesions in Korsakoff's syndrome neuropsychological and neuropathological data on two patients. *Cortex, 24*, 367–388.

Mayser, P. (1879). Eine Erwiederung an Herrn Professor P. Flechsig in Leipzig [A rejoinder to Professor P. Flechsig in Leipzig]. *Archiv für Psychiatrie und Nervenkrankheiten, 9*, 105–121.

McBurney, C., & Starr, M.A. (1893). A contribution to cerebral surgery. Diagnosis, localization, and operation for removal of thre tumors of the brain: with some comments upon the surgical treatment of brain tumors. *American Journal of the Medical Sciences, 105*, 361–387.

McGeoch, J.A. (1928). Memory. *Psychological Bulletin, 25*, 513–549.

McGeoch, J.A. (1930). Memory. *Psychological Bulletin, 27*, 514–563.

McHenry, L.C. (1969). *Garrison's history of neurology. Revised and enlarged with a bibliography of classical, original and standard works in neurology*. Springfield, IL: C.C. Thomas.

McKendree, C.A., & Feinier, L. (1927). Somnolence: Its occurrence and significance in cerebral neoplasms. *A.M.A. Archives of Neurology and Psychiatry, 17*, 44–56.

McKissock, W. (1943). The technique of prefrontal leucotomy. *Journal of Mental Science, 89*, 194–198.

McKissock, W. (1951). Rostral leucotomy. *Lancet, ii*, 91–94.

McKissock, W., & Paine, K.W.E. (1958). Primary tumours of the thalamus. *Brain 81*, 41–63.

McLardy, T., & Davis, T.L. (1949). Clinical and pathological observations on relapse after successful leucotomy. *Journal of Neurology, Neurosurgery, and Psychiatry, 12*, 231–238.

McLardy, T., & Meyer, A. (1949). Anatomical correlates of improvement after leucotomy. *Journal of Mental Science, 95*, 182–196.

Meggendorfer, E. (1923). Die psychischen Störungen bei der Huntingtonschen Chorea, klinische und genealogische Untersuchungen. (Zugleich Mitteilung 11 neuer Huntingtonfamilien) [The psychic disturbances in Huntington's chorea, clinical and genealogical investigations]. *Zeitschrift für die gesamte Neurologie und Psychiatrie, 87*, 1–49.

Meggendorfer, E. g. (1928). Intoxikationspsychosen. Die exogenen Reaktionsformen und die organischen Psychosen [Psychoses after intoxication. The exogenic forms of reaction and the organic psychoses]. In O. Bumke (Ed.), *Handbuch der Geisteskrankheiten (Vol. 7, Pt. 3)* (pp. 151–400). Berlin: Springer.

Meinecke, G. (1951). Der organisatorische Ort. Über Prinzipien der biologischen Lokalisation [The locus of organization. On principles of biological localization]. *Archiv für Psychiatrie und Zeitschrift Neurologie, 186*, 516–526.

Meischner, W., & Eschler, E. (1979). *Wilhelm Wundt*. Leipzig: Urania-Verlag.

Mengech, H.N.K. arap (1983). Strangulation as a cause of Korsakoff psychosis. *East African Medical Journal 60*, 343–345.

Menninger, K. (1969). *Number words and number symbols. A cultural history of numbers*. Cambridge, MA: MIT Press.

Menninger-Lerchenthal, E. (1946). *Der eigene Doppelgänger* [One's own double]. Bern: Huber. (Supplement to the *Schweizer Zeitschrift für Psychologie, 11*, 1–96, 1946.)

Mesulam, M.-M. (1985). Patterns in behavioral neuroanatomy: association areas, the limbic system, and hemispheric specialization. In M.-M. Mesulam (Ed.), *Principles of behavioral neurology* (pp. 1–70). Philadelphia: F.A. Davis.

Mettler, F. (Ed.). (1949). *Selective partial ablation of the frontal cortex*. New York: Hoeber.

Meumann, E. (1912). *Ökonomie und Technik des Gedächtnisses* [Economy and technique of memory] (3rd ed). Leipzig: Julius Klinkhardt.

Meyer, A. (1904). The anatomical facts and clinical varieties of traumatic insanity. *American Journal of Insanity, 60*, 373–441.

Meyer, A., & Beck, E. (1954). *Prefrontal leucotomy and related operations: Anatomical aspects of success and failure*. Edinburgh: Oliver & Boyd.

Meyer, A., Beck, E., & McLardy, T. (1947). Prefrontal leucotomy: neuro-anatomical report. *Brain 70*, 18–49.

Meyer, A., & McLardy, T. (1948). Posterior cuts in prefrontal leucotomy: a clinico-pathological study. *Journal of Mental Science, 94*, 555–564.

Meyer, E. (1899). Sarcom des III. Ventrikels mit Metastasen im IV. Ventrikel [Sarcoma of the III. ventricle with metastates in the IV. ventricle]. *Archiv für Psychiatrie und Nervenkrankheiten, 32*, 320–329.

Meyer, E. (1904). Korsakowscher Symptomenkomplex nach Gehirnerschütterung [Korsakoff's symptom complex after cerebral concussion]. *Neurologisches Zentralblatt, 23*, 710–716.

Meyer, E. (1910). Psychische Störungen nach Strangulation [Psychic disturbances after strangulation]. *Medizinische Klinik, No. 38*, 1482–1486.

Meyer, E., & Raecke, J. (1903). Zur Lehre vom Korsakow'schen Symptomenkomplex [On the theory of the Korsakoff's symptom complex]. *Archiv für Psychiatrie und Nervenkrankheiten, 37*, 1–44.

Meyer, L. (1868). Aneurysmatische Entartung der Gehirnrinde nach übermässiger Anstrengung [Aneurysmic degeneration of the cerebral cortex after excessive exertion]. *Archiv für Psychiatrie und Nervenkrankheiten, 1*, 279–298.

Meynert, T. (1867). Das Gesammtgewicht und die Theilgewichte des Gehirns in ihren Beziehungen zum Geschlechte, dem Lebensalter und dem Irrsinn, untersucht nach einer neuen Wägungsmethode an den Gehirnen der in der Wiener Irrenanstalt im Jahre 1866 Verstorbenen [The total and the partial weights of the brain and their relations to gender, age and insanity, investigated with a new weighing method on the brains of those who died in the Vienna lunatic asylum in the year 1866]. *Vierteljahresschrift für Psychiatrie, Psychologie und gerichtliche Medicin*, 125–170.

Meynert, T. (1878). *Ueber Fortschritte im Verständnis der krankhaften psychischen Gehirnzustände* [On progress in understanding pathological psychic brain conditions]. Wien: Wilhelm Braumüller.

Meynert, T. (1884). *Psychiatrie. Klinik der Erkrankungen des Vorderhirns, begründet auf dessen Bau, Leistungen und Ernährung* [Psychiatry. Clinical description of diseases of the telencephalon, based on its construction, performance and nutrition]. Wien: Braumüller.

Michel, H. (1948). Erfahrungen über die Wirksamkeit der präfrontalen Leukotomie bei chronischen Schizophrenien [Experience on the efficiency of prefrontal leucotomy in chronic schizophrenia]. *Schweizer Archiv für Neurologie und Psychiatrie, 61*, 256–279.

Mickle, W.J. (1897). Atypical and unusual brainforms, especially in relation to mental status: A study on brain-surface morphology. *Journal of Mental Science (London)*, 798–803.

Mickle, W.J. (1898). Atypical and unusual brainforms, especially in relation to mental status: A study on brain-surface morphology. *Journal of Mental Science (London)*, 17–45.

Miller, L. (1985). Cognitive risk-taking after frontal or temporal lobectomy – I. The synthesis of fragmented visual information. *Neuropsychologia, 23*, 359–369.

Miller, L., & Milner, B. (1985). Cognitive risk-taking after frontal or temporal lobectomy – II. The synthesis of phonemic and semantic information. *Neuropsychologia, 23*, 371–379.

Mills, C.K., & Spiller, W.G. (1907). The symptomatology of lesions of the lenticular zone with some discussion of the pathology of aphasia. *Journal of Nervous and Mental Disease, 34*, 624–650.

Mills, C.K., & Weisenburg, T.H. (1906). The localization of the higher psychic functions, with special reference to the prefrontal lobe. *Journal of the American Medical Association, 46*, 337–341.

Milner, B. (1959). The memory defect in bilateral hippocampal lesions. *American Psychiatric Association. Psychiatric Research Reports, 11*, 43–58.

Milner, B. (1966). Amnesia following operation on the temporal lobes. In C.W.M. Whitty & O.L. Zangwill (Eds.), *Amnesia* (pp. 109–132). London: Butterworths.

Milner, B. (1970). Memory and the medial temporal regions of the brain. In K.H. Pribram & D.E. Broadbent (Eds.), *Biology of memory* (pp. 29–50). New York: Academic Press.

Minabe, Y., Kadono, Y., & Kurachi, M. (1990). A schizophrenic syndrome associated with a midbrain tegmental lesion. *Biological Psychiatry, 27*, 661–663.

Mingazzini, G. (1901). Klinische und pathologisch-anatomische Beiträge zur Diagnose und Therapie der Gehirngeschwülste [Clinical and pathologic-anatomical contributions to the diagnosis and therapy of brain tumors]. *Deutsche Zeitschrift für Nervenheilkunde, 19*, 1–62 (and 2 tables).

Mingazzini, G. (1922). *Der Balken. Eine anatomische, physiologische und klinische Studie* [The corpus callosum. An anatomical, physiological, and clinical study]. *(Monographien aus dem Gesamtgebiete der Neurologie und Psychiatrie, No. 28)*. Berlin: Springer.

Minski, L. (1936). Non-alcoholic polyneuritis with Korsakow syndrome. *Journal of Neurology and Psychopathology, 16*, 219–224.

Mishkin, M. (1978). Memory in monkeys severely impaired by combined, but not by separate removal of amygdala and hippocampus. *Nature, 273*, 297–298.

Mitchell-Heggs, N., Kelly, D. & Richardson, A. (1976). Stereotactic limbic leucotomy – A follow-up at 16 months. *British Journal of Psychiatry, 128*, 226–240.

Mixter, W.J., Tillotson, K.J., & Wies, D. (1941). Reports of partial frontal lobectomy and frontal lobotomy performed on three patients: One chronic epileptic and two cases of chronic agitated depression. *Psychosomatic Medicine, 3*, 26–37.

Möbius, P.J. (1900). *Ueber die Anlage zur Mathematik* [On the disposition for mathematics]. Leipzig: J.A. Barth.

Möbius, P.J. (1922). Über den physiologischen Schwachsinn des Weibes [On the physiological feeblemindedness of woman]. (12th ed.). Halle: Carl Marhold.

Moeli, C. (1883). Statistisches und Klinisches über Alcoholismus [Statistical and clinical facts on alcoholism]. *Königliches Charité-Krankenhaus (Berlin): Charité-Annalen, 9*, 524–548.

Moeli, C. (1891 a). Einige abnorme Schädel mit Demonstrationen [Some abnormal skulls with demonstrations]. *Allgemeine Zeitschrift für Psychiatrie, 47*, 411–412.

Moeli, C. (1891 b). Veränderungen des Tractus und Nervus opticus bei Erkrankungen des Occipitalhirns [Changes in the optic tract and nerve after diseases of the occipital lobe]. *Archiv für Psychiatrie und Nervenkrankheiten, 22*, 73–120 (and 2 tables).

Moll, J.M. (1915). "Amnestic" or "Korsakow's" syndrome with alcoholic etiology: An analysis of 30 cases. *Journal of Mental Science, 61*, 424–443.

Monakow, C. von (1881). Beitrag zur Lokalisation von Hirnrindentumoren [Contribution to the localization of cerebral cortical tumors]. *Archiv für Psychiatrie und Nervenkrankheiten, 11*, 613–635 (and 1 Table).

Monakow, C. von (1892). Experimentelle und pathologisch-anatomische Untersuchungen über die optischen Centren und Bahnen nebst klinischen Beiträgen zur corticalen Hemianopsie und Alexie [Experimental and pathological-anatomical investigations on the optic centers and fibers, with clinical contributions on cortical hemianopia and alexia]. *Archiv für Psychiatrie und Nervenkrankheiten, 23*, 669–671 (and 2 tables).

Monakow, C. von (1893). Experimentelle und pathologisch-anatomische Untersuchungen über die optischen Centren und Bahnen nebst klinischen Beiträgen zur corticalen Hemianopsie und Alexie [Experimental and pathological-anatomical investigations on the optic centers and fibers, with clinical contributions on cortical hemianopia and alexia]. *Archiv für Psychiatrie und Nervenkrankheiten, 24*, 229–268.

Monakow, C. von (1895). Experimentelle und pathologisch-anatomische Untersuchungen über die Haubenregion, den Sehhügel und die Regio subthalamica, nebst Beiträgen zur Kenntnis früh erworbener Gross- und Kleinhirndefekte [Experimental and pathological-anatomical investigations on the pontine tegmentum, the thalamus and the subthalamic region, with contributions on early acquired defects of the cerebrum and cerebellum]. *Archiv für Psychiatrie und Nervenkrankheiten, 27*, 1–128 and 386–479.

Monakow, C. von (1902). Ueber den gegenwärtigen Stand der Frage nach der Lokalisation im Grosshirn [On the current state of the question on the localization in the cerebrum]. *Ergebnisse der Physiologie, 1*, 534–665.

Monakow, C. von (1904). Ueber den gegenwärtigen Stand der Frage nach der Lokalisation im Grosshirn [On the current state of the question on the localization in the cerebrum]. *Ergebnisse der Physiologie, II. Abt.: Biophysik und Psychophysik*, 3–122.

Monakow, C. von (1909). Neue Gesichtspunkte in der Frage nach der Lokalisation im Grosshirn [New views on the question of localization in the cerebrum]. *Zeitschrift für Psychologie, 54*, 161–182.

Monakow, C. von (1910 a). Neue Gesichtspunkte in der Frage nach der Lokalisation im Grosshirn [New views on the question of localization in the cerebrum]. *Zeitschrift für Psychologie und Physiologie der Sinnesorgane. I. Abteilung: Zeitschrift für Psychologie, 54*, 161–182.

Monakow, C. von (1910 b). Über Lokalisation der Hirnfunktionen [On localization of brain functions]. Wiesbaden: Bergmann.

Monakow, C. von (1914). *Die Lokalisation im Grosshirn und der Abbau der Funktion durch kortikale Herde* [Localization in the cerebral cortex and the diminution of function by focal cortical damage]. Wiesbaden: Bergmann.

Moniz, E. (1936). *Tentatives opèratoires dans le traitement des certaines psychoses* [Tentative surgery for the treatment of certain psychoses]. Paris: Masson.

Moniz, E. (1937). Prefrontal leucotomy in the treatment of mental disorders. *American Journal of Psychiatry, 93*, 1379–1385.

Moniz, E. (1948) Mein Weg zur Leukotomie. *Deutsche medizinische Wochenschrift, 73*, 581–583.

Moniz, E. (1956). How I succeeded in performing the prefrontal leukotomy. In A.M. Sackler (Ed.), *The great psychodynamic therapies in psychiatry* (pp. 131–137). New York: Hoeber-Harper.

Moniz, E., & Lima, A. (1936). Premier essais de psychochirurgia technique et résultats [First essay on a psychosurgical technique and results]. *Lisboa Medica 38*, 725.

Mönkemöller, O., & Kaplan, L. (1899). Symptomatischer Korsakoff und Rückenmarkserkrankung bei Hirntumor [Symptomatic Korsakoff syndrome and spinal cord disease after brain tumor]. *Allgemeine Zeitschrift für Psychiatrie und ihre Grenzgebiete, 56*, 706–724.

Moore, B.E., Friedman, S., Simon, B., & Farmer, J. (1948). Connecticut lobotomy committee. A cooperative clinical study of lobotomy. In J.F. Fulton, W.C. Aring, & S.B. Wortis (Eds.), *The frontal lobes. (Research publications of the association for research in nervous and mental disease, Vol. 27)* (pp. 769–794). Baltimore: Williams & Wilkins.

Moore, M.T., & Lutz, W.M. (1951). Transorbital leucotomy in a state hospital program. *Journal of the American Medical Association, 146*, 324–330.

Moore, M.T., & Winkelmann, N.W. (1951). Some experiences with transorbital leucotomy. A review of results in 110 cases. *American Journal of Psychiatry, 107*, 801–87.

Moranska-Oscherovitsch, V. (1910). Über einen Fall von rein amnestischer Aphasie mit amnestischer Apraxie [On a case of pure amnesic aphasia with amnesic apraxia]. *Deutsche Zeitschrift für Nervenheilkunde, 40*, 37–55.

Mörchen, (n.n.g.) (1904). Epileptische Bewusstseinsveränderungen von ungewöhnlicher Dauer und forensischen Folgen [Epileptic changes of consciousness of unusual duration and forensic consequences]. *Monatsschrift für Psychiatrie und Neurologie, 17*, 15–28.

Morgagni, G.B. (1761/1967). *Sitz und Ursachen der Krankheiten aufgespürt durch die Kunst der Anatomie (Venedig 1761)* [Location and origins of diseases traced through the art of anatomy]. Bern: Huber.

Morgan, W.P. (1896). A case of congenital word blindness. *British Medical Journal, Nov. 7*, 1378.

Morsier, G. de (1929). Le syndrome prèfrontal de l'amnèsie de fixation [The prefrontal syndrome of fixation amnesia]. *Encephale, 24*, 19–49.

Morsier, G. de, & Rey, A. (1945). Le syndrome psychologique dans les tumeurs des lobes frontaux et dans les tumeurs du diencéphale [The psychological syndrome in frontal lobe tumors and in diencephalic tumors]. *Monatschrift für Psychiatrie und Neurologie, 110*, 293–308.

Mott, F.W., & Schaefer, E.A. (1890). On associated eye-movements produced by cortical faradization of the monkey brain. *Brain, 13*, 165–173.

Muhr, (n.n.g.) (1875). Anatomische Befunde bei einem Falle von Verrücktheit [Anatomical results in a case of madness]. *Archiv für Psychiatrie und Nervenkrankheiten, 6*, 733–754 (and tables IX and X).

Müller, C. (1960). Gottlieb Burckhardt, the father of topectomy. *American Journal of Psychiatry, 117*, 461–463.

Müller, E. (1902 a). Kritische Beiträge zur Frage nach den Beziehungen des Stirnhirns zur Psyche [Critical contributions on the question of the relations of the frontal lobe to the psyche]. *Allgemeine Zeitschrift für Psychiatrie und ihre Grenzgebiete, 57*, 830–875.

Müller, E. (1902 b). Ueber psychische Störungen bei Geschwülsten und Verletzungen des Stirnhirns [On psychic disturbances after tumors and injuries of the frontal lobe]. *Deutsche Zeitschrift für Nervenheilkunde, 21*, 177–208.

Müller, E. (1902 c). Zur Symptomatologie und Diagnostik der Geschwülste des Stirnhirns [On the symptomatology and diagnosis of tumors of the frontal lobe]. *Deutsche Zeitschrift für Nervenheilkunde, 22*, 375–427.

Müller, E. (1903). Zur Aetiologie und pathologischen Anatomie der Geschwülste des Stirnhirns [On the etiology and pathological anatomy of tumors of the frontal lobe]. *Deutsche Zeitschrift für Nervenheilkunde, 23*, 378–416.

Müller, E. (1904). Erwiderung auf die vorstehenden Bemerkungen von S. Auerbach [Reply to the preceding remarks of S. Auerbach]. *Deutsche Zeitschrift für Nervenheilkunde, 24*, 322–324.

Müller, F. (1892). Ein Beitrag zur Kenntniss der Seelenblindheit [A contribution to the knowledge of optic agnosia]. *Archiv für Psychiatrie und Nervenkrankheiten, 24*, 856–917.

Müller, G.E. (1911–1917). *Zur Analyse der Gedächtnistätigkeit und des Vorstellungsverlaufes* [On the analysis of memory performance and imagination] *(3 Vols.)*. Leipzig: Barth.

Müller, G.E., & Pilzecker, A. (1900). Experimentelle Beiträge zur Lehre vom Gedächtnis [Experimental contribution on the concept of memory]. *Zeitschrift für Psychologie, Ergänzungsband 1.*

Müller, G.E., & Schumann, F. (1894). Experimentelle Beiträge zur Untersuchung des Gedächtnisses [Experimental contribution on the concept of memory]. *Zeitschrift für Psychologie, 6*, 81–190 and 257–339.

Müller-Freienfels, R. (1915). Studien zur Lehre vom Gedächtnis [Studies on the concept of memory]. *Archiv für die gesamte Psychologie, 34*, 65–105.

Müller-Suur, H. (1949). Beitrag zur Frage des Korsakow-Syndroms und zur Analyse der amnestischstrukturellen Demenz [Contribution to the question of Korsakoff's syndrome and to the analysis of amnesic-structural dementia]. *Archiv für Psychiatrie und Nervenkrankheiten, 181*, 683–711.

Munk, H. (1877). Zur Physiologie der Grosshirnrinde [On the physiology of the cerebral cortex]. *Berliner klinische Wochenschrift, 14*, 505–506.

Munk, H. (1878). Weiteres zur Physiologie der Grosshirnrinde [Further remarks on the physiology of the cerebral cortex]. *Archiv für Anatomie und Physiologie, Physiologische Abteilung*, 547–563.

Munk, H. (1881). *Ueber die Functionen der Grosshirnrinde. Gesammelte Mittheilungen aus den Jahren 1877–80* [On the functions of the cerebral cortex. Collected contributions of the years 1877–80]. Berlin: Hirschwald.

Munk, H. (1882). Ueber die Stirnlappen des Grosshirns [On the frontal lobes of the cerebrum]. *Sitzungsberichte der königlich preussischen Akademie der Wissenschaften, 36*, 753–789.

Munk, H. (1890). *Ueber die Functionen der Grosshirnrinde* [On the functions of the cerebral cortex]. (2nd ed.). Berlin: Hirschwald.

Munk, H. (1894). Ueber den Hund ohne Grosshirn [On the dog without a cerebral cortex]. *Archiv für Anatomie und Physiologie, Physiologische Abteilung*, 355–369.

Münsterberg, H. (1900). *Grundzüge der Psychologie, Vol. 1. Die Prinzipien der Psychologie* [Fundamentals of psychology, Vol.1. Principles of psychology]. Leipzig: J.A. Barth.

Murawieff, W. (1897). Zwei Fälle von Polioencephalitis acuta haemorrhagica superior (Wernicke) [Two cases of Polioencephalitis acuta haemorrhagica superior (Wernicke)]. *Neurologisches Centralblatt, 16*, 2403–2405.

Näcke, P. (1893). Untersuchungen von 16 Frauenschädeln, darunter solche von 12 Verbrecherinnen (incl. einer Selbstmörderin) [Investigations on the skulls of 16 women, including 12 criminals (and one suicide)]. *Archiv für Psychiatrie und Nervenkrankheiten, 25*, 227–247.

Naef, M. (1897). Ein Fall von temporärer, totaler, theilweise retrograder Amnesie (durch Suggestion geheilt) [A case of temporary, total, partial retrograde amnesia (treated by suggestion)]. *Zeitschrift für Hypnotismus, 6*, 321–355.

Namba, M. (1958). Über die feineren Strukturen des medio-dorsalen Supranucleus und der Lamella medialis des Thalamus beim Menschen [On the more minute structures of the human mediodorsal supra-nucleus and the lamella medialis of the thalamus]. *Journal für Hirnforschung, 4*, 1–42.

Nathan, P.W., & Smith, M.C. (1950). Normal mental activity associated with maldeveloped "rhinencephalon". *Journal of Neurology, Neurosurgery, and Psychiatry, 13*, 191–197.

Netschajeff, A. (1900). Experimentelle Untersuchungen über die Gedächtnisentwicklung bei Schulkindern [Experimental investigations on the development of memory in school-age children]. *Zeitschrift für Psychologie, 24*, 321–351.

Netschajeff, A. (1902). *Über Memorieren. Eine Skizze aus dem Gebiete der experimentellen pädagogischen Psychologie* [On memorizing. A sketch from the area of experimental pedagogical psychology]. Berlin: Reuther & Reichard.

Neubürger, K. (1929). Demonstration von Hirnveränderungen bei Alkoholintoxikationen [Documentation of brain changes after alcoholic intoxication]. *Allgemeine Zeitschrift für Psychiatrie und ihre Grenzgebiete, 91*. (Cited after Kant, 1932, and after Neubürger, 1931.)

Neubürger, K. (1931). Über Hirnveränderungen nach Alkoholmissbrauch (unter Berücksichtigung einiger Fälle von Wernickescher Krankheit mit anderer Ätiologie) [On brain changes after alcohol abuse (including some cases with Wernicke's disease of different etiology)]. *Zeitschrift für die gesamte Neurologie und Psychiatrie, 135*, 159–209.

Neubürger, K. (1937). Wernickesche Krankheit bei chronischer Gastritis. Ein Beitrag zu den Beziehungen zwischen Magen und Gehirn [Wernicke disease in chronic gastritis. A contribution on the relations between stomach and brain]. *Zeitschrift für die gesamte Neurologie und Psychiatrie, 160*, 208–225.

Newcombe, R.L. (1973). Anatomical placement of lesions in the ventromedial segment of the frontal lobe. In L.V. Laitinen & K.E. Livingston (Eds.), *Surgical approaches in psychiatry* (pp. 83–89). Lancaster, UK: Medical and Technical Publ. Comp.

Nichols, I.C., & Hunt, J. McV. (1940). A case of partial bilateral frontal lobectomy. *American Journal of Psychiatry, 96*, 1063–1087.

Nickel, B. (1990). Das Korsakow-Konzept bei Karl Bonhoeffer und sein Bezug zur Psychometrie mnestischer Störungen [The Korsakoff-concept of Karl Bonhoeffer and its relation to the psychometrics of mental disturbances]. *Psychiatrie, Neurologie und medizinische Psychologie, 42*, 42–50.

Nicolai, G.F. (1908). Die physiologische Methodik zur Erforschung der Tierpsyche, ihre Möglichkeit und ihre Anwendung [The physiological methods for investigating the animal soul, their possibilities and their application]. *Journal für Psychologie und Neurologie, 10*, 1–27.

Niessl von Mayendorf, E. (1905). Zur Theorie des corticalen Sehens [On the theory of cortical vision]. *Archiv für Psychiatrie und Nervenkrankheiten, 39*, 1070–1105.

Niessl von Mayendorf, E. (1908). Casuistische Mittheilungen zu Pathologie des Stirnhirns [Casuistic contributions on the pathology of the frontal lobe]. *Archiv für Psychiatrie und Nervenkrankheiten, 43*, 1175–1192.

Niessl von Mayendorf, E. (1910). Ein Fall von motorischer Aphasie mit Intaktheit der linken dritten Stirnwindung [A case of motoric aphasia with intactness of the left third frontal gyrus]. *Deutsche Zeitschrift für Nervenheilkunde, 38*, 314–315.

Niessl von Mayendorf, E. (1922). Ueber die Wiederherstellbarkeit der Grosshirnfunktion [On recovery of cerebral cortical function]. *Münchener medizinische Wochenschrift, 69*, 1040–1041.

Niessl von Mayendorf, E. (1930). Aphasie und Balken [Aphasia and corpus callosum]. *Zentralblatt für die gesamte Neurologie und Psychiatrie, 56*, 142–143.

Nissl, F. (1904). Zur Histopathologie der paralytischen Rindenerkrankung [On the histopathology of the paralytic cortical disease]. *Histologische und histopathologische Arbeiten über die Grosshirnrinde mit besonderer Berücksichtigung der pathologischen Anatomie der Geisteskrankheiten, 1*, 315–494.

Nissl, F. (1919). Korbinian Brodmann. *Zeitschrift für die gesamte Neurologie und Psychiatrie, 45*, 338–349.

Nitta, M., & Symon, L. (1985). Colloid cysts of the third ventricle. A review of 36 cases. *Acta Neurochirurgica, 76*, 99–104.

Nothnagel, H. (1879). *Topische Diagnostik der Gehirnkrankheiten. Eine klinische Studie* [Topical diagnosis of brain diseases. A clinical study]. Berlin: Hirschwald.

Obersteiner, H. (1879). Experimental researches on attention. *Brain, 1*, 439–453.

Oeser, E., & Seitelberger, F. (1988). *Gehirn, Bewusstsein und Erkenntnis* [Brain, consciousness and epistomology]. Darmstadt: Wissenschaftliche Buchgesellschaft.

Offner, M. (1924). *Das Gedächtnis. Die Ergebnisse der experimentellen Psychologie und ihre Anwendungen in Unterricht und Erziehung* [Memory. The results of experimental psychology and their applications to teaching and education]. Berlin: Reuther & Reichard.

Ogden, R.M. (1903). Untersuchungen über den Einfluss der Geschwindigkeit des lauten Lesens auf das Erlernen und Behalten von sinnlosen und sinnvollen Stoffen [Investigations on the influence of the speed of reading aloud on learning and remembering meaningless and meaningful material]. *Archiv für die gesamte Psychologie, 2*, 93–189.

Ogden, R.M. (1904). Memory and the economy of learning. *Psychological Bulletin, 1*, 177–184.

Oltman, J.E., Brody, B.S., Friedman, S., & Green, W.J. (1949). Frontal lobotomy: Clinical experiences with 107 cases in a state hospital. *American Journal of Psychiatry, 105*, 742–751.

Omorokow, L. (1914). Zur pathologischen Anatomie der Dementia praecox [On the pathological anatomy of dementia praecox]. *Archiv für Psychiatrie und Nervenkrankheiten, 54*, 1031–1055 (and 2 tables).

Onufrowicz, W. (1887). Das balkenlose Mikrocephalengehirn Hofmann. Ein Beitrag zur pathologischen und normalen Anatomie des menschlichen Gehirnes [The acollosal microcephalic brain Hofmann. A contribution to the pathological and normal anatomy of the human brain]. *Archiv für Psychiatrie und Nervenkrankheiten, 18*, 305–328.

Oppenheim, H. (1890a). Zur Pathologie der Grosshirngeschwülste [On the pathology of cerebral tumors]. *Archiv für Psychiatrie und Nervenkrankheiten, 21*, 560–587.

Oppenheim, H. (1890b). Zur Pathologie der Grosshirngeschwülste [On the pathology of cerebral tumors]. *Archiv für Psychiatrie und Nervenkrankheiten, 21*, 705–745.

Oppenheim, H. (1891). Zur Pathologie der Grosshirngeschwülste [On the pathology of cerebral tumors]. *Archiv für Psychiatrie und Nervenkrankheiten, 22*, 27–72.

Oppenheim, H. (1902). *Die Geschwülste des Gehirns* [Tumors of the brain]. (2nd ed.). Wien: Hölder.

Oppenheim, H. (1907). *Beiträge zur Diagnostik und Therapie der Geschwülste im Bereich des zentralen Nervensystems* [Contributions to diagnosis and therapy of tumors in the region of the central nervous system]. Berlin: Karger.

Orr, D., & Rows, R.G. (1901). The nerve cells of the human posterior root ganglia and their changes in general paralysis of the insane. *Brain 24*, 286–309.

Oscar-Berman, M. (1988). Links between clinical and experimental neuropsychology. *Journal of Clinical and Experimental Neuropsychology, 11*, 571–588.

Otuszewski, W. (1898). Von der Bedeutung der Associationscentren von Flechsig zur Erforschung der Entwickelung des Geistes, der Sprache, der Psychologie der Sprache, wie auch der Lehre von der Sprachlosigkeit [On the role of Flechsig's association centers for the investigation of the development of the mind, the psychology of language, as well as of speechlessness]. *Neurologisches Centralblatt, 17*, 163–170 and 203–211.

Owen, R. (1868). *On the anatomy of vertebrates (Vol. III. Mammals)*. London: Longmans, Green & Co.

Pakkenberg, B. (1989). What happens in the leucotomised brain? A postmortem morphological study of brains from schizophrenic patients. *Journal of Neurology, Neurosurgery, and Psychiatry, 52*, 156–161.

Pakkenberg, B. (1990). Pronounced reduction of total neuron number in mediodorsal thalamic nucleus and nucleus accumbens in schizophrenics. *Archives of General Psychiatry, 47*, 1023–1028.

Papez, J.W. (1937). A proposed mechanism of emotion. *A.M.A. Archives of Neurology and Psychiatry, 38*, 725–743.

Pappenheim, M. (1907). Über die Kombination allgemeiner Gedächtnisschwäche und amnestischer Aphasie nach leichtem zerebralem Insult [On the combination of general memory weakness and amnesic aphasia after a minor cerebral insult]. *Journal für Psychologie und Neurologie, 9*, 201–214.

Pappenheim, M. (1908 a). Über die Kombination allgemeiner Gedächtnisschwäche und amnestischer Aphasie nach leichtem zerebralen Insult [On the combination of general memory weakness and amnesic aphasia after a minor cerebral insult]. *Journal für Psychologie und Neurologie, 10*, 55–82.

Pappenheim, M. (1908 b). Merkfähigkeit und Assoziationsversuch [Ability to memorize and an association experiment]. *Zeitschrift für Psychologie, 46*, 161–173.

Parkin, A.J., Blunden, J., Rees, J.E., & Hunkin, N.M. (1991). Wernicke-Korsakoff syndrome of nonalcoholic origin. *Brain and Cognition, 15*, 69–82.

Parkinson, J. (1817). *An essay on the shaking palsy*. London: Nelly and Jones.

Partridge, M. (1949). *Pre-frontal leucotomy. A survey of 300 cases personally followed over $1^1/_2$ – 3 years*. Oxford: Blackwell.

Parwatikar, S. (1990). Medicolegal aspects of transient global amnesia. In H.J. Markowitsch (Ed.), *Transient global amnesia and related disorders* (pp. 191–205). Toronto: Hogrefe & Huber Publs.

Passingham, R.E. (1981). Broca's area and the origin of human vocal skill. *Philosophical Transactions of the Royal Society, B 292*, 167–175.

Passingham, R.E. (1982). *The human primate*. Oxford: W.H. Freeman and Comp.

Patten, B.M. (1972). The ancient art of memory: usefulness in treatment. *Archives of Neurology, 26*, 25–31.

Patten, B.M. (1990). The history of memory arts. *Neurology, 40*, 346–352.

Paul, M. (1899). Beiträge zur Frage der retrograden Amnesie [Contributions to the question of retrograde amnesia]. *Archiv für Psychiatrie und Nervenkrankheiten, 32*, 251–282.

Paul, N.L., Fitzgerald, E., & Greenblatt, M. (1956). Five-year follow up of patients subjects to three different lobotomy procedures. *Journal of the American Medical Association, 161*, 815–819.

Pawlow, I.P. (1953). *Sämtliche Werke* [Complete works]. Berlin: Akademie-Verlag.

Pearce, J.M.S. (1982). The first attempts at removal of brain tumors. In F.C. Rose & W.F. Bynum (Eds.), *Historical aspects of the neurosciences* (pp. 239–242). New York: Raven Press.

Pearlson, G.D., Kim, W.S., Kubos, K.L., Moberg, P.J., Jayaram, G., Bascom, M.J., Chase, G.A., Goldfinger, A.D., & Tune, L.E. (1989). Ventricle-brain ratio, computed tomographic density, and brain area in 50 schizophrenics. *Archives of General Psychiatry, 46*, 690–697.

Penfield, W., & Evans, J. (1935). The frontal lobe in man: A clinical study of maximum removals. *Brain, 38*, 115–133.

Peraita, P., & Lerma, J.L. de (1977). Frontal psychosurgery: A review of 424 cases. In W.H. Sweet, S. Obrador, & J.G. Martín-Rodríguez (Eds.), *Neurosurgical treatment in psychiatry, pain and epilepsy* (pp. 211–216). Baltimore: University Park Press.

Perecman, E. (Ed.). (1987). *The frontal lobes revisited*. New York: IRBN Press.

Peritz, G. (1918). Zur Psychopathologie des Rechnens [On the psychopathology of calculating]. *Deutsche Zeitschrift für Nervenheilkunde, 61*, 234–340.

Perry, R.B. (1904). Conceptions and misconceptions of consciousness. *Psychological Review, 11*, 282–296.

Pestronk, A. (1989). The first neurology book written in English (1650) by Robert Pemell. *Archives of Neurology, 46*, 215–220.

Peters, F. (1912). Untersuchungen der Gedächtnisstörungen paralytisch Geisteskranker mit der „Zahlenmethode“ [Investigations of memory disturbances in paralytic mental patients with the "method of figures“]. *Zeitschrift für die gesamte Neurologie und Psychiatrie, 11*, 173–217.

Petrie, A. (1949). Preliminary report of changes after prefrontal leucotomy. *Journal of Mental Science, 95*, 449–455.

Petrie, A. (1950). Personality changes after pre-frontal leucotomy. *British Journal of Medical Psychology, 22*, 200–207.

Petrie, A. (1952). A comparison of the psychological effects of different types of operations on the frontal lobes. *Journal of Mental Science, 98*, 326–329.

Petrina, T. (1912). Ein Sarkom des linken Stirnlappens. Kasuistischer Beitrag zur Pathologie des Stirnhirns [A sarcoma of the left frontal lobe. Casuistic contribution to the pathology of the frontal lobe]. *Prager medizinische Wochenschrift, 37*, 217–220.

Pfänder, A. (1904). *Einführung in die Psychologie* [Introduction to psychology]. Leipzig: J.A. Barth.

Pfeifer, B. (1910). Psychische Störungen bei Hirntumoren [Psychic disturbances after brain tumors]. *Archiv für Psychiatrie und Nervenkrankheiten, 47*, 558–738.

Pfeifer, B. (1922). Die Bedeutung psychologischer Leistungs- und Arbeitsprüfungen für die Topik der Grosshirnrinde [On the role of psychological tests of performance and work for the topical arrangement of the cerebral cortex]. *Zeitschrift für die gesamte Neurologie und Psychiatrie, 30*, 139–142.

Pfeifer, B. (1928). Zur Symptomatologie der progressiven Paralyse (Korsakowsche Psychose und delirante Zustände) [On the symptomatology of progressive paralysis (Korsakoff's psychosis and delirious states]. *Journal für Psychologie und Neurologie, 37*, 274–281.

Pfuhl, W. (1954). Anatomische Stellungnahme zum Problem der präfrontalen Leukotomie [Anatomical opinion on the problem of prefrontal leucotomy]. *Nervenarzt, 25*, 20–25.

Phelps, C. (1894). The differential diagnosis of traumatic intracranial lesions. *New York Medical Journal, 60*, 577–582, 710–716, 741–745, 779–785, and 807–815.

Phelps, C. (1902). Cases illustrative of the localization of the mental faculties in the left prefrontal lobe. *American Journal of the Medical Sciences, 123*, 563–594 and 751–771.

Phelps, C. (1906). The function of the left prefrontal lobe. *American Journal of the Medical Sciences, 131*, 457–480.

Piazza, A. (1909). Ein Fall von Hirntumor [A case of brain tumor]. *Berliner klinische Wochenschrift, 46*, 1599–1604.

Pichot, P. (1983). *Ein Jahrhundert Psychiatrie* [A century of psychiatry]. Basel: Roche.

Pick, A. (1876). Zur Casuistik der Erinnerungstäuschungen [On the casuistry of illusions of remembrance]. *Archiv für Psychiatrie und Nervenkrankheiten, 6*, 568–574.

Pick, A. (1878). Beiträge zur normalen und pathologischen Anatomie des Centralnervensystems [Contributions on the normal and pathological anatomy of the central nervous system]. *Archiv für Psychiatrie und Nervenkrankheiten, 8*, 283–309.

Pick, A. (1886). Zur Pathologie des Gedächtnisses [On the pathology of memory]. *Archiv für Psychiatrie und Nervenkrankheiten, 17*, 83–98.

Pick, A. (1892). Ueber die Beziehungen der senilen Hirnatrophie zur Aphasie [On the relations of senile brain atrophy and aphasia]. *Prager medicinische Wochenschrift, 17*, 165–167.

Pick, A. (1893). Ueber allgemeine Gedächtnisschwäche als Folge cerebraler Herderkrankung, mit einem Beitrage zur Lehre von der topischen Diagnostik der Sehhügel-Läsionen [On general memory weakness as a consequence of focal cerebral disease, with a contribution on the topical diagnosis of optic thalamus lesions]. *Prager medicinische Wochenschrift, 18*, 451–452 and 465–466.

Pick, A. (1901). Senile Hirnatrophie als Grundlage von Herderscheinungen [Senile brain atrophy as basis of focal phenomena]. *Wiener klinische Wochenschrift, 14*, 403–404.

Pick, A. (1903 a). Fortgesetzte Beiträge zur Pathologie der sensorischen Aphasie [Consecutive contributions on the pathology of sensory aphasia]. *Archiv für Psychiatrie und Nervenkrankheiten, 37*, 468–487.

Pick, A. (1903 b). Zur Pathologie des Bekanntheitsgefühls (Bekanntheitsqualität) [On the pathology of the feeling of knowing (quality of familiarity)]. *Neurologisches Zentralblatt, 22*, 2–7.

Pick, A. (1905 a). Zur Analyse der Elemente der Amusie und deren Vorkommen im Rahmen aphasischer Störungen [On the analyis of the elements of amusia and their occurrence in the framework of aphasic disturbances]. *Monatsschrift für Psychiatrie und Neurologie, 18*, 87–96.

Pick, A. (1905 b). Zur Psychologie des Vergessens bei Geistes- und Nervenkranken [The psychology of forgetting in psychiatric and neurological patients]. *Archiv für kriminologische Anthropologie, 18*, 251–261.

Pick, A. (1906). Ueber einen weiteren Symptomenkomplex im Rahmen der Dementia senilis, bedingt durch umschriebene stärkere Hirnatrophie (gemischte Apraxie) [On a further symptom complex within the framework of senile dementia, caused by circumscribed major brain atrophy (mixed apraxia)]. *Monatsschrift für Psychiatrie und Neurologie, 19*, 97–108.

Pick, A. (1915). Beitrag zur Pathologie des Denkverlaufes beim Korsakow [Contribution on the pathology of the course of thought in Korsakoff's syndrome]. *Zeitschrift für die gesamte Neurologie und Psychiatrie, 28*, 344–383.

Pick, A. (1921). Die Palilalie, ein Teilstück striärer Motilitätsstörungen [The palilaly, a part of striatal disturbances of motility]. *Neurologische Forschungsrichtungen in der Psychopathologie und andere Aufsätze. Abhandlungen aus der Neurologie und Psychiatrie (Berlin), Heft 13*, 178- 224.

Pilleri, G. (1960). Studien über die thalamo-kortikalen Verbindungen des Menschen: Histologische Analyse von Fällen mit orbitalen Rindenläsionen [Studies on thalamo-cortical connections in humans: Histological analysis of cases with orbital cerebral lesions]. *Psychiatrica et Neurologica, 140*, 369–381.

Pintner, R. (1915). The standardization of Knox's cube test. *Psychological Review, 22*, 377–401.

Pippard, J. (1955). Rostral leucotomy: a report on 240 cases personally followed up after 1 1/2 to 5 years. *Journal of Mental Science, 101*, 756–773.

Pitt, G.N. (1898). The accurate localisation of intracranial tumours, excluding tumours of the motor cortex, motor tract, pons and medulla. *Brain, 21*, 329–332.

Poeck, K., Pilleri, G., & Risso, M. (1962). *Katamnestische Untersuchungen nach frontaler Leukotomie (Teil II: Anatomisch-klinische Korrelationen* [Catamnestic investigations after frontal leucotomy (Part II: Anatomical-clinical correlations)] (pp. 77–111). Basel: Karger.

Poltyrew, S., & Zeliony, G. (1930). Grosshirnrinde und Assoziationsfunktion [Cerebral cortex and associative functions]. *Zeitschrift für Biologie, 90*, 157–160.

Ponitus, A.A., & Ruttiger, K. (1976). Frontal lobe system maturational lag in juvenile deliquents shown in narratives test. *Adolescence, 11*, 509–518.

Ponitus, A.A., & Yudowitz, B.S. (1980). Frontal lobe system dysfunction in some criminal actions as shown in the narratives test. *The Journal of Nervous and Mental Disease, 168*, 111–117.

Pool, J.L. (1949). Topectomy. The treatment of mental illness by frontal gyrectomy or bilateral subtotal ablation of frontal cortex. *Lancet, 2*, 776–781.

Pool, J.L. (1951). Topectomy, 1946–1951 – Report on 106 consecutive non-project topectomy operations. *Transactions and Studies of the College of Physicians of Philadelphia, 19*, 49–67.

Popoff, L. (1875). Ueber Veränderungen im Gehirn bei Abdominaltyphus und traumatischer Entzündung [On changes in the brain with abdominal typhoid fever and traumatic infections]. *Virchow's Archiv, 63*, 421–446.

Poppelreuter, W. (1912). Nachweis der Unzweckmässigkeit die gebräuchlichen Assoziationsexperimente mit sinnlosen Silben nach dem Erkennungs- und Trefferverfahren zur exakten Gewinnung elementarer Reproduktionsgesetze zu verwenden [Proof of the inexpediency of using the common association experiments with nonsense syllables made with recognition and hit procedures for an exact acquisition of elementary laws of reproduction] . *Zeitschrift für Psychologie, 61*, 1–24.

Poppelreuter, W. (1915). Ueber psychische Ausfallerscheinungen nach Hirnverletzungen [On psychic deficits after brain damage]. *Münchener medicinische Wochenschrift, 62*, 489–491.

Poppelreuter, W. (1917). *Die psychischen Schädigungen durch Kopfschuss im Kriege 1914/16 (Band I)* [Psychic disturbances caused by head shots in the War of 1914/16 (Vol. I)]. Leipzig: Voss.

Poppelreuter, W. (1918). *Die psychischen Schädigungen durch Kopfschuss im Kriege 1914/17. Band II. Die Herabsetzung der körperlichen Leistungsfähigkeit und des Arbeitswillens durch Hirnverletzungen im Vergleich zu Normalen und Psychogenen* [Psychic disturbances caused by head shots in the War of 1914/17. Vol. II: The deterioration of somatic performance and will to work after brain injuries in comparison to normals and psychogenic patients]. Leipzig: Voss.

Porter, J.P. (1904). A preliminary study of the psychology of the English sparrow. *American Journal of Psychology, 15*, 313–346.

Porter, J.P. (1906 a). Further studies of the psychology of the English sparrow. *American Journal of Psychology, 17*, 248–271.

Porter, J.P. (1906 b). The habits, instincts, and mental powers of spiders, genera, argiope and epeira. *American Journal of Psychology, 17*, 306–357.

Porteus, S.D. (1952). A survey of recent results obtained with the Porteus maze test. *British Journal of Medical Psychology, 23*, 180–188.

Porteus, S.D., & Kepner, R. de M. (1942). Mental changes after bi-lateral pre-frontal lobotomy. *American Journal of Psychiatry, 99*, 426–430.

Porteus, S.D., & Kepner, R. de M. (1944). Mental changes after bilateral prefrontal lobotomy. *Genetic Psychology Monographs 29*, 1–115.

Porteus, S.D., & Peters, H.N. (1947). Psychosurgery and test validity. *Journal of Abnormal and Social Psychology, 42x , 473–475.*

Potwin, E.B. (1901). Study of early memories. *Psychological Review, 8*, 596–601.

Pötzl, O. (1938). Zwischenhirn und periodisches Irresein [Diencephalon and periodic insanity]. *Wiener klinische Wochenschrift, 51*, 845–849.

Pötzl, O. (1939). Physiologisches und Pathologisches über das persönliche Tempo [Physiologic and pathologic findings on the personal tempo]. *Wiener klinische Wochenschrift, 52*, 569–573.

Pötzl, O. (1942). Alterserkrankungen im Gehirn [Age-related diseases in the brain]. *Wiener klinische Wochenschrift, 55*, 3–8.

Pötzl, O. (1951). Weiteres über das Zeitraffer-Erlebnis [More on the experience of speeded-up motion]. *Wiener Zeitschrift für Nervenheilkunde, 4*, 9–39.

Pötzl, O. (1958). Zur Hirnphysiologie des Zeiterlebens [On the brain physiology of the experience of time]. *Wiener Zeitschrift für Nervenheilkunde, 15*, 370–393.

Prager, J.J. (1912). Experimenteller Beitrag zur Psychopathologie der Merkfähigkeitsstörungen [Experimental contribution to the psychopathology of disturbances of memorizing]. *Journal für Psychologie und Neurologie, 18*, 1–22.

Prawdicz-Neminski, W.W. (1925). Zur Kenntnis der elektrischen und der Innervationsvorgänge in den funktionellen Elementen und Geweben des tierischen Organismus. Electrocerebrogramm der Säugetiere [On the knowledge of electrical and innervation processes in the functional elements and tissue of the animal organism. Electrocerebrogram of mammals]. *Pflüger's Archiv für die gesamte Physiologie, 209*, 362–382.

Preyer, W. (1882). *Die Seele des Kindes. Beobachtungen über die geistige Entwickelung des Menschen in den ersten Lebensjahren* [The soul of the child. Observations on human mental development during the first years of life]. Leipzig: Th. Grieben.

Price, D.L. (1986). New perspectives in Alzheimer's disease. *Annual Review of Neuroscience, 9*, 489–512.

Prince, M. (1906 a). *The dissociation of a personality*. London: Longmans, Green & Co.

Prince, M. (1906 b). Hysteria from the point of view of dissociated personality. *Journal of Abnormal Psychology, 1*, 170–187.

Prince, M. (1908 a). Experiments to determine co-conscious (subconscious) ideation. *Journal of Abnormal Psychology, 3*, 33–42.

Prince, M. (1908 b). My life as a dissociated personality. *Journal of Abnormal Psychology, 3*, 240–260 and 311–334.

Prince, M. (1910). Cerebral localisation from the point of view of function and symptoms. *Journal of Nervous and Mental Disease, 37*, 337–354.

Prince, M. (1924). *The unconscious*. (2nd ed.). New York: Macmillan.

Prince, M. (1929). Miss Beauchamp: The theory of the psychogenesis of multiple personality. *Journal of Abnormal Psychology, 15*, 65–135.

Probst, M. (1901 a). Ueber das Gehirn der Taubstummen [On the brain of deaf-mutes]. *Archiv für Psychiatrie und Nervenkrankheiten, 34*, 584–590.

Probst, M. (1901 b). Ueber den Bau des vollständig balkenlosen Grosshirnes sowie über Mikrogyrie und Heterotopie der grauen Substanz [On the construction of the completely acallosal cerebrum, as well as on microgyry and heterotopy of the gray matter]. *Archiv für Psychiatrie und Nervenkrankheiten, 34*, 709–786 (and 6 tables).

Probst, M. (1903). Ueber durch eigenartigen Rindenschwund bedingten Blödsinn [On idiocy caused by a peculiar loss of the cerebral cortex]. *Archiv für Psychiatrie und Nervenkrankheiten, 36*, 762–792 (and 2 tables).

Pussep, L.M. (1900). Ueber den Einfluss der Unterbindung und der Compression der Abdominalaorta auf das Rückenmark [On the influence of ligating or compressing of the abdominal aorta on the spinal cord]. *Neurologisches Zentralblatt, 19*, 991.

Puusepp, L. (1914). *Etat actuel et problèmes prochains sur la question du traitement des maladies mentales* [Actual state and coming problems on the question of the treatment of mental diseases]. Congrès International, Moscou.

Puusepp, L. (1937). Alcune considerazioni sugli interventi chirurgici nelle malattie mentali [Some considerations on surgical interventions in mental diseases]. *Giornale della accademia di medicina di Torino, 100*, 3–16.

Rabagliati, A. (1878). Luciani and Tamburini on the functions of the brain. *Brain 1*, 529–544.

Rabagliati, A. (1879). Luciani and Tamburini on the functions of the brain. The psycho-sensory cortical centres. *Brain, 2*, 234–250.

Rabinowitsch, A. (1925). Ein Fall von Hirntumor unter dem Bilde einer epidemischen Encephalitis [A case of brain tumor appearing as epidemical encephalitis]. *Deutsche Zeitschrift für Nervenheilkunde, 88*, 67–74.

Rademaker, G.G. & Winkler, C. (1928). Physiology. – Annotations on the physiology and the anatomy of a dog, living 38 days, without both hemispheres of the cerebrum and without cerebellum. *Proceedings of the Royal Academy of Sciences (Amsterdam), 31*, 332–338.

Raecke, J. (1903). *Die transitorischen Bewusstseinsstörungen der Epileptiker* [The transitory disturbances of consciousness of epileptics]. Halle: Carl Marhold.

Raecke, J. (1906). Psychische Störungen bei der multiplen Sklerose [Psychic disturbances in multiple sclerosis]. *Archiv für Psychiatrie und Nervenkrankheiten, 41*, 482–518.

Raecke, J. (1908). Ueber epileptische Wanderzustände (Fugues, Poriomanie) [On epileptic states of wandering (fugues, poriomania)]. *Archiv für Psychiatrie und Nervenkrankheiten, 43*, 398–423.

Raimann, E. (1900). Polioencephalitis superior acuta und Delirium alkoholicum als Einleitung einer Korsakow'schen Psychose ohne Polyneuritis [Polioencephalitis superior acuta and alcoholic delirium initiating Korsakoff's psychosis without polyneuritis]. *Wiener klinische Wochenschrift, 13*, 31–37.

Raimann, E. (1901). Beiträge zur Lehre von den alkoholischen Augenmuskellähmungen [Contributions on alcoholic paralysis of the eye muscles]. *Jahrbücher für Psychiatrie, 20*, 36–76.

Raimann, E. (1902). Ein Fall von Cerebropathia psychica toxaemica (Korsakoff), gastro-intestinalen Ursprunges [A case of cerebropathia psychica toxaemica (Korsakoff) of gastro-intestinal origin]. *Monatsschrift für Psychiatie und Neurologie, 12*, 329–339.

Ranschburg, P. (1901 a). Apparat und Methode zur Untersuchung des (optischen) Gedächtnisses für medicinisch- und pädagogisch-psychologische Zwecke [Apparatus and method for the investigation of (optic) memory for medical and pedagogical-psychological purposes]. *Monatsschrift für Psychiatrie und Neurologie, 10*, 321–333.

Ranschburg, P. (1901 b). Studien über die Merkfähigkeit der Normalen, Nervenschwachen und Geisteskranken [Studies on the ability to memorize in normals, neurasthenics, and mental patients]. *Monatsschrift für Psychiatrie und Neurologie, 9*, 241–259.

Ranschburg, P. (1905). Über die Bedeutung der Ähnlichkeit beim Erlernen, Behalten und bei der Reproduktion [On the importance of similarity for learning, memory and reproduction]. *Journal für Psychologie und Neurologie, 5*, 94–127.

Ranschburg, P. (1911). *Das kranke Gedächtnis. Ergebnisse und Methoden der experimentellen Erforschung der alltäglichen Falschleistungen und der Pathologie des Gedächtnisses* [The diseased memory. Results and methods of experimental research on common misperformance and the pathology of memory]. Leipzig: Barth.

Ranschburg, P. (1930). Experimentelle Beiträge zur Lehre von Gedächtnis, Urteil und Schlussfolgerung an Gesunden und Kranken [Experimental contributions to the study of memory and reasoning in healthy and ill subjects]. *Archiv für die gesamte Psychologie, 77*, 437–526.

Ransohoff, (n.n.g.) (1897). Ueber Erinnerungstäuschungen bei Alkoholparalyse [On delusions of remembrance in alcoholic paralysis]. *Allgemeine Zeitschrift für Psychiatrie, 53*, 933–943.

Ratig, H. (1923). Erfahrungen über die Bedeutung von Fremdkörpern im Gehirn [Experiences on the role of foreign bodies in the brain]. *Zeitschrift für die gesamte Neurologie und Psychiatrie, 85*, 98–119.

Raue, G. (1850). *Die neue Seelenlehre Dr. Beneke's nach methodischen Grundsätzen in einfach entwickelnder Weise für Lehrer bearbeitet* [The new theory of the soul of Dr. Beneke, processed for teachers after methodical principles in a simple developing method]. (2nd ed.). Bautzen: Weller.

Ray, W.S. (1937). The relationship of retroactive inhibition, retrograde amnesia and the loss of recent memory. *Psychological Review, 44*, 339–345.

Read, C.F. (1923). Hysterical amnesia following physical injury. A case study. *Journal of Nervous and Mental Disease, 58*, 513–524.

Redlich, E. (1898). Ueber miliare Sklerose der Hirnrinde bei seniler Atrophie [On miliary sclerosis of the cerebral cortex in senile atrophy]. *Jahrbücher für Psychiatrie, 17*, 208–216.

Rehmke, J. (1891). Die Seelenfrage [The question of the soul]. *Zeitschrift für Psychologie und Physiologie der Sinnesorgane, 2*, 180–218.

Reihnert, R. (1950). Leukotomie bei schwerer Psychopathie [Leucotomy in severe psychopathy]. *Archiv für Psychiatrie und Zeitschrift Neurologie, 184*, 385–392.

Reinhard, C. (1886). Zur Frage der Hirnlocalisation mit besonderer Berücksichtigung der cerebralen Sehstörungen [On the question of brain localization with special consideration of cerebral visual disturbances]. *Archiv für Psychiatrie und Nervenkrankheiten, 17*, 717–756.

Reinhard, C. (1887 a). Zur Frage der Hirnlocalisation mit besonderer Berücksichtigung der cerebralen Sehstörungen [On the question of brain localization with special consideration of cerebral visual disturbances]. *Archiv für Psychiatrie und Nervenkrankheiten, 18*, 240–258.

Reinhard, C. (1887 b). Zur Frage der Hirnlocalisation mit besonderer Berücksichtigung der cerebralen Sehstörungen [On the question of brain localization with special consideration of cerebral visual disturbances]. *Archiv für Psychiatrie und Nervenkrankheiten, 18*, 449–486.

Reitman, F. (1946). Orbital cortex syndrome following leucotomy. *American Journal of Psychiatry, 103*, 238–241.

Reitman, F. (1947). Observations on personality changes after leucotomy. *Journal of Nervous and Mental Disease, 105*, 582–589.

Reitman, F. (1948). Evaluation of leucotomy results. *American Journal of Psychiatry, 105*, 86–89.

Remy, M. (1942). Contribution à l'étude de la maladie de Korsakow. *Monatsschrift für Psychiatrie und Neurologie, 106*, 128–144.

Retzius, G. (1898). Das Gehirn des Astronomen Hugo Gyldens (The brain of the astronomer Hugo Gyldens]. *Biologische Untersuchungen (Neue Folge), 8*, 1–22 (and 6 tables).

Retzius, G. (1900 a). Das Gehirn des Mathematikers Sonja Kowalewski [The brain of the mathematician Sonja Kowalewski]. *Biologische Untersuchungen (Neue Folge), 9*, 1–16 (and 4 tables).

Retzius, G. (1900 b). Vier Mikrocephalen-Gehirne [Four microcephalic brains]. *Biologische Untersuchungen (Neue Folge), 9*, 17–44 (and 5 tables).

Retzius, G. (1902). Das Gehirn des Physikers und Pädagogen Per Adam Siljeström [The brain of the physicist and educationalist Per Adam Siljeström]. *Biologische Untersuchungen (Neue Folge), 10*, 1–14 (and 3 tables).

Retzius, G. (1904). Das Gehirn eines Staatsmannes [The brain of a statesman]. *Biologische Untersuchungen (Neue Folge), 11*, 89–102 (and 5 tables).

Retzius, G. (1905). Das Gehirn des Histologen und Physiologen Christian Loven [The brain of the historian and physiologist Christian Loven]. *Biologische Untersuchungen (Neue Folge), 12*, 33–49 (and 4 tables).

Reuther, F. (1905). Beiträge zur Gedächtnisforschung [Contributions on memory research]. *Psychologische Studien, 1*, 4–101.

Reynolds, E.H. (1988). Hughlings Jackson. A Yorkshireman's contribution to epilepsy. *Archives of Neurology, 45*, 675–678.

Reynolds, G.P., Czudek, C., & Andrews, H.B. (1990). Deficit and hemispheric asymmetry of GABA uptake sites in the hippocampus in schizophrenia. *Biological Psychiatry, 27*, 1038–1044.

Ribot, T. (1882). *Diseases of memory*. New York: D. Appleton and Co. [French original: Ribot, T. (1881). *Les maladies de la mémoire* [The disturbances of memory]. Paris; German translation, cited after Kalberlah (1904): Ribot, T. (1882). *Das Gedächtnis und seine Störungen*. Hamburg, Leipzig].

Richter, H. (1918). Eine besondere Art von Stirnhirnschwund mit Verblödung [A peculiar kind of frontal lobe atrophy with idiocy]. *Archiv für Psychiatrie und Nervenkrankheiten, 38*, 127–160 (and 3 tables).

Riddoch, G. (1936). Progressive dementia, without headache or changes in the optic discs, due to tumours of the third ventricle. *Brain 59*, 225–233.

Ridewood, H.E., & Jones, R. (1903). A case of cerebral tumour complicated with alcoholic confusional insanity. *Journal of Mental Science, 49*, 511–516.

Riechert,lT. (1950). Klinisches zur Leukotomie [Clinical arguments on leucotomy]. *Archiv für Psychiatrie und Nervenkrankheiten, 184*, 282–284.

Rieger, C. (1889). Beschreibung der Intelligenzstörungen in Folge einer Hirnverletzung; nebst einem Entwurf zu einer allgemein anwendbaren Methode der Intelligenzprüfung [Description of disturbances of intelligence after brain damage; with a sketch of a generally applicable method of testing intelligence]. *Verhandlungen der Physikalisch-Medizinischen Gesellschaft zu Würzburg (Neue Folge), 22*, 1–70.

Rieger, C. (1890). Beschreibung der Intelligenzstörungen in Folge einer Hirnverletzung; nebst einem Entwurf zu einer allgemein anwendbaren Intelligenzprüfung [Description of disturbances of intelligence after brain damage; with a sketch of a generally applicable method of testing intelligence]. *Verhandlungen der Physikalisch-medicinischen Gesellschaft zu Würzburg (Neue Folge), 23*, 1–56.

Riggs, H.E., & Boles, R.S. (1944). Wernicke's disease. A clinical and pathological study of 42 cases. *Quarterly Journal of Studies on Alcohol, 5*, 361–370.

Ringo, J.L. & Guttmacher, L.B. (1988). Amnesia for the McCullough effect following unilateral electroconvulsive therapy: Implications for laterality. *Biological Psychiatry, 24*, 384–390.

Rinkel, M., Greenblatt, M., Coon, G.P., & Solomon, H.C. (1947). The effect of bilateral frontal lobotomy upon the autonomic nervous system. *American Journal of Psychiatry, 104*, 81–82.

Risso, M., Poeck, K., & Creutzfeldt, O. (1962). *Katamnestische Untersuchungen nach frontaler Leukotomie (Teil I: Klinische Beobachtungen* [Catamnestic investigations after prefrontal leucotomy (Part I: Clinical observations)] (pp. 1–76). Basel: Karger.

Rittershain, G. Ritter von (1871). *Geistesleben* [Life of the mind]. Wien: Wilhelm Braumüller.

Roberts, G.W. (1991). Schizophrenia: A neuropathological perspective. *British Journal of Psychiatry, 158*, 8–17.

Robin, A.A. (1958). A retrospective controlled study of leucotomy in schizophrenia and affective disorders. *Journal of Mental Science, 104*, 1025–1042.

Robin, A.A., & Macdonald, D. (1975). *Lessons of leucotomy*. London: Henry Kimpton Publs.

Robinson, C.H. (1877). Cirrhosis of the liver: Alcoholic paralysis. *British Medical Journal, 1*, 352–353.

Robinson, M.F. (1946). What price lobotomy? *Journal of Abnormal and Social Psychology 41*, 421–436.

Robinson, M.F., & Freeman, W. (1954). *Psychosurgery and the self.* New York: Grune and Stratton.

Rodrigues, N. (1906). La psychose polyneuritique et le beri-beri [Polyneuritic psychosis and beri-beri]. *Annales medico-psychiatrique (Mars-Avril)* (Cited after Serbsky, 1907).

Roemheld, (n.n.g.) (1906). Uber den Korsakowschen Symptomenkomplex bei Hirnlues [On Korsakoff's symptom complex in cerebral lues]. *Archiv für Psychiatrie und Nervenkrankheiten, 41*, 703–711.

Rolleston, H.D. (1888). Description of the cerebral hemispheres of an adult Australian male. *Journal of the Anthropological Institute of Great Britain and Ireland, 17*, 32–43.

Rollett, A. (1900). Die Localisation psychischer Vorgänge im Gehirne [The localization of psychic processes in the brain]. *Pflüger's Archiv für die gesamte Physiologie des Menschen und der Tiere, 79*, 303–311.

Rolls, E. (1990). Spatial memory, episodic memory, and neuronal network functions in the hippocampus. In L.R. Squire & E. Lindenlaub (Eds.), *The biology of memory* (pp. 445–470). Stuttgart: Schattauer.

Roman-Campos, G., Poser, C.M., & Wood, F.B. (1980). Persistent retrograde memory deficit after transient global amnesia. *Cortex, 16*, 509–518.

Rose, F.C. (Ed.). (1989). *James Parkinson: His life and times.* Basel: Birkhäuser.

Rose, M. (1926). Der Allocortex bei Tier und Mensch. I. Teil [The allocortex of animals and man. First part]. *Journal für Psychologie und Neurologie, 34*, 1–111 (and 30 tables).

Rose, M. (1927). Die sog. Riechrinde beim Menschen und beim Affen. II. Teil des „Allocortex bei Tier und Mensch". [The socalled brain of smell in the human and the monkey. Second part of "The allocortex of animals and man"]. *Journal für Psychologie und Neurologie, 34*, 261–401 (and 35 tables).

Rosenfeld, M. (1917). Ueber psychische Störungen bei Schussverletzung beider Frontallappen [On psychic disturbances after gunshot wounds of both frontal lobes]. *Archiv für Psychiatrie und Nervenkrankheiten, 57*, 84–90.

Rosenfeld, M. (1928). Ueber Stirnhirnpsychosen [On frontal lobe psychoses]. *Deutsche medizinische Wochenschrift, 54*, 85–87

Rosenthal, (n.n.g.) (1881). Ueber anatomische Veränderungen im Gehirn bei infectiösen Krankheiten [On anatomical changes in the brain after infectious diseases]. *Centralblatt für die medicinischen Wissenschaften, No. 20.*

Rossi, A., Stratta, P., D'Albenzio, L., Tartaro, A., Schiazza, G., di Michele, V., Bolino, F., & Casacchia, M. (1990). Reduced temporal lobe areas in schizophrenia: Preliminary evidences from a controlled multiplanar magnetic resonance imaging study. *Biological Psychiatry, 27*, 61–68.

Rossi, A., Stratta, P., Dimichelle, V., Gallucci, M., Splendiani, A., DeCataldo, S., & Casacchia, M. (1991). Temporal lobe structure by magnetic resonance in bipolar affective disorders and schizophrenia. *Journal of Affective Disorders, 21*, 19–22.

Rosvold, H.E., & Mishkin, M. (1950). Evaluation of the effects of prefrontal lobotomy on intelligence. *Canadian Journal of Psychology, 4*, 122–126.

Rothmann, H. (1911). Zur Funktion der Stirnlappen [On the function of the frontal lobes]. *Medizinische Klinik, No. 52*, 2041–2042.

Rothmann, H. (1923). Zusammenfassender Bericht über den Rothmannschen grosshirnlosen Hund nach klinischer und anatomischer Untersuchung [Summarizing report on Rothmann's dog without cerebrum after clinical and anatomical investigation]. *Zeitschrift für die gesamte Neurologie und Psychiatrie, 87*, 247–313.

Rothmann, M. (1914). Zur Symptomatologie der Stirnhirnschüsse [On the symptomatology of frontal lobe shots]. *Berliner klinische Wochenschrift, 51*, 1923–1924.

Rothschild, D., & Kaye, A. (1949). The effects of prefrontal lobotomy on the symptomatology of schizophrenic patients. *American Journal of Psychiatry, 105*, 752–759.

Roussy, G. (1907). *La couche optique. Le syndrome thalamique* [The optic thalamus. The thalamic syndrome]. Paris: G. Steinheil.

Rowe, S.N., & Moyar, J.B. (1950). Experiences with unilateral prefrontal lobotomies for pain. *Journal of Neurosurgery, 7*, 121–126.

Ruckert, A. (1909). Ein Stirnhirntumor unter dem klinischen Bild eines Tumors der hinteren Schädelgrube [A frontal lobe tumor with the clinical picture of the posterior cranial fossa]. *Berliner Klinische Wochenschrift, 27*, 1248–1250.

Ruffin, H. (1939). Stirnhirnsymptomatologie und Stirnhirnsyndrome [Frontal lobe symptomatology and frontal lobe syndromes]. *Fortschritte der Neurologie und Psychiatrie, 11*, 34–52.

Rüsken, W. (1950). Über die Beeinflussung schizophrener Krankheitszustände durch die Leukotomie [On the influence of leucomoty on schizophrenic states of illness]. *Nervenarzt, 21*, 508–514.

Russell, W.R. (1948). Functions of the frontal lobes. *Lancet, ii*, 356–360.

Russell, W.R., & Nathan, P.W. (1946). Traumatic amnesia. *Brain, 69*, 280–300.

Rutishauser, F. (1899). Experimenteller Beitrag zur Stabkranzfaserung im Frontalhirn des Affen [Experimental contribution to the fibers of the thalamic radiations in the monkey's frontal lobe]. *Monatsschrift für Psychiatrie und Neurologie, 5*, 161–180.

Rylander, G. (1939). Personality changes after operations on the frontal lobes. A clinical study of 32 cases. *Acta Psychiatrica et Neurologica, Suppl. 20*, 1–327.

Rylander, G. (1943). Mental changes after excision of cerebral tissue. *Acta Psychiatrica et Neurologica, 25*, 4–81.

Rylander, G. (1948). Personality analysis before and after frontal lobotomy. In J.F. Fulton, W.C. Aring, & S.B. Wortis (Eds.), *The frontal lobes. (Research publications of the association for research in nervous and mental disease, Vol. 27)* (pp. 691–705). Baltimore: Williams & Wilkins.

Rylander, G. (1950). Persönlichkeitsveränderungen nach verschiedenen Formen der Leukotomie [Personality changes after different forms of leucotomy]. *Zeitschrift für die gesamte Neurologie und Psychiatrie, 108*, 303–305.

Rylander, G. (1973). The renaissance of psychosurgery. In L.V. Laitinen & K.E. Livingston (Eds.), *Surgical approaches in psychiatry* (pp. 3–12). Lancaster, UK: Medical and Technical Publ. Comp.

Sachdev, P., Smith, J.S., & Matheson, J. (1990). Is psychosurgery antimanic? *Biological Psychiatry, 27*, 363–371.

Sachs, B. (1907). Discussion of aphasia, with presentation of cases. *Journal of Nervous and Mental Disease, 34*, 602–609.

Sachs, E. (1927). Symptomatology of a group of frontal lobe lesions. *Brain, 50*, 474–479.

Sachs, E. (1930). Lesions of the frontal lobe. A review of forty-five cases. *Archives of Neurological Psychiatry, 24*, 735–742.

Sachs, E., Avman, N., & Fisher, R.R. (1962). Meningiomas of pineal region and posterior part of 3rd ventricle. *Journal of Neurosurgery, 19*, 325–331.

Sackeim, H.A., Prohovnik, I., Moeller, J.E., Brown, R.P., Apter, S., Prudic, J., Devanand, D.P., & Mukherjee, S. (1990). Regional cerebral blood flow in mood disorders. *Archives of General Psychiatry, 47*, 60–70.

Saelan, Th. (1886). Zur Casuistik der Hirntumoren. – Ein Beitrag zur Kenntniss der Gehirnlocalisationen [On the casuistry of brain tumors. – A contribution to our knowledge of brain localizations]. *Allgemeine Zeitschrift für Psychiatrie und psychisch-gerichtliche Medicin, 42*, 247–253.

Salomonsohn, H. (1891). Ueber Polioencephalitis acuta superior [On polioencephalitis acuta superior]. *Deutsche medizinische Wochenschrift, 17*, 849–852.

Sander, J. (1868a). Beschreibung zweier Mikrocephalen-Gehirne mit einigen Bemerkungen [Description of two brains of microcephalics with some remarks]. *Archiv für Psychiatrie und Nervenkrankheiten, 1*, 299–307.

Sander, J. (1868b). Ueber Balkenmangel im menschlichen Gehirn [On callosal lack in the human brain]. *Archiv für Psychiatrie und Nervenkrankheiten, 1*, 128–142.

Sander, J. (1875). Ueber eine affenartige Bildung am Hinterhauptslappen eines menschlichen Gehirns [On a monkey-like formation in the occipital lobes of a human brain]. *Archiv für Psychiatrie und Nervenkrankheiten, 5*, 842–849.

Sands, S.L., & Malamud, W. (1949). A rating scale analysis of the clinical effects of lobotomy. *American Journal of Psychiatry, 105*, 760–766.

Sankey, H.R.O. (1878). Two cases of microcephalic idiotcy in one family – convulsions of mother during pregnancy. *Brain, 1*, 391–399.

Sarbo, A. v. (1925). Ein Fall von Stirnhirngeschwulst mit Beteiligung des Zwischen- und Mittelhirngebietes. Ein neuer histopathologisch unterstützter Beitrag zur rubralen Ataxie [A case of frontal lobe tumor with involvement of the areas of the diencephalon and the brain stem. A new histopathologically supported contribution to rubral ataxia]. *Klinische Wochenschrift, 4*, 168–170.

Sargant, W. (1951). Leucotomy in psychosomatic disorders. *Lancet, ii*, 87–91.

Sargant, W., & Stewart, A. (1947). Chronic battle neurosis treated with leucotomy. *British Medical Journal 2*, 866–869.

Saubidet, R, Lyonnet, J., & Brichetti, D. (1977). Undercutting of lateral aspect of frontal lobes for treatment in the chronic paranoid psychosis, paraphrenia. In W.H. Sweet, S. Obrador, & J.G. Martín-Rodríguez (Eds.), *Neurosurgical treatment in psychiatry, pain and epilepsy* (pp. 225–228). Baltimore: University Park Press.

Savage, G.H. (1878). Acute mania associated with abscess of the brain. *Brain, 1*, 265–269.

Scarff, J.E. (1950). Unilateral prefrontal lobotomy for the relief of intractable pain. Report of 58 cases with special consideration of failures. *Journal of Neurosurgery, 7*, 330–336.

Schacter, D.L. (1986). Amnesia and crime. *American Psychologist, 41*, 286–295.

Schäfer, E.A. (1888a). Experiments on the electrical excitation of the visual area of the cerebral cortex in the monkey. *Brain, 11*, 1–6.

Schäfer, E.A. (1888b). On the functions of the temporal and occipital lobes: a reply to Dr. Ferrier. *Brain, 11*, 145–165.

Schäfer, E.A. (1900). *Textbook of physiology (Vol. II)*. Edinburgh and London: Y.J. Pentland.

Schaffer, K. (1892). Beitrag zur Histologie der Ammonshornformation [Contribution to the histology of the Ammon's horn formation]. *Archiv für mikroskopische Anatomie, 39*, 611–632.

Schaffer, K. (1905). Weitere Beiträge zur pathologischen Histologie der familiären amaurotischen Idiotie [Further contributions to the pathological histology of familiar amaurotic idiocy]. *Journal für Psychologie und Neurologie, 6*, 84–107.

Scheid, W. (1935). Zur Pathopsychologie des Korsakow-Syndroms [On the psychopathology of Korsakoff's syndrome]. *Zeitschrift für die gesamte Neurologie und Psychiatrie, 151*, 346–369.

Scheller, H. (1961). Korsakow-Syndrom und Zeitlichkeit [Korsakoff's syndrome and temporality]. *Zentralblatt für die gesamte Neurologie und Psychiatrie 159*, 5–6.

Scherer, I.W., Klett, C.J., & Winne, J.F. (1957). Psychological changes over a five year period following bilateral prefrontal lobotomy. *Journal of Consulting Psychology, 21*, 291–295.

Scherer, I.W., Winne, J.F., & Baker, R.W. (1955). Psychological changes over a three year period following bilateral prefrontal lobotomy. *Journal of Consulting Psychology, 19*, 291–298.

Scherer, I.W., Winne, J.F., Clancy, D.D., & Baker, R.W. (1953). Psychological changes during the first year following prefrontal lobotomy. *Psychological Monographs, 67*, No.7 (Whole No. 357).

Schiff, M. (1880). Ueber die Erregbarkeit des Rückenmarks. Dritter Artikel: Das Rückenmark im Ganzen [On the excitability of the spinal cord. Third article: The spinal cord in toto]. *Pflüger's Archiv für die gesammte Physiologie des Menschen und der Thiere, 30*, 199–275.

Schilder, P. (1924). Zur Lehre von den Amnesien Epileptischer, von der Schlafmittelhypnose und vom Gedächtnis [On the study of the amnesias of epileptics, on barbiturate hypnosis and on memory]. *Archiv für Psychiatrie und Nervenkrankheiten, 72*, 326–340.

Schiller, F. (1985). The mystique of the frontal lobes. *Gesnerus, 42*, 415–424.

Schiller, F. (1986). Rigidity and drooling in Parkinson's disease. *Neurology, 36*, 1583.

Schlesinger, H. (1916). Hochgradige retrograde Amnesie nach Gehirnverletzung [Severe retrograde amnesia after brain damage]. *Muenchener medicinische Wochenschrift, Nr. 1*, 18.

Schmidt, R. & Shashoua, V.E. (1981). A radioimmunoassay for ependymins ß and γ : Two goldfish brain proteins involved in behavioral plasticity. *Journal of Neurochemistry, 36*, 1368–1377.

Schmidt, R. & Shashoua, V.E. (1983). Structural and metabolic relations between goldfish brain glycoproteins participating in functional plasticity of the central nervous system. *Journal of Neurochemistry, 40*, 652–660.

Schneider, H. (1901). Ueber Auffassung und Merkfähigkeit beim Altersblödsinn [On comprehension and ability to memorize in senile dementia]. In E. Kraepelin (Ed.), *Psychologische Arbeiten (Vol. 3)* (pp. 458–481). Leipzig. Engelmann.

Schneider, K. (1912). Über einige klinisch-psychologische Untersuchungsmethoden und ihre Ergebnisse. Zugleich ein Beitrag zur Psychopathologie der Korsakowschen Psychose [On some clinical-pathological methods of investigation and their results. Simultaneously a contribution to the psychopathology of Korsakoff's psychosis]. *Zeitschrift für die gesamte Neurologie und Psychiatrie/ Originalien, 8*, 553–615.

Schneider, K. (1928). Die Störungen des Gedächtnisses [Disturbances of memory]. In O. Bumke (Ed.), *Handbuch der Geisteskrankheiten, (Vol. 1)* (pp. 508–529). Berlin: Springer.

Schob, (n.n.g.) (1921). Über psychische Störungen nach Durchschuss beider Stirnlappen [On psychic disturbances after a shot-through both frontal lobes]. *Allgemeine Zeitschrift für Psychiatrie, 77*, 281–294.

Scholz, W. (1923). Josef Harder. *Nissls Beiträge zur Frage nach der Beziehung zwischen klinischem Verlauf und anatomischem Befund bei Nerven- und Geisteskrankheiten, 2*, 101–128.

Scholz, W. (1961). *50 Jahre Neuropathologie in Deutschland 1885–1935*| [50 years of neuropathology in Germany 1885–1935]. Stuttgart: Georg Thieme.

Schrader, P.J., & Robinson, M.F. (1945). An evaluation of prefrontal lobotomy through ward behavior. *Journal of Abnormal and Social Psychology, 40*, 61–69.

Schreiber, F.R. (1973). *Sybil*. Chicago: Regnery.

Schröder, P. (1930). Paul Flechsig. *Archiv für Psychiatrie und Nervenkrankheiten, 91*, 1–7.

Schüle, A. (1899). Zur Lehre von den Grosshirntumoren und den Rückenmarksveränderungen bei denselben [On cerebral cortical tumors and changes in the spinal cord accompanying them]. *Neurobiologisches Zentralblatt, 18*, 290–294.

Schulman, S. (1956). Bilateral symmetrical degeneration of the thalamus: clinicopathological study. *Journal of Neuropathology and Experimental Neurology, 15*, 208.

Schulman, S. (1957). Bilateral symmetrical degeneration of the thalamus. A clinico-pathological study.

Journal of Neuropathology and Experimental Neurology, 16, 446–470.
Schultz, J.H. (1915). Fünf neurologisch bemerkenswerte Hirnschüsse [Five neurologically remarkable brain shots]. *Monatsschrift für Psychiatrie und Neurologie, 38*, 319–328.
Schultz, J.H. (1917). Zur Klinik der Nachbehandlung Kopfverletzter [On the clinical appearance of postoperative care of head injured]. *Monatsschrift für Psychiatrie und Neurologie, 42*, 327–348.
Schultz, J.H. (1924). Zur Psychopathologie und Psychotherapie amnestischer Zustände [On the psychopathology and psychotherapy of amnesic conditions]. *Zeitschrift für die gesamte Neurologie und Psychiatrie, 89*, 107–129.
Schultze, E. (1898). Beitrag zur pathologischen Anatomie des Thalamus opticus bei der progressiven Paralyse [Contribution to the pathological anatomy of the optic thalamus in progressive paralysis]. *Monatsschrift für Psychiatrie und Neurologie, 4*, 300–317.
Schultze, E. (1903). Ueber krankhaften Wandertrieb [On poriomania]. *Allgemeine Zeitschrift für Psychologie, 60*, 795–814.
Schulz, (n.n.g.) (1908). Korsakoff'sches Syndrom bei CO-Vergiftungen [Korsakoff's syndrome after CO-intoxications]. *Berliner Klinische Wochenschrift, No. 45*, 1621–1623.
Schuster, J. (1930). Beitrag zur Histopathologie der Dementia praecox [Contribution to the histopathology of dementia praecox]. *Archiv für Psychiatrie und Nervenkrankheiten, 90*, 457–516.
Schuster, P. (1902). *Psychische Störungen bei Hirntumoren* [Psychic disturbances in brain tumors]. Stuttgart: Enke.
Schuster, P. (1936a). Beiträge zur Pathologie des Thalamus opticus I [Contributions to the pathology of the optic thalamus I]. *Archiv für Psychiatrie und Nervenkrankheiten, 105*, 358–432.
Schuster, P. (1936b). Beiträge zur Pathologie des Thalamus opticus II [Contributions to the pathology of the optic thalamus II]. *Archiv für Psychiatrie und Nervenkrankheiten, 105*, 550–622.
Schuster, P. (1937a). Beiträge zur Pathologie des Thalamus opticus III [Contributions to the pathology of the optic thalamus II]. *Archiv für Psychiatrie und Nervenkrankheiten, 106*, 13–53.
Schuster, P. (1937b). Beiträge zur Pathologie des Thalamus opticus IV [Contributions to the pathology of the optic thalamus IV]. *Archiv für Psychiatrie und Nervenkrankheiten, 106*, 201–233.
Schwab, S.I. (1927). Changes in personality in tumours of the frontal lobe. *Brain, 50*, 480–487.
Schwab, (n.n.g.) (1925). Zur Diagnose der Schläfenlappentumoren [On diagnosing tumors of the temporal lobe]. *Deutsche Zeitschrift für Nervenheilkunde, 84*, 38–44.
Scoville, W.B. (1954a). The limbic lobe in man. *Journal of Neurosurgery, 11*, 64–66.
Scoville, W.B. (1954b). Orbital undercutting in the treatment of psychoneurosis, depressions and senile emotional states. *Diseases of the Nervous System, 15*, 1–12.
Scoville, W.B. (1960). Late results of orbital undercutting. *American Journal of Psychiatry, 117*, 525–532.
Scoville, W.B. (1968). Amnesia after bilateral mesial temporal-lobe excision: Introduction to case H.M. *Neuropsychologia 6*, 211–213.
Scoville, W.B. (1971). The effect of surgical lesions of the brain on psyche and behavior in man. In A. Winter (Ed.), *Symposium on the surgical control of behavior* (pp. 53–68). Springfield, IL: C.C. Thomas.
Scoville, W.B. (1972). Introduction. In E. Hitchcock, L. Laitinen & K. Vaernet (Eds.), *Psychosurgery* (pp. XIX-XXIII). Springfield, IL: C.C. Thomas.
Scoville, W.B. (1973). Surgical locations for psychiatric surgery with special reference to orbital and cingulate operations. In L.V. Laitinen & K. Livingston (Eds.), *Surgical appraoches in psychiatry* (pp. 29–38). Lancaster, UK: Medical and Technical Publ. Comp.
Scoville, W.B., & Bettis, D.B. (1977). Results of orbital undercutting today: A personal series. In W.H. Sweet, S. Obrador, & J.G. Martín-Rodríguez (Eds.), *Neurosurgical treatment in psychiatry, pain and epilepsy* (pp. 189–202). Baltimore: University Park Press.
Scoville, W.B., Dunsmoore, R.H., Liberson, W.T., Henry, C.E., & Pepe, A. (1953). Observations on medial temporal lobotomy and uncotomy in the treatment of psychotic states. Preliminary view of 19 operative cases compared with 60 frontal lobotomy and undercutting cases. *Research Publications of the Association for Research in Nervous and Mental Disease, 31*, 347–369.
Scoville, W.B., & Milner, B. (1957). Loss of recent memory after bilateral hippocampal lesions. *Journal of Neurology, Neurosurgery, and Psychiatry, 20*, 11–21.
Scoville, W.B., Wilk, E.K., & Pepe, A.J. (1951). Selective cortical undercutting. Results in new method of fractional lobotomy. *American Journal of Psychiatry, 107*, 730–738.
Seidman, L.J. (1983). Schizophrenia and brain dysfunction: an integration of recent neurodiagnostic findings. *Psychological Bulletin, 94*, 195–238.
Seidemann, H. (1926). Einfache klinische Testmethode zur Prüfung der Merkfähigkeit [Simple

clinical method for testing the ability of memorizing]. *Archiv für Psychiatrie und Nervenkranheiten, 77*, 614–635.

Seiffer, W. (1905). Ueber psychische, insbesondere Intelligenzstörungen bei multipler Sklerose [On psychic, particularly intelligence disturbances in multiple sclerosis]. *Archiv für Psychiatrie und Nervenkrankheiten, 40*, 252–303.

Seletzky, W., & Gilula, J. (1928). Zur Frage der Funktionen des Balkens bei Tieren [On the question of the functions of the corpus callosum in animals]. *Archiv für Psychiatrie und Nervenkrankheiten, 86*, 57–73.

Semon, R. (1904). *Die Mneme als erhaltendes Prinzip im Wechsel des organischen Geschehens* [Mnemis as conservation principle in the change of organic action]. Leipzig: Wilhelm Engelmann.

Semon, R. (1920). *Bewusstseinsvorgang und Gehirnprozess* [The processes of consciousness and of the brain]. Wiesbaden: J.F. Bergmann.

Serbsky, W. (1907). Die Korsakowsche Krankheit [Korsakoff's disease]. *Arbeiten aus dem neurologischen Institut der Wiener Universität, 15*, 389–424.

Serog, M. (1911). Die psychischen Störungen bei Stirnhirntumoren und die Beziehungen des Stirnhirns zur Psyche [Psychic disturbances in frontal lobe tumors and the relations of the frontal lobe to the psyche]. *Allgemeine Zeitschrift für Psychiatrie, 68*, 583–612.

Shakespeare, W. (1599–1601). Hamlet. In H. Jenkins (Ed.), *Hamlet. The Arden Shakespeare*. London: Routledge.

Sharkey, S.J. (1898). The accurate localisation of intracranial tumours, excluding tumours of the motor cortex, motor tract, pons and medulla. *Brain, 21*, 319–328.

Sharpey, W. (1879). The re-education of the adult brain. *Brain, 2*, 1–9.

Shashoua, V.E. (1982). Molecular and cell biological aspects of learning: toward a theory of memory. *Advances in Cell Neurobiology, 3*, 97–141.

Sheer, D.E. (1966). Brain and behavior: the background of interdisciplinary research. In D.E. Sheer (Ed.), *Electrical stimulation of the brain* (pp. 3–21). Austin, TX: University of Texas Press.

Shenkin, H.A., Woodford, R.B., Freyhan, F.A. & Kety, S.S. (1948). Effects of frontal lobotomy on cerebral blood flow and metabolism. In J.F. Fulton, W.C. Aring, & S.B. Wortis (Eds.), *The frontal lobes. (Research publications of the association for research in nervous and mental disease, Vol. 27)* (pp. 823–831). Baltimore: Williams & Wilkins.

Shimamura, A.P., & Squire, L.R. (1988). Long-term memory in amnesia: Cued recall, recognition memory, and confidence ratings. *Journal of Experimental Psychology: Learning, Memory, and Cognition, 14*, 763–770.

Shraberg, D., & Weisberg, G.L. (1978). The Klüver-Bucy syndrome in man. *Journal of Nervous and Mental Disease, 166*, 130–134.

Sibelius, C. (1905). Die psychischen Störungen nach akuter Kohlenmonoxydvergiftung [Psychic disturbances after acute carbon monoxide poisoning]. *Monatsschrift für Psychiatrie und Neurologie, 18 (Suppl.)*, 39–178.

Sidis, B., & Goodhart, S.P. (1905). *Multiple personality: an experimental investigation into the nature of human individuality*. New York: Appleton.

Siebert, H. (1933). Über den nicht ungünstigen Verlauf von amnestischen und polyneuritischen Alkoholpsychosen [On the favorable course of amnesic and polyneuritic alcoholic psychoses]. *Allgemeine Zeitschrift für Psychiatrie, 99*, 219–220.

Siemerling, (n.n.g.) (1887). Casuistischer Beitrag zur Localisation im Grosshirn [Casuistric contribution on the localization in the cerebrum]. *Archiv für Psychiatrie und Nervenkrankheiten, 18*, 877–881.

Siemerling, (n.n.g.) (1890). Ein Fall von sogenannter Seelenblindheit nebst anderweitigen cerebralen Symptomen [A case of socalled optic agnosia, with further cerebral symptoms]. *Archiv für Psychiatrie und Nervenkrankheiten, 21*, 284–299.

Simmel, G. (1890). Zur Psychologie der Frauen [On the psychology of women]. *Zeitschrift für Völkerkunde und Sprachwissenschaft, 20*, 6–46.

Simon, A., Margolis, L.H., Adams, J.E., & Bowman, K.M. (1951). Unilateral and bilateral lobotomy. A controlled evaluation. *A.M.A. Archives of Neurology and Psychiatry, 66*, 494–505.

Singelmann, (n.n.g.) (1919). *Über einen Fall von Tumor cerebri im rechten Schläfenlappen* [On a case of cerebral tumor in the right temporal lobe]. Unpublished doctoral dissertation, Königliche Christian-Albrechts-Universität, Kiel. (cited after Artom, 1923).

Singer, H.D., & Low, A.A. (1933). Acalculia (Henschen). A clinical study. *A.M.A. Archives of Neurology and Psychiatry, 29*, 476–498.

Sittig, O. (1914). Ein Fall von Korsakowscher Psychose auf Grund diabetischer Acidose [A case of Korsakoff's psychosis due to diabetic acidosis]. *Monatsschrift für Psychiatrie und Neurologie, 32*, 241–251.

Sittig, O. (1916). Zur Symptomatologie der Stirnhirnschüsse [On the symptomatology of frontal lobe shots]. *Medizinische Klinik, 41*, 1076.

Sittig, O. (1921). Störungen des Ziffernschreibens und Rechnens bei einem Hirnverletzten [Disturbances in writing digits and in calculating in a brain damaged patient]. *Monatsschrift für Psychiatrie und Neurologie, 49*, 299–306.

Smith, A., & Kinder E.F. (1959). Changes in psychological test performances of brain-operated schizophrenics after 8 years. *Science, 129*, 149–150.

Smith, H. (1906). A case of cerebral tumour; operation; recovery. *Lancet, i*, 1688–1690.

Smith, J.S., & Kiloh, L.G. (1980). The psychosurgical treatment of anxiety. In G.D. Burrows & B. Davies (Eds.), *Handbook of studies on anxiety* (pp. 377–398). Amsterdam: Elsevier.

Smith, J.S., Kiloh, L.G., & Boots, J.A. (1977). Prospective evaluation of prefrontal leucotomy: Results at 30 months' follow-up. In W.H. Sweet, S. Obrador, & J.G. Martín-Rodríguez (Eds.), *Neurosurgical treatment in psychiatry, pain and epilepsy* (pp. 217–224). Baltimore: University Park Press.

Smith, W.G. (1895). The relation of attention to memory. *Mind (New Series), 4*, 47–73.

Smyth, G.E., & Stern, K. (1938). Tumours of the thalamus – a clinico-pathological study. *Brain, 61*, 339–374.

Soemmerring, S.T. (1796). *Ueber das Organ der Seele* [On the organ of the soul]. (Reprint 1966 [of the Koenigsberg edition].) Amsterdam: E.J. Bonset.

Sölder, (n.n.g.) von (1895). Ueber Perseverationen [On perseverations]. *Neurologisches Centralblatt*, 958.

Sollier, P. (1900). *Le problème de la mémoire* [Problems of memory]. Paris: F. Alcan.

Solly, S. (1836). *The human brain*. London: Longman, Rees, Orme, Brown, Green & Longman.

Soltmann, O. (1875). Experimentelle Studien über die Functionen des Grosshirns der Neugeborenen [Experimental studies on the functions of the cerebrum in new-borns]. *Jahrbuch für Kinderheilkunde und physische Erziehung (Neue Folge), 9*, 106–148.

Sommer, M. (1903). Zur Kenntnis der amnestischen Störungen nach Strangulationsversuchen [On amnesic disturbances after attempts of strangulation]. *Monatsschrift für Psychiatrie und Neurologie, 14*, 221–230.

Sommer, R. (1891). Zur Pathologie der Sprache [On the pathology of language]. *Zeitschrift für Psychologie und Physiologie der Sinnesorgane, 2*, 143–163.

Sommer, R. (1899). *Lehrbuch der psychopathologischen Untersuchungs-Methoden* [Textbook of psychopathological methods of investigation]. Berlin: Urban & Schwarzenberg.

Sommer, W. (1880). Erkrankung des Ammonshorns als aetiologisches Moment der Epilepsie [Disease of Ammon's horn as an etiological cause of epilepsy]. *Archiv für Psychiatrie und Nervenkrankheiten, 10*, 631–675.

Sommer, W. (1897). Nervöse Veranlagung und Schädeldifformität [Nervous predisposition and deformation of the skull]. *Allgemeine Zeitschrift für Psychiatrie, 53*, 686–694.

Sondhaus, E., & Finger, S. (1988). Aphasia and the CNS from Imhotep to Broca. *Neuropsychology, 2*, 87–110.

Soukhanoff, S., & Boutenko, J. (1903). A study of Korsakoff's disease. *Journal of Mental Pathology, 4*, 1–33.

Souplet, (n.n.g.) (1871). Aliénation mentale par cause traumatique; guérison [Mental changes of traumatic origin; curation]. *Bulletin de la Societé de Medicine de l'Yonne. Auxerre, 12*, 69–86.

Soury, J. (1899). *Le système nerveux central. Structure et fonctions, Histoire critique des théories et des doctrines (2 vols)* [The central nervous system. Structure and functions. Historical critique of theories and doctrines (2 vols.)]. Paris: Masson.

Spatz, H. (1929). Über den mikroskopisch-anatomischen Befund bei Polioencephalitis Wernicke [On the microscopical-anatomical findings after Wernicke's polioencephalitis]. *Allgemeine Zeitschrift für Psychiatrie und ihre Grenzgebiete, 91*. (cited after Kant, 1932).

Spatz, H. (1930). Über den Entzündungsbegriff im allgemeinen [General remarks on the term infection]. In In O. Bumke (Ed.), *Handbuch der Geisteskrankheiten, Vol. 7. Die Anatomie der Psychosen* (pp.157–288). Berlin: Springer.

Spatz, H. (1937). Über die Bedeutung der basalen Rinde. Auf Grund von Beobachtungen bei Pickscher Krankheit und bei gedeckten Hirnverletzungen [On the importance of the basal cerebral cortex. Based on observations in Pick's disease and after covered injuries of the brain]. *Zeitschrift für die gesamte Neurologie und Psychiatrie, 158*, 208–232.

Spatz, H. (1941). Gehirnpathologie im Kriege. Von den Gehirnwunden [Brain pathology during war. About brain wounds]. *Zentralblatt für Neurochirurgie, 6*, 162–211.

Spatz, H. (1950). Diskussionsbemerkung [Comment]. *Archiv für Psychiatrie und Nervenkrankheiten, 184*, 285–286.

Sperling, E. (1957). Thalamusveränderungen bei Stirnhirnverletzungen. (Zugleich ein Beitrag zum Problem hirnorganischen Wesenswandels) [Thalamic changes in frontal lobe injuries. (At the same time a contribution to the problem of personality changes in the organic brain syndrome]. *Archiv für Psychiatrie und Zeitschrift für die gesamte Neurologie, 195*, 589–606.

Sperry, R.W. (1988). Psychology's mentalist paradigm and the religion/science tension. *American Psychologist, 43*, 607–613.

Spiegel, E.A., & Wycis, H.T. (1949). Mesencephalothalamotomy for relief of pain (Principles of the method). In H.J. Urban (Ed.), *Festschrift zum 70. Geburtstag von Prof. Dr. Otto Pötzl* (pp. 437–443). Innsbruck: Universitätsverlag Wagner.

Spiegel, E.A., & Wycis, H.T. (1955). Mesencephalotomy in treatment of "intractable" facial pain. *A.M.A. Archives of Neurology and Psychiatry, 69*, 1–13.

Spiegel, E.A., Wycis, H.T., Freed, H., & Orchinik, C. (1953). Thalamotomy and hypothalamotomy for the treatment of psychoses. In S.B. Wortis, M. Herman, & C.C. Hare (Eds.), *Research publications for research in nervous and mental disease, Vol. 31. Psychiatric treatment* (pp. 379–391). Baltimore, MD: Williams & Wilkins.

Spiegel, E.A., Wycis, H.T., Orchinik, C., & Freed, H. (1956). Thalamic chronotaraxis. *American Journal of Psychiatry, 113*, 97–105.

Spielmeyer, W. (1904). Ueber die Prognose der akuten haemorrhagischen Polioencephalitis superior (Wernicke) [On the prognosis of acute hemorrhagical polioencephalitis superior (Wernicke)]. *Centralblatt für Nervenheilkunde und Psychiatrie, 27*, 673–691.

Spitzka, E. (1901). The redundancy of the preinsula in the brains of distinguished educated men. *Medical Record, 59*, 940–943.

Spitzka, E. (1903). A study of the brain of the late Major J.W. Powell. *American Anthropologist (New Series), 5*, 585–643.

Spitzka, E. (1907). A study of the brains of six eminent scientists and scholars belonging to the American Anthropometric Society, together with a description of the skull of Professor E.D. Cope. *Transactions of the American Philosophical Society (New series), 21*, 175–308.

Sprofkin, B.E., & Sciarra, D. (1952). Korsakoff's psychosis associated with cerebral tumors. *Neurology, 2*, 427–434.

Squire, L.R. (1981). Two forms of human amnesia: An analysis of forgetting. *Journal of Neuroscience, 1*, 635–640.

Squire, L.R. (1982). Comparisons between forms of amnesia: some deficits are unique to Korsakoff's syndrome. *Journal of Experimental Psychology, 8*, 560–571.

Squire, L.R. (1987). *Memory and brain*. New York: Oxford University Press.

Squire, L.R., Cohen, N.J., & Zouzounis, J.A. (1984). Preserved memory in retrograde amnesia: Sparing of recently acquired skill. *Neuropsychologia, 22*, 145–152.

Squire, L.R., Slater, P.C., & Chase, P.M. (1975). Retrograde amnesia: Temporal gradient in very long term memory following electroconvulsive therapy. *Science, 187*, 77–79.

Stafiniak, P., Saykin, A.J., Sperling, M.R., Kester, D.B., Robinson, L.J., O'Connor, M.J., & Gur, R.C. (1990). Acute naming deficits following dominant temporal lobectomy: Prediction by age at 1st risk for seizures. *Neurology, 40*, 1509–1512.

Stämpfli, K. (1952). Leukotomieversager bei indizierten Fällen von chronischer Schizophrenie [Failures of leucotomy in assumed cases of chronic schizophrenia]. *Nervenarzt, 23*, 241–248.

Stanley, C.E. (1909/10). A report of three cases of Korsakow's psychosis. *American Journal of Insanity, 66*, 613–622.

Starr, A. (1894). *Hirnchirurgie* [Brain surgery]. (Transl. by M. Weiss). Leipzig and Wien: Franz Deuticke.

Steegmann, A.T. (1962). Dr. Harlow's famous case: The "impossible" accident of Phineas P. Gage. *Surgery, 52*, 952–958.

Steffens, L. (1900). Experimentelle Beiträge zur Lehre vom ökonomischen Lernen [Experimental contributions to the theory of economical learning]. *Zeitschrift für Psychologie und Physiologie der Sinnesorgane, 22*, 321–382.

Stein, J. (1931/33). Zur Symptomatologie der Stirnhirnläsionen [On the symptoms of frontal lobe shots]. *Deutsche Zeitschrift für Nervenheilkunde, 117/119*, 623–629.

Steinthal, E. (1921). Ein eigenartiger Fall Korsakowscher Psychose [A peculiar case of Korsakoff's syndrome]. *Zeitschrift für die gesamte Neurologie und Psychiatrie, 67*, 287–310.

Stengel, E. (1949). Die Läsionen im Stirnhirn nach praefrontaler Leukotomie [Lesions in the frontal lobe after prefrontal leucotomy]. In H.J. Urban (Ed.), *Festschrift zum 70. Geburtstag von Prof. Dr. Otto Pötzl* (pp. 446–452). Innsbruck: Universitätsverlag Wagner.

Stern, A. (1914). Die psychischen Störungen bei Hirntumoren und ihre Beziehungen zu den durch Tumorwirkung bedingten diffusen Hirnveränderungen [Psychic disturbances in brain tumors and their relation to brain changes caused by the effects of tumors]. *Archiv für Psychiatrie und Nervenkrankheiten, 54*, 565–657 and 663–927 (and 2 tables).

Stern, A. (1915). Beobachtungen bei Schussverletzungen des Gehirns [Observations in gunshot wounds of the brain]. *Deutsche Medizinische Wochenschrift, 36*, 1067–1070.

Stern, E. (1917). Experimentelle Untersuchungen über die Assoziation bei Gehirnverletzten [Experimental investigations on association in brain injured]. *Archiv für Psychiatrie und Nervenkrankheiten, 57*, 725–771.

Stern, K. (1939). Severe dementia associated with bilateral symmetrical degeneration of the thalamus. *Brain, 62*, 157–171.

Stertz, G. (1910). Ueber psychogene Erkrankungen und Querulantenwahn nach Trauma nebst ihrer Bedeutung für die Begutachtungspraxis [On psychogenic diseases and delusions of querulous persons after trauma and their importance for the practice of expert reports. *Zeitschrift für ärztliche Fortbildung, 7*, 201–211.

Stertz, G. (1928). Störungen der Intelligenz [Disturbances of intelligence]. In O. Bumke (Ed.), *Handbuch der Geisteskrankheiten (Vol. 1)* (pp. 689–711). Berlin: Springer.

Stertz, G. (1931). Über den Anteil des Zwischenhirns an der Symptomgestaltung organischer Erkrankungen des Zentralnervensystems: Ein diagnostisch brauchbares Zwischenhirnsyndrom [On the contribution of the diencephalon to the development of organic diseases of the central nervous system: A diagnostically usable syndrome of the diencephalon]. *Deutsche Zeitschrift für Nervenheilkunde, 117–119*, 630–665.

Stertz, G. (1933). Probleme des Zwischenhirns [Problems of the diencephalon]. *Archiv für Psychiatrie und Nervenkrankheiten, 98*, 441–445.

Stevens, J.W. (1907). Korsakoff's psychosis superimposed upon melancholia. *Journal of Nervous and Mental Disease, 34*, 447–458.

Stewart, T.G. (1906). The diagnosis and localisation of tumours of the frontal regions of the brain. *Lancet, ii*, 1209–1211.

Stieda, L. (1908). Das Gehirn eines Sprachkundigen [The brain of a polyglot]. *Zeitschrift für Morphologie und Anthropologie, 11*, 83–138.

Stier, E. (1903). Zur pathologischen Anatomie der Huntingtonschen Chorea [On the pathological anatomy of Huntington's chorea]. *Archiv für Psychiatrie und Nervenkrankheiten, 37*, 62–85 (and 1 Table).

Stier, E. (1912). *Wandertrieb und pathologisches Fortlaufen bei Kindern* [Poriomania and pathological running away in children]. Jena: Gustav Fischer.

Stockert, F.G. von (1932). Subcorticale Demenz. Ein Beitrag zur encephalitischen Denkstörung [Subcortical dementia. A contribution to the encephalitic disturbance of thought]. *Archiv für Psychiatrie und Nervenkrankheiten, 97*, 77–100.

Stoddart, W.H.B. (1903). The evolution of consciousness. *Brain, 26*, 432–439.

Stoll, W.A. (1954). Leukotomie-Erfahrungen der Psychiatrischen Universitätsklinik Zürich [Experiences with leucotomy in the Psychiatric University Clinic Zurich]. *Nervenarzt, 25*, 195–197.

Störring, G.E. (1931). Über den ersten reinen Fall eines Menschen mit völligem, isoliertem Verlust der Merkfähigkeit. (Gleichzeitig ein Beitrag zur Gefühls-, Willens- und Handlungspsychologie) [On the first pure case of a man with complete, isolated loss of memory. (At the same time a contribution to the psychology of emotions, will, and action)]. *Archiv für die gesamte Psychologie, 81*, 257–384.

Stransky, E. (1905 a). Zur Lehre von der Amentia [On amentia]. *Journal für Psychologie und Neurologie, 4*, 158–171.

Stransky, E. (1905 b). Zur Lehre von der Amentia [On amentia]. *Journal für Psychologie und Neurologie, 5*, 18–36.

Stransky, E. (1905 c). Zur Lehre von der Amentia [On amentia]. *Journal für Psychologie und Neurologie, 6*, 37–83, and 155–191.

Strauss, I., & Keschner, M. (1935). Mental symptoms in cases of tumor of the frontal lobe. *A.M.A. Archives of Neurology and Psychiatry, 33*, 986–1007.

Sträussler, E. (1902). Zur Aetiologie der acuten hämorrhagischen Encephalitis [On the etiology of acute hemorrhagic encephalitis]. *Wiener klinische Wochenschrift, 15*, 61–65.

Strecker, E.A., Palmer, H.D., & Grant, F.C. (1942). A study of frontal lobotomy. *American Journal of Psychiatry, 98*, 524–532.

Ström-Olsen, R. (1946). Discussion of prefrontal lobotomy. *Proceedings of the Royal Society of Medicine, 39*, 451–453.

Ström-Olsen, R., & Carlisle, S. (1971). Bi-frontal stereotactic tractotomy. A follow-up study of its effects on 210 patients. *British Journal of Psychiatry, 118*, 141–154.

Ström-Olsen, R., & Carlisle, S. (1972). Bifrontal stereotaxic tractotomy. In E. Hitchcock, L. Laitinen, & K. Vaernet (Eds.), *Psychosurgery. Proceedings of the Second International Conference on Psychosurgery* (pp. 278–288). Springfield, IL: C.C. Thomas.

Ström-Olsen, R., Last, S.L., Brody, M.B., & Knight, G.G. (1943). Results of pre-frontal leucotomy in thirty cases of mental disorder, with observations. *Journal of Mental Science, 89*, 165–174.

Ström-Olsen, R., & Tow, P.M. (1949). Late social results of prefrontal leucotomy. *Lancet, i*, 87–90.

Stroop, J.R. (1935). Studies of interference in serial verbal reactions. *Journal of Experimental Psychology, 18*, 643–662.

Strümpell, A. (1891). Ueber primäre acute Encephalitis [On primary acute encephalitis]. *Deutsches Archiv für klinische Medicin, 47*, 53–74.

Strümpell, A. (1897). Ueber Störungen des Wortgedächtnisses und der Verknüpfung der Vorstellungen bei einem Kranken mit rechtsseitiger Hemiplegie [On disturbances of word memory and the combination of imaginations in a patient with right-sided hemiplegia]. *Deutsche Zeitschrift für Nervenheilkunde*, 397–415.

Stuss (1991 a). Self, awareness and the frontal lobes: A neuropsychological perspective. In G.R. Goethals & J. Strauss (Eds.), *The self: An interdisciplinary approach.* (in press). New York: Springer-Verlag.

Stuss (1991 b). Disturbance of self-awareness after frontal system damage. In G.P. Prigatano & D.L. Schacter (Eds.), Awareness of deficit after brain injury. (in press). New York: Oxford University Press.

Stuss, D.T., & Benson, D.F. (1983). Emotional concomitants of psychosurgery. In K.M. Heilman & P. Satz (Eds.), *Neuropsychology of human emotion* (pp. 111–140). New York: Guilford Press.

Stuss, D.T., & Benson, D.F. (1986). *The frontal lobes.* New York: Raven Press.

Stuss, D.T., Benson, D.F., Clermont, R., Della Malva, C.L., Kaplan, E.F. & Weir, W.S. (1986). Language functioning after bilateral prefrontal leucotomy. *Brain and Language, 28*, 66–70.

Stuss, D.T., Benson, D.F., Kaplan, E.F., Weir, W.S., & Della Malva, C.L. (1981). Leucotomized and nonleucotomized schizophrenics: Comparison on tests of attention. *Biological Psychiatry, 16*, 1085–1100.

Stuss, D.T., Benson, D.F., Kaplan, E.F., Weir, W.S., Naeser, M.A., Lieberman, I. & Ferrill, D. (1983). The involvement of orbitofrontal cerebrum in cognitive tasks. *Neuropsychologia, 21*, 235–248.

Stuss, D.T., Kaplan, E.F, Benson, D.F., Weir, W.S., Chiulli, S. & Sarazin, F.F. (1982). Evidence for the involvement of orbitofrontal cortex in memory functions: An interference effect. *Journal of Comparative and Physiological Psychology, 96*, 913–925.

Sullivan, W.C. (1911). Note on two cases of tumour of the prefrontal lobe in criminals; with remarks on disorders of social conduct in cases of cerebral tumour. *Lancet, ii*, 1004–1006.

Sweet, W.H., Cotzias, G.C., Seed, J., & Yakovlev, P.I. (1948). Gastro-intestinal hemorrhages, hyperglycemia, azotemia, hyperchloremia and hypernatremia following lesions of the frontal lobe in man. In J.F. Fulton, W.C. Aring, & S.B. Wortis (Eds.), *The frontal lobes. (Research publications of the association for research in nervous and mental disease, Vol. 27)* (pp. 795–822). Baltimore: Williams & Wilkins.

Sweet, W.H., Obrador, S., & Martín-Rodriguez, J.G. (Eds.), (1977). *Neurosurgical treatment in psychiatry, pain, and epilepsy*. Baltimore: University Park Press.

Sykes, M.K., & Tredgold, R.F. (1964). Restricted orbital undercutting. A study of its effects on 350 patients over the ten years 1951–1960. *British Journal of Psychiatry, 110*, 609–640.

Symonds, C.P. (1931). Mental symptoms associated with tumours of the frontal lobes. *Proceedings of the Royal Society of Medicine, 24*, 1007.

Symonds, C.P. (1937). The assessment of symptoms following head injury. *Guy's Hospital Gazette, 51*, 461–468.

Syz, H. (1937). Recovery from loss of mnemonic retention after head trauma. *Journal of General Psychology, 17*, 355–387.

Szymanski, J.S. (1913). Lernversuche bei Hunden und Katzen [Learning experiments in dogs and cats]. *Pflüger's Archiv für die gesamte Physiologie des Menschen und der Tiere, 152*, 307–338.

Takács, A. (1880). Antwort und Selbstvertheidigung gegenüber den Angriffen des Herrn Prof. Erb [Response and self-defense against the attacks of Prof. Erb]. *Archiv für Psychiatrie und Nervenkrankheiten, 10*, 815–818.

Talbot, E.B. (1897). An attempt to train the visual memory. *American Journal of Psychology, 8*, 414–417.

Tan, E., Marks, I.M., & Marset, P. (1971). Bimedial leucotomy in obsessive-compulsive neurosis: a controlled serial enquiry. *British Journal of Psychiatry, 118*, 155–164.

Tanzi, E. (1893). I fatti e le induzioni nell'odierna istologia del sistema nervoso [Facts and inductions in the actual histology of the nervous system]. *Rivista sperimentale di Freniatria e di Medicina Legale, 19*, 419–472.

Taylor, L., Tomphins, R., Demers, R., & Anderson, D. (1982). Electroconvulsive therapy and memory dysfunction? Is there evidence for prolonged defects? *Biological psychiatry, 17*, 1169–1193.

Teahan, J.E. (1987). It's a sin to tell a lie if you don't believe it yourself. *American Psychologist, 42*, 604–605.

Terman, L.M. (1916). *The measurement of intelligence*. Boston: Houghton Migglin.

Terzian, H., & Dalle Ore, G. (1955). Syndrome of Klüver and Bucy. Reproduced in man by bilateral removal of the temporal lobes. *Neurology, 5*, 373–381.

Teuber, H.L. (1972). Unity and diversity of frontal lobe functions. *Acta Neurobiologiae Experimentalis, 32*, 615–656.

Teuber, H.L. (1975). Effects of focal brain injury on human behavior. In D.B. Tower (Ed.), *The nervous system. Vol. 2. The clinical neurosciences* (pp. 457–480). New York: Raven Press.

Theissen, A. (1924). Eine Mehrleistung auf dem Gebiete des Gedächtnisses bei einem Schwachsinnigen [An improved performance in the area of memory in an imbecile]. *Zeitschrift für Kinderforschung, 29*, 198–250.

Thiele, R. (1924). Polyneuritis und Korsakow bei schwerer Inanition (Demonstration) [Polyneuritis and Korsakoff's disease in severe inanition (illustration)]. *Zentralblatt für die gesamte Neurologie und Psychiatrie, 36*, 258–259.

Thompson, R.F., & Berry, S.D. (1988). Learning and motivation, a historical overview. In G.C. Galbraith, M.L. Kletzman, & E. Donchin (Eds.), *Neurophysiology and psychophysiology: Experimental and clinical applications* (pp. 270–297). Hillsdale, NJ: LEA.

Thomsen, R. (1888). Zur Pathologie und pathologischen Anatomie der acuten completen (alkoholischen) Augenmuskellähmung (Polioencephalitis acuta superior Wernicke) [On the pathology and pathological anatomy of acute complex (alcoholic) paralysis of the eye muscles (Polioencephalitis acuta superior Wernicke)]. *Archiv für Psychiatrie und Nervenkrankheiten, 19*, 185–199.

Thomsen, R. (1890). Zur Klinik und pathologischen Anatomie der multiplen „Alkohol-Neuritis" [On the clinical picture and pathological anatomy of multiple "alcohol neuritis"]. *Archiv für Psychiatrie und Nervenkrankheiten, 21*, 806–835.

Thyssen, E.-H.-M. (1888). *Contribution a l'etude de l'hystérie traumatique* [Contribution on the study of traumatic hystery]. Paris: A. Davy.

Tiling, T. (1890). Ueber die bei der alkoholischen Neuritis multiplex beobachteten Geistesstörungen [On the mental disturbances observed in alcoholic neuritis multiplex]. *Allgemeine Zeitschrift für Psychiatrie, 46*, 233–257.

Tiling, T. (1892). Ueber die amnestische Geistesstörung [On the amnesic disturbance of mind]. *Allgemeine Zeitschrift für Psychiatrie, 48*, 549–565.

Titchener, E.B. (1895 a). *The investigation of memory and association.* New York: Macmillan.

Titchener, E.B. (1895 b). Affective memory. *Philosophical Review, 4*, 65–76.

Tomkins, J.B. (1948). A summary of 36 cases of lobotomy. *American Journal of Psychiatry, 105*, 443–444.

Torvik, A. (1987). Topographic distribution and severity of brain lesions in Wernicke's encephalopathy. *Clinical Neuropathology, 6*, 25–29.

Tow, P.M. (1955). *Personality changes following frontal leucotomy.* New York: Oxford University Press.

Tow, P.M., & Lewin, W. (1953). Orbital leucotomy (isolation of the orbital cortex by open operation). *Lancet, ii*, 644–649.

Trautscholdt, M. (1882). Experimentelle Untersuchungen über die Association der Vorstellungen [Experimental investigations on the association of imaginations]. *Philosophische Studien 1*, 213–250.

Treitel, L. (1892). Ueber Sprachstörung und Sprachentwicklung hauptsächlich auf Grund von Sprachuntersuchungen in den Berliner Kindergärten [On language disturbance and language development on the basis of investigations of language in the Berlin kindergartens]. *Archiv für Psychiatrie und Nervenkrankheiten, 24*, 578–611.

Trescher, J.H., & Ford, F.R. (1937). Colloid cyst of the third ventricle: report of a case; operative removal with section of the posterior half of the corpus callosum. *A.M.A. Archives of Neurology and Psychiatry, 37*, 959–973.

Triarhou, L.C., & del Cerro, M. (1985). Freud's contribution to neuroanatomy. *Archives of Neurology, 42*, 282–287.

Troemner, E. (1899). Pathologisch-anatomische Befunde bei Delirium tremens, nebst Bemerkungen zur Structur der Ganglienzellen [Pathological-anatomical results in delirium tremens, with remarks on the structure of ganglion neurons]. *Archiv für Psychiatrie und Nervenkrankheiten, 31*, 700–735.

Tsiminakis, Y. (1931). Beitrag zur Pathologie der alkoholischen Erkrankungen des Zentral-Nervensystems [Contribution to the pathology of alcoholic diseases of the central nervous system]. *Arbeiten aus dem Neurologischen Institut der Universität Wien, 33*, 24–62.

Tulving, E. (1985). How many memory systems? *American Psychologist, 40*, 385–398.

Tulving, E. (1987). Multiple memory systems and consciousness. *Human Neurobiology, 6*, 67–80.

Tulving, E. (1989). Remembering and knowing the past. *American Scientist, 77*, 361–366.

Tuwim, R.I., jun. (1914). Zur Frage der Pathogenese und Therapie des chronischen Alkoholismus [On the question of the pathogenesis and therapy of chronic alcoholism]. *Archiv für Psychiatrie und Nervenkrankheiten, 54*, 970–1014.

Turner, E. (1973). Custom psychosurgery. *Postgraduate Medical Journal, 49*, 834–844.

Turner, J. (1903 a). An account of the nerve-cells in thirty-three cases of insanity. *Brain, 26*, 27–72.

Turner, J. (1903 b). Clinical notes and cases. Twelve cases of "Korsakow's disease" in women. *Journal of Mental Science, 49*, 673–686.

Tyler, K.L. & Tyler, H.R. (1986). The secret life of James Parkinson (1755–1825): The writings of Old Hubert. *Neurology, 36*, 222–224.

Uchimura, J. (1928). Über die Gefässversorgung des Ammonshornes [On the vascular supply of Ammon's horn]. *Zeitschrift für die gesamte Neurologie und Psychiatrie, 112*, 1–19.

Ule, G. (1951). Korsakow-Psychose nach doppelseitiger Ammonshornzerstörung mit transneuronaler Degeneration der Corpora mamillaria [Korsakoff's psychosis after bilateral destruction of Ammon's horn with transneuronal degeneration of the mammillary bodies]. *Deutsche Zeitschrift für Nervenheilkunde, 165*, 446–456.

Ulrich, A. (1910). Über einen Tumor im rechten Temporalhirn [On a tumor in the right temporal brain]. *Zeitschrift für Nervenheilkunde, 40*, 1–23.

Valenstein, E.S. (1973). *Brain control: A critical examination of brain stimulation and psychosurgery*. New York: Wiley.

Valenstein, E.S. (1980 a). Historical perspective. In E.S. Valenstein (Ed.), *The psychosurgery debate. Scientific, legal, and ethical perspectives* (pp. 11–54). San Francisco: W.H. Freeman.

Valenstein, E.S. (1980 b). Review of the literature on postoperative evaluation. In E.S. Valenstein (Ed.), *The psychosurgery debate. Scientific, legal, and ethical perspectives* (pp. 141–163). San Francisco: W.H. Freeman.

Valenstein, E. S. (Ed.). (1980 c). *The psychosurgery debate. Scientific, legal, and ethical perspectives*. San Francisco: W.H. Freeman.

Van Buren, J.M., & Borke, R.C. (1972). *Variations and connections of the human thalamus. Vol. 1. The nuclei and cerebral connections of the human thalamus*. Berlin: Springer.

Van der Horst, L. (1928). Over de psychologie van het syndroom van Korsakow [On the psychology of Korsakoff's syndrome]. *Psychiatric en Neurologic Bladen, 32 (Wiersam-Festschrift)*, 59–77.

Van der Horst, L. (1932). Über die Psychologie des Korsakowsyndroms [On the psychology of Korsakoff's syndrome]. *Monatsschrift für Psychiatrie und Neurologie, 83*, 65–94.

Van der Kolk, J., & Jansens, J.B.A. (1905). Kasuistischer Beitrag: Aussergewöhnliche Hypermnesie für Kalenderdaten bei einem niedrigstehenden Imbezillen [Casuistric contribution: Exceptional hypermnesia for calendar dates in a severe imbecile]. *Allgemeine Zeitschrift für Psychiatrie und ihre Grenzgebiete, 62*, 347–363.

Veraguth, O., & Cloetta, G. (1907). Klinische und experimentelle Beobachtungen an einem Fall von traumatischer Läsion des rechten Stirnhirns [Clinical and experimental observations in a case with traumatic lesion of the right frontal lobe]. *Deutsche Zeitschrift für Nervenheilkunde, 32*, 407–476.

Vicente, K.J., & de Groot, A.D. (1990). The memory recall paradigm: straightening out the historical record. *American Psychologist, 45*, 285–287.

Victor, M., Adams, R.D., & Collins, G.H. (1989). *The Wernicke-Korsakoff syndrome and related neurological disorders due to alcoholism and malnutrition*. (2nd ed.). Philadelphia: F.A. Davis.

Victor, M., & Yakovlev, P.I. (1955). Translations of S.S. Korsakoff's psychic disorder in conjunction with peripheral neuritis. *Neurology, 5*, 394–406.

Viedenz, (n.n.g.) (1903). Ueber psychische Störungen nach Schädelverletzungen [On psychic disturbances after cranial damage]. *Archiv für Psychiatrie und Nervenkrankheiten, 36*, 863–888.

Vieregge, C. (1908). Prüfung der Merkfähigkeit Gesunder und Geisteskranker mit einfachen Zahlen [Testing of the ability to memorize by the use of simple figures]. *Allgemeine Zeitschrift für Psychiatrie und ihre Grenzgebiete, 65*, 207–239.

Viner, N. (1931). Amnesia. Dual personality. With special reference to a case recalled by hypnotism. *Canadian Medical Association Journal 25*, 147–152.

Voegelin, H. (1897). Beitrag zur Kenntnis der Stirnhirn-Erkrankungen [Contribution on frontal lobe diseases]. *Allgemeine Zeitschrift für Psychiatrie und ihre Grenzgebiete, 54*, 588–599.

Vogt, C. (1900). *Etude sur la myèlinisation des hemispheres cèrèbraux* [Study on the myelination of the cerebral hemispheres]. Paris: Steinheil.

Vogt, C., & Vogt, O. (1937). *Sitz und Wesen der Krankheiten im Lichte der topischen Hirnforschung und des Variierens der Tiere. Erster Teil: Befunde der topistischen Hirnforschung als Beitrag zur Lehre vom Krankheitssitz* [Locus and nature of the illnesses in the light of topical brain research and of the variation among animals. First part: Results of topical brain research as contribution to the doctrine of the locus of the illnesses]. Leipzig: Barth.

Vogt, C., & Vogt, O. (1948). Über anatomische Substrate. Bemerkungen zu patho-anatomischen Befunden bei Schizophrenen [On anaotmical substrates. Remarks on patho-anatomical findings in schizophrenics]. *Ärztliche Forschung, 2*, 101–108.

Vogt, H. (1905). Über Balkenmangel im menschlichen Grosshirn [On the lack of the corpus callosum in the human brain]. *Journal für Psychologie und Neurologie, 5*, 1–17.

Vogt, O. (1897). Flechsig's Associationscentrenlehre, ihre Anhänger und Gegner [Flechsig's teachings on association centers, its followers and opponents]. *Zeitschrift für Hypnotisismus [Suggestionstherapie, Suggestionslehre und verwandte psychologische Forschung], 5*, 347–361.

Vogt, O. (1900a). Flechsig's Associationscentrenlehre im Lichte vergleichend-anatomischer Forschung [Flechsig's teachings on association centers in the light of comparative-anatomical research]. *Neurologisches Zentralblatt, 19*, 334–335.

Vogt, O. (1900b). Zur Kritik der sog. entwickelungsgeschichtlichen anatomischen Methode [Critique of the so-called ontogenetic anatomical method]. *Neurologisches Zentralblatt, 19*, 480–481.

Vogt, O. (1910). Die myeloarchitektonische Felderung des menschlichen Stirnhirns [The myelo-architectonic regionalization of the human frontal lobe]. *Journal für Psychiatrie und Neurologie, 15*, 221- 232.

Vogt, O. (1929). 1. Bericht über die Arbeiten des Moskauer Staatsinstituts für Hirnforschung [First report on the work of the Moscow State Institute for Brain Research]. *Journal für Psychologie und Neurologie, 40*, 108–118.

Vogt, O. (1951). Die anatomische Vertiefung der menschlichen Hirnlokalisation [Anatomical deepening of human brain localization]. *Klinische Wochenschrift, 29*, 111–125.

Volkelt, H. (1914). *Über die Vorstellungen der Tiere (Arbeiten zur Entwicklungspsychologie, Vol. 1)* [On the imaginations of animals (Work on developmental psychology. Vol. 1)]. Leipzig: W. Engelmann.

Volkmar, W.V. von (1875). *Lehrbuch der Psychologie vom Standpunkte des Realismus und nach genetischer Methode (Vol. 1)* [Textbook of psychology from the view of realism and following the genetic method (Vol. 1)]. (2nd ed.). Cöthen: Otto Schulze.

Volkmar, W.V. von (1876). *Lehrbuch der Psychologie vom Standpunkte des Realismus und nach genetischer Methode (Vol. 2)* [Textbook of psychology from the view of realism and following the genetic method (Vol. 2)]. (2nd ed.). Cöthen: Otto Schulze.

Voris, H.C., Adson, A.W., & Moersch, F.P. (1934). Tumors of the frontal lobe. Clinical observations in a series verified microscopically. *Journal of the American Medical Association, 104*, 93–99.

Wachsmuth, H. (1907). Schussverletzung des Gehirns (Selbstmordversuch?) mit retrograder Amnesie und unrichtiger Ergänzung der Erinnerungslücke (Beschuldigung eines Andern) [Shot-caused damage of the brain (attempt of suicide?) with retrograde amnesia and incorrect completion of the memory gaps (accusation of someone else)]. *Archiv für Psychiatrie und Nervenkrankheiten, 42*, 311–317.

Waddington, J.L., O'Callaghan, E., Larkin, C., Redmond, O., Stack, J., & Ennis, J.T. (1990). Magnetic resonance imaging spectroscopy in schizophrenia. *British Journal of Psychiatry, 157 (Suppl. 9)*, 56–65.

Wagner, J. (1889). Ueber einige Erscheinungen im Bereiche des Centralnervensystems, welche nach Wiederbelebung Erhängter beobachtet werden [On some phenomena within the central nervous system, observed after reanimation of hanged persons]. *Jahrbücher für Psychiatrie, 8*, 313–332.

Wagner, J. (1891). Psychische Störungen nach Wiederbelebung eines Erhängten [Psychic disturbances after reanimation of a hanged person]. *Wiener Klinische Wochenschrift, 53*, 998–1002.

Wagner, R. (1860). *Ueber die typischen Verschiedenheiten der Windungen der Hemisphären und über die Lehre vom Hirngewicht mit besondrer Rücksicht auf die Hirnbildung intelligenter Männer* [On the typical differences in the gyri of the hemispheres and on teachings of brain weight with special consideration of the brain construction of intelligent men]. Göttingen: Dietrichsche Buchhandlung.

Wagner, R. (1862). *Vorstudien zu einer wissenschaftlichen Morphologie und Physiologie des menschlichen Gehirns als Seelenorgan* [Preliminary studies on a scientific morphology and physiology of the human brain as organ of the soul]. Göttingen: Dietrichsche Buchhandlung.

Wahle, R. (1885). Bemerkungen zur Beschreibung und Eintheilung der Ideenassociationen [Remarks on the description and classification of associations of ideas]. *Vierteljahresschrift für wissenschaftliche Philosophie, 9*, 404–432.

Waldschmidt, J. (1887). Beitrag zur Anatomie des Taubstummengehirns [Contribution to the anatomy of the deaf-mute brain]. *Allgemeine Zeitschrift für Psychiatrie*, 371–379.

Walker, A. (1834). *The nervous system.* London: Smith, Elder & Co.

Walker, A.E. (1940). The medial thalamic nucleus. A comparative anatomical, physiological and clinical study of the nucleus medialis dorsalis thalami. *Journal of Comparative Neurology, 73*, 87–115.

Wallace, A.R. (1905). *My life: A record of events and opinions.* New York: Dodd Mead.

Walsh, K.W. (1977). Neuropsychological aspects of modified leucotomy. In W.H. Sweet, S. Obrador, & J.G. Martìn-Rodrìguez (Eds.), *Neurosurgical treatment in psychiatry, pain, and epilepsy* (pp. 163–174). Baltimore: University Park Press.

Walshe, F. (1964). An attempted correlation of the diverse hypotheses of functional localization in the cerebral cortex. *Journal of the Neurological Sciences, 1*, 111–128.

Wasmann, E. (1899). Die psychischen Fähigkeiten der Ameisen [The psychic abilities of ants]. *Zoologica. Original-Abhandlungen aus dem Gesammtgebiete der Zoologie, Nr. 26*, 1–133 (and 3 tables). Stuttgart: Nägele.

Wasmann, E. (1909). *Vergleichende Studien über das Leben und die Seele von Ameisen und höheren Thieren* [Comparative studies on the life and the soul of ants and higher animals] (2nd ed.). Stuttgart: Nägele.

Watanabe, T. (1923). Zur Pathologie der Spinalganglien mit besonderer Berücksichtigung der Zystenbildung [On the pathology of the spinal ganglion with special consideration of the development of cysts]. *Deutsche Zeitschrift für Nervenheilkunde, 78*, 146–192.

Watson, J. (1913). Psychology as the behaviorist views it. *Psychological Review, 20*, 158–177.

Watts, J.W., & Freeman, W. (1938). Psychosurgery, effect on certain mental symptoms of surgical interruption of pathways in the frontal lobe. *Journal of Nervous and Mental Disease, 88*, 589–601.

Watts, J.W., & Freeman, W. (1945). Intelligence following prefrontal lobotomy in obsessive tension states. *A.M.A. Archives of Neurology and Psychiatry, 53*, 244.

Watts, J.W., & Freeman, W. (1948 a). Frontal lobotomy in the treatment of unbearable pain. In J.F. Fulton, W.C. Aring, & S.B. Wortis (Eds.), *The frontal lobes. (Research publications of the association for research in nervous and mental disease, Vol. 27)* (pp. 715–722). Baltimore: Williams & Wilkins.

Watts, J.W., & Freeman, W. (1948 b). Prefrontal lobotomy: Indications and results in schizophrenia. *American Journal of Surgery, 75*, 227–230.

Weber, (n.n.g.) (1906). Rudimentäre Formen der Korsakowschen Psychose [Rudimentary forms of Korsakoff's psychosis]. *Deutsche Medizinische Wochenschrift, 32*, 485–486.

Weber, E. (1907). Zur Frage der Funktion des Stirnhirns. Rindenreizungen bei Katzen [On the question of the function of the frontal lobe. Cortical stimulations in cats]. *Zentralblatt für Physiologie*, 531–533.

Wechsler, I.S. (1933). Etiology of polyneuritis. *A.M.A. Archives of Neurology and Psychiatry, 29*, 813–827.

Wehrlin, K. (1904). Diagnostische Assoziationsstudien. I. Beitrag: Über Assoziationen von Imbezillen und Idioten [Diagnostic studies of association. First contribution: On the association of imbeciles and idiots]. *Journal für Psychologie und Neurologie, 4*, 109–123.

Wehrlin, K. (1905). Diagnostische Assoziationsstudien. II. Beitrag: Über Assoziationen von Imbezillen und Idioten [Diagnostic studies of association. Second contribution: On the association of imbeciles and idiots]. *Journal für Psychologie und Neurologie, 4*, 129–143.

Wehrung, G. (1905). Beitrag zur Lehre von der Korsakoff'schen Psychose mit besonderer Berücksichtigung der pathologischen Anatomie. Ein weiterer Fall [Contribution on Korsakoff's psychosis with special consideration of pathological anatomy. A further case]. *Archiv für Psychiatrie und Nervenkrankheiten, 39*, 627–675.

Weigl, E. (1927 a). Zur Psychologie sogenannter Abstraktionsprozesse. I. Untersuchungen über das Ordnen [On the psychology of so-called processes of abstraction. I. Investigations on sorting]. *Zeitschrift für Psychologie und Physiologie der Sinnesorgane, 103*, 1–45.

Weigl, E. (1927 b). Zur Psychologie sogenannter Abstraktionsprozesse. II. Wiedererkennungsversuche mit Umrissfiguren [On the psychology of so-called processes of abstraction. II. Experiments on recognition, using contour-figures]. *Zeitschrift für Psychologie und Physiologie der Sinnesorgane, 103*, 257–322.

Weigner, K. (1906). Kurze Bemerkung zu Herrn E. Handmanns: "Ueber das Hirngewicht des Menschen auf Grund von 1414 im pathologischen Institut zu Leibzig vorgenommenen Hirnwägungen„ [Short remarks on Mr. E. Handmann's: "On the human brain weight on the basis of 1414 brain weights, done at the pathological institute of the University of Leibzig]. *Archiv für Anatomie und Physiologie, Anatomische Abteilung*, 195–196.

Weinberg, R. (1905). Zur Lehre von den Varietäten der Gehirnwindungen [On the study of variations in the cerebral convolutions]. *Monatsschrift für Psychiatrie und Neurologie, 18*, 4–62.

Weiner, R.D. (1984). Does electroconvulsive therapy cause brain damage? *Behavioral and Brain Sciences, 7*, 1–53.

Weir Mitchell, S. (1889). *Mary Reynolds, a case of double consciousness*. Philadelphia (cited after Janet, 1894, p. 74).

Weisenberg, T.H. (1910). Tumours of the third ventricle. With the establishment of a symptom-complex. *Brain, 33*, 236–260.

Welt, L. (1888). Ueber Charakterveränderungen des Menschen infolge von Läsionen des Stirnhirns [On character changes of man as a consequence of lesions of the frontal lobe]. *Deutsches Archiv für klinische Medicin, 42*, 339–390 (and 1 Table).

Wendt, F.M. (1891). *Die Seele des Weibes* [The soul of woman]. Korneuburg: Kühkopf.

Wernick, F. (1918). *Zur Symptomatologie der Stirnhirntumoren (Sarkom des rechten Stirnhirns)* [Symptomatology of frontal tumors (Sarcoma of the right frontal side)]. (Doctoral dissertation, Königliche Christian-Albrechts-Universität Kiel). Kiel: Schmidt & Klaunig.

Wernicke, C. (1874). *Der aphasische Symptomenkomplex* [The aphasic symptom complex]. Breslau, Germany: Cohn & Weigert.

Wernicke, C. (1881). *Lehrbuch der Gehirnkrankheiten für Aerzte und Studirende. (Vols. I and II)* [Textbook of brain diseases for physicians and students. (Vols. I and II)]. Kassel: Fischer.

Wernicke, C. (1889). Herderkrankung des unteren Scheitelläppchens [Focal disease of the inferior parietal lobulus]. *Archiv für Psychiatrie und Nervenkrankheiten, 20*, 243–275.

Wernicke, C. (1893 a). Ueber das Bewusstsein [On consciousness]. In C. Wernicke (Ed.), *Gesammelte Aufsätze und kritische Referate zur Pathologie des Nervensystems* (pp. 130–140). Berlin: Fischer's Medicinische Buchhandlung.

Wernicke, C. (1893 b). Nochmals das Bewusstsein (an Herrn Koch aus Zwiefalten addressiert) [Again on consciousness (Addressed to Mr. Koch from Zwiefalten)]. In C. Wernicke (Ed.), *Gesammelte Aufsätze und kritische Referate zur Pathologie des Nervensystems* (pp. 141–145). Berlin: Fischer's Medicinische Buchhandlung.

Wernicke, C. (1900). *Grundriss der Psychiatrie* [Principles of psychiatry]. Leipzig: Thieme.

Westphal, C. (1874). Einige Bemerkungen zu der vorstehenden Mittheilung des Herrn Dr. Bernhardt [Some remarks on the foregoing contribution of Dr. Bernhardt]. *Archiv für Psychiatrie und Nervenkrankheiten, 4*, 482–484.

Wilbrand, H. (1881). *Ueber Hemianopsie und ihr Verhältnis zur topischen Diagnose der Gehirnkrankheiten* [On hemianopia and its relation to the topical diagnosis of brain diseases]. Berlin: Hirschwald.

Wilbrand, H. (1887). *Die Seelenblindheit als Herderscheinung und ihre Beziehungen zur homonymen Hemianopsie, zur Alexie und Agraphie* [Optic agnosia as a focal phenomenon and its relations to homonymous hemianopia, alexia, and agraphia]. Wiesbaden: J.F. Bergmann.

Wilbrand, H. (1892). Ein Fall von Seelenblindheit und Hemianopsie mit Sectionsbefund [A case of optic agnosia and hemianopia with post-mortem findings]. *Deutsche Zeitschrift für Nervenheilkunde, 2*, 361–387.

Wilbrand, H. (1907). Über die makulär-hemianopische Lesestörung und die von Monakow'sche Projektion der Makula auf die Sehsphäre [On the macular-hemianopic disturbance in reading and the von Monakow-projection of the macula to the visual cortex]. *Klinische Monatsblätter für Augenheilkunde, 45*, 1–39.

Wilbrand, H. (1917). *Die Neurologie des Auges, Vol. 7. Die Erkrankungen der Sehbahn vom Tractus bis in den Cortex – Die homonyme Hemianopsie nebst ihren Beziehungen zu den anderen cerebralen Herderscheinungen* [Neurology of the eye, Vol. 7. Diseases of the visual pathway from the tract to the cortex – The homonymous hemianopia with its relations to other focal cerebral disturbances]. Wiesbaden: Bergmann.

Wilkins, R.H., & Brody, I.A. (1971). Down's syndrome. *Archives of Neurology, 25*, 88.

Willett, R.A. (1961). The effects of psychosurgical procedures on behaviour. In H.J. Eysenck (Ed.), *Handbook of abnormal psychology. An experimental approach.* (1st ed.) (pp.566–610). London: Pitman.

Williams, J.M., & Freeman, W. (1953). Evaluation of lobotomy with special reference to children. In S.B. Wortis, M. Herman, & C.C. Hare (Eds.), *Psychiatric treatment. (Research Publications of the Association for Research in Nervous and Mental Disease, Vol. 31)*, 311–340.

Williamson, R.T.C. (1891). A case of abscess in right frontal lobe of the brain. *Medicale Chronicle, 13*, 423–427.

Williamson, R.T.C. (1896). On the symptomatology of gross lesions (tumours and abscesses) involving the prae-frontal region of the brain. *Brain, 19*, 346–365.

Wilson, A. (1903). A case of double consciousness. *Journal of Mental Science, 49*, 640–658.

Wilson, B.A., Baddeley, A.D., & Cockburn, J.M. (1989). How do old dogs learn new tricks: teaching a technological skill to brain injured people. *Cortex, 25*, 115–119.

Wilson, B.A., Cockburn, J., & Baddeley, A.D. (1985). *The Rivermead behavioural memory test.* Reading: Thames Valley Test Comp.

Wilson, B.A., Cockburn, J., Baddeley, A., & Hiorns, R. (1989). The development and validation of a test battery for detecting and monitoring everyday memory problems. *Journal of Clinical and Experimental Neuropsychology, 11*, 855–870.

Wilson, S.A.K. (1906). Ectopia pupillae in certain mesencephalic lesions. *Brain, 29*, 524–536.

Wilson, S.A.K. (1931). Discussion on the mental symptoms associated with cerebral tumours. *Proceedings of the Royal Society of Medicine, 24*, 997–1008.

Wilson, W.W., Pittman, A.R., Bennett, R.E., & Garber, R.S. (1951). Transorbital lobotomy in chronically disturbed patients. *American Journal of Psychiatry, 108*, 444–449.

Wilson, W.W., Pittman, A.R., Bennett, R.E., & Garber, R.S. (1953). Results of transorbital lobotomy in 400 state hospital patients. *Neurology, 3*, 879–885.

Wimmer, A. (1926). Über Charakter- und Temperamentsänderungen nach Stirnhirnverletzungen [On changes in character and temperament after lesions of the frontal lobes]. *Allgemeine Zeitschrift für Psychiatrie und psychisch-gerichtliche Medizin, 84 (Festschrift Kraepelin)*, 451–459.

Winne, J.F., & Scherer, I.W. (1956). A second study of psychological changes during the first year following prefrontal lobotomy. *Journal of Consulting Psychology, 20*, 281–285.

Winocur, G., Kinsbourne, M., & Moscovitch, M. (1981). The effect of cuing on release from proactive interference in Korsakoff amnesic patients. *Journal of Experimental Psychology, 7*, 56–65.

Wirth, W. (1902). Ein neuer Apparat für Gedächtnisversuche mit sprungweise fortschreitender Exposition ruhender Gesichtsobjekte [A new apparatus for memory experiments, based on the exposition of resting face-objects, progressing by bounds]. *Philosophische Studien, 18*, 701–714.

Witkowski, A. (1887). Zur Klinik der multiplen Alkoholneuritis [On the clinical picture of multiple alcoholic neuritis]. *Archiv für Psychiatrie und Nervenkrankheiten, 18*, 809–818.

Wittenborn, J.R., & Mettler, F.A. (1951). Some psychological changes following psychosurgery. *Journal of Abnormal and Social Psychology, 46*, 548–556.

Witter, M.P., Groenewegen, H.J., Lopes da Silva, F.H., & Lohman, A.H.M. (1989). Functional organization of the extrinsic and intrinsic circuitry of the parahippocampal region. *Progress in Neurobiology, 33*, 161–253.

Wizel, A. (1904). Ein Fall von phänomenalem Rechentalent bei einem Imbecillen [A case of phenomenal calculation talent in an imbecile]. *Archiv für Psychiatrie und Nervenkrankheiten, 38*, 122–155.

Wollenberg, R. (1897). Weitere Bemerkungen über die bei wiederbelebten Erhängten auftretenden Krankheitserscheinungen [Further remarks on the pathological symptoms occuring in reanimated strangulated]. *Archiv für Psychiatrie und Nervenkrankheiten, 31*, 241–257.

Woltär, O. (1906). Über den Bewusstseinszustand während der Fugue [On the state of consciousness during a fugue state]. *Jahrbücher für Psychiatrie und Neurologie, 27*, 125–143.

Wood, F.B., Brown, I.S., & Felton, R.H. (1989). Long-term follow-up of a childhood amnesic syndrome. *Brain and Cognition, 10*, 76–86.

Worchel, P., & Lyerly, J.G. (1941). Effects of prefrontal lobotomy on depressed patients. *Journal of Neurophysiology, 4*, 62–67.

Worster-Drought, C. (1931). Mental symptoms associated with tumours of the frontal lobes. *Proceedings of the Royal Society of Medicine, 24*, 1007.

Wreschner, A. (1900). Eine experimentelle Studie über die Association in einem Falle von Idiotie [An experimental study on association in a case of idiocy]. *Allgemeine Zeitschrift für Psychiatrie, 57*, 241–339.

Wundt, W. (1874). *Grundzüge der Physiologischen Psychologie (Vols. 1–3)* [Principles of physiological psychology (Vols.1–3)]. Leipzig: W. Engelmann.

Wundt, W. (1888). Bemerkungen zur Assoziationslehre (Remarks on the theory of association]. *Philosophische Studien, 7*, 329–361.

Wundt, W. (1901). *Grundriss der Psychologie* [Principles of psychology]. (4th ed.). Leipzig: W. Engelmann.

Wundt, W. (1908). *Grundzüge der Physiologischen Psychologie. (Vol. 1)* [Principles of physiological psychology. (Vol. 1)]. (6th ed.). Leipzig: W. Engelmann.

Wundt, W. (1910). *Grundzüge der Physiologischen Psychologie. (Vol 2)* [Principles of physiological psychology. (Vol. 2)]. (6th ed.). Leipzig: W. Engelmann.

Wundt, W. (1911 a). *Grundzüge der Physiologischen Psychologie. (Vol. 3)* [Principles of physiological psychology. (Vol. 3)]. (6th ed.). Leipzig: W. Engelmann.

Wundt, W. (1911 b). *Vorlesungen über die Menschen- und Tierseele* [Lectures on the soul of man and animals]. (5th ed.). Hamburg: L. Voss.

Wurtman, R.J. (1985). Alzheimer's disease. *Scientific American*, Jan., 48–56.

Wycis, H.T. (1972). The role of stereotaxic surgery in the compulsive state. In E. Hitchcock, L. Laitinen & K. Vaernet (Eds.), *Psychosurgery* (pp. 115–116). Springfield, IL: C.C. Thomas.

Wyeth, J.A. (1904). A case of gunshot wound of the brain. *Medical Record (New York)*, 195.

Yacorzynski, G.K., Boshes, B., & Davis, L. (1948). Psychological changes produced by frontal lobotomy. In J.F. Fulton, W.C. Aring, & S.B. Wortis (Eds.), *The frontal lobes. (Research publications of the association for research in nervous and mental disease, Vol. 27)* (pp. 642–657). Baltimore: Williams & Wilkins.

Yahr, M.D. (1978). A physician for all seasons. *Archives of Neurology, 35*, 185–188.

Yakovlev, P.I. (1954). Anatomical studies in frontal leucotomies: II – Cortical origin of the fronto-pontine tract and organization of the thalamo-frontal projections. *Transactions of the American Neurological Association, 79*, 53–56.

Yakovlev, P.I., Hamlin, H., & Sweet, W.H. (1950). Frontal lobotomy. Neuroanatomical observations. *Journal of Neuropathology and Experimental Neurology, 9*, 250–285.

Yates, F.A. (1966). *The art of memory*. London: Routledge & Kegan.

Yeo, J.B. (1878). A case of large tumour of the left cerebral hemisphere, with remarkable remissions in the symptoms. *Brain, 1*, 273–276.

Yoshikawa, I. (1905). Ein Fall von Idiotie mit Erweichungsherd in den Zentral-Ganglien des Gehirns [A case of idiocy with focal softening in the basal ganglia of the brain]. *Monatsschrift für Neurologie und Psychiatrie, 18 (Suppl.)*, 282–292.

Young, A.H., Blackwood, D.H.R., Roxborough, H., McQueen, J.K., Martin, M.J., & Kean, D. (1991). A magnetic resonance imaging study of schizophrenia. Brain structure and clinical symptoms. *British Journal of Psychiatry, 158*, 158–164.

Zagari, G. (1893). Ueber Veränderungen im Sehhügel bei der progressiven Paralyse [On changes in the optic thalamus in progressive paralysis]. *Neurologisches Zentralblatt, 10*, 103–106.

Zahn, T. (1903). Eine merkwürdige Gedächtnisleistung in einem epileptischen Dämmerzustande [A peculiar memory performance in an epileptic somnolent condition]. *Allgemeine Zeitschrift für Psychiatrie und ihre Grenzgebiete, 60*, 889–984.

Zangwill, O.L. (1941). On a peculiarity of recognition in three cases of Korsakow's psychosis. *British Journal of Psychology, 31*, 230–248.

Zangwill, O.L. (1943). Clinical tests of memory impairment. *Proceedings of the Royal Society of Medicine, 36*, 576–580.

Zeliony, G. (1929). Effets de l'ablation des hémisphères cérébraux [Effects of ablation of the cerebral hemispheres]. *Revue de Medicine, No. 2*, 191–214.

Ziehen, T. (1891). *Leitfaden der Physiologischen Psychologie* [Textbook of physiological psychology]. Jena: G. Fischer.

Ziehen, T. (1901 a). Ueber die Furchen und Lappen des Kleinhirns bei Echidna [On the sulci and gyri of the cerebellum in Echidna]. *Monatsschrift für Psychiatrie und Neurologie, 10*, 143–149.

Ziehen, T. (1901 b). Gehirngewichte [Weights of brains]. *Monatsschrift für Psychiatrie und Neurologie, 10*, 473.

Ziehen, T. (1901 c). Ueber die Affektstörung der „Ergriffenheit" bei akuten Psychosen [On affective disturbances during emotion in acute psychoses]. *Monatsschrift für Psychiatrie und Neurologie, 10*, 310–320.

Ziehen, T. (1902). *Psychiatrie für Aerzte und Studirende* [Psychiatry for physicians and students]. (2nd ed.). Leipzig: S. Hirzel.

Ziehen, T. (1903). Ueber den Bau des Gehirns bei den Halbaffen und bei *Galeopithecus* [On the construction of the brain of the prosimians and of *Galeopithecus*]. *Anatomischer Anzeiger, 22*, 506–522.

Ziehen, T. (1905). Carl Wernicke. *Monatsschrift für Psychiatrie und Neurologie, 18*, I-IV.

Ziehen, T. (1906). *Leitfaden der Physiologischen Psychologie* [Textbook of physiological psychology]. (7th ed.). Jena: G. Fischer.

Ziehen, T. (1907). *Psychophysiologische Erkenntnistheorie* [Psychophysiological theory of cognition]. (2nd ed.). Jena: Fischer.

Ziehen, T. (1908 a). *Leitfaden der Physiologischen Psychologie* [Textbook of physiological psychology]. (8th ed.). Jena: G. Fischer.

Ziehen, T. (1908 b). Das Gedächtnis [Memory]. Berlin: A. Hirschwald.

Ziehen, T. (1909). *Die Prinzipien und Methoden der Intelligenzprüfung* [Principles and methods of testing intelligence]. Berlin: Karger.

Ziehen, T. (1911). *Die Prinzipien und Methoden der Intelligenzprüfung* [Principles and methods of testing intelligence]. (3rd ed.). Berlin: Karger.

Ziehen, T. (1913). *Erkenntnistheorie auf psychophysiologischer und physikalischer Grundlage* [Theory of cognition on a psychophysiological and physical basis]. Jena: Fischer.

Ziehen, T. (1921). *Die Beziehungen der Lebenserscheinungen zum Bewusstsein* [The relations of life phenomena to consciousness]. Berlin: Borntraeger.

Ziehen, T. (1924). *Leitfaden der Physiologischen Psychologie in 16 Vorlesungen* [Textbook of physiological psychology in 16 lectures]. (12th ed.). Jena: Fischer.

Ziehen, T. (1934). *Erkenntnistheorie, Teil I: Allgemeine Grundlagen der Erkenntnistheorie. Spezielle Erkenntnistheorie der Empfindungstatsachen einschliesslich Raumtheorie* [Theory of cognition.

Part I: General bases of the theory of cognition. Special theory of cognition of perceptual facts including a spatial theory]. (2nd ed.). Jena: Fischer.

Ziehen, T. (1939). *Erkenntnistheorie, Teil II: Zeittheorie. Wirklichkeitsproblem. Erkenntnistheorie der anorganischen Natur (erkenntnistheoretische Grundlagen der Physik). Kausalität* [Theory of cognition.Part II: Theory of time. Problem of reality. Theory of cognition of inorganic nature (principles of physics, based on the theory of cognition)]. Jena: Fischer.

Zingerle, H. (1898). Ueber die Bedeutung des Balkenmangels im menschlichen Grosshirn [On the meaning of the lack of the callosum in the human brain]. *Archiv für Psychiatrie und Nervenkrankheiten, 30*, 400–440.

Zingerle, H. (1900). Zur Symptomatik der Geschwülste des Balkens [On the symptoms of the tumors of the corpus callosum]. *Jahrbücher für Psychiatrie und Neurologie, 19*, 367–379.

Zingerle, H. (1912 a). Über einseitigen Schläfenlappendefekt beim Menschen [On a unilateral defect of the temporal lobe in man]. *Journal für Psychologie und Neurologie, 18*, 205–235.

Zingerle, H. (1912 b). *Ueber transitorische Geistesstörungen und deren forensische Beurteilung. Juristisch-psychiatrische Grenzfragen* [On transitory mental disturbances and their forensic evaluation. Borderline or minor juridical-psychiatric cases]. Jena: Gustav Fischer.

Zipursky, R.B., Lim, K.O., & Pfefferbaum, A. (1991). Brain size in schizophrenia. *Archives of General Psychiatry, 48*, 179–180.

Zola-Morgan, S., Cohen, N.J., & Squire, L.R. (1983). Recall of remote episodic memory in amnesia. *Neuropsychologia, 21*, 487–500.

Zola-Morgan, S., & Öberg, R.G.E. (1980). Recall of life experiences in an alcoholic Korsakoff patient: a naturalistic approach. *Neuropsychologia, 18*, 549–557.

Zola-Morgan, S., Squire, L.R., & Amaral, D.G. (1986). Human amnesia and the medial temporal region: enduring memory impairment following a bilateral lesion limited to field CA1 of the hippocampus. *Journal of Neuroscience, 6*, 2950–2967.

Zola-Morgan, S., Squire, L.R., & Amaral, D.G. (1989). Lesions of the amygdala that spare adjacent cortical regions do not impair memory of exacerbate the impairment following lesions of the hippocampal formation. *Journal of Neuroscience, 9*, 1922–1936.

Zola-Morgan, S., Squire, L.R., Amaral, D.G., & Suzuki, W.A. (1989). Lesions of perirhinal and parahippocampal cortex that spare the amygdala and hippocampal formation produce severe memory impairment. *Journal of Neuroscience, 9*, 4355–4370.

Zola-Morgan, S., Squire, L.R., & Mishkin, M. (1982). The neuroanatomy of amnesia: The amygdala-hippocampus vs. temporal stem. *Science, 218*, 1337–1339.

Zubenko, G.S., Sullivan, P., Nelson, J.P., Belle, S.H., Huff, J., & Wolf, G.L. (1990). Brain imaging abnormalities in mental disorders of late life. *Archives of Neurology, 47*, 1107–1111.